PATTERNS OF PLAGUE

MCGILL-QUEEN'S/ASSOCIATED MEDICAL SERVICES STUDIES IN THE HISTORY OF MEDICINE, HEALTH, AND SOCIETY

Series editors: J.T.H. Connor and Erika Dyck

This series presents books in the history of medicine, health studies, and social policy, exploring interactions between the institutions, ideas, and practices of medicine and those of society as a whole. To begin to understand these complex relationships and their history is a vital step to ensuring the protection of a fundamental human right: the right to health. Volumes in this series have received financial support to assist publication from Associated Medical Services, Inc. (AMS), a Canadian charitable organization with an impressive history as a catalyst for change in Canadian healthcare. For eighty years, AMS has had a profound impact through its support of the history of medicine and the education of healthcare professionals, and by making strategic investments to address critical issues in our healthcare system. AMS has funded eight chairs in the history of medicine across Canada, is a primary sponsor of many of the country's history of medicine and nursing organizations, and offers fellowships and grants through the AMS History of Medicine and Healthcare Program (www.amshealthcare.ca).

1 Home Medicine
The Newfoundland Experience
John K. Crellin

2 A Long Way from Home
The Tuberculosis Epidemic among the Inuit
Pat Sandiford Grygier

3 Labrador Odyssey
The Journal and Photographs of Eliot Curwen on the Second Voyage of Wilfred Grenfell, 1893
Ronald Rompkey

4 Architecture in the Family Way
Doctors, Houses, and Women, 1870–1900
Annmarie Adams

5 Local Hospitals in Ancien Régime France
Rationalization, Resistance, Renewal, 1530–1789
Daniel Hickey

6 Foisted upon the Government?
State Responsibilities, Family Obligations, and the Care of the Dependent Aged in Nineteenth-Century Ontario
Edgar-André Montigny

7 A Young Man's Benefit
The Independent Order of Odd Fellows and Sickness Insurance in the United States and Canada, 1860–1929
George Emery and J.C. Herbert Emery

8 The Weariness, the Fever, and the Fret
The Campaign against Tuberculosis in Canada, 1900–1950
Katherine McCuaig

9 The War Diary of Clare Gass, 1915–1918
Edited by Susan Mann

10 Committed to the State Asylum
Insanity and Society in Nineteenth-Century Quebec and Ontario
James E. Moran

11 Jessie Luther at the Grenfell Mission
Edited by Ronald Rompkey

12 Negotiating Disease
Power and Cancer Care, 1900–1950
Barbara Clow

13 For Patients of Moderate Means
A Social History of the Voluntary Public General Hospital in Canada, 1890–1950
David Gagan and Rosemary Gagan

14 Into the House of Old
A History of Residential Care in British Columbia
Megan J. Davies

15 St Mary's
The History of a London Teaching Hospital
E.A. Heaman

16 Women, Health, and Nation
Canada and the United States since 1945
Edited by Georgina Feldberg, Molly Ladd-Taylor, Alison Li, and Kathryn McPherson

17 The Labrador Memoir of Dr Henry Paddon, 1912–1938
Edited by Ronald Rompkey

18 J.B. Collip and the Development of Medical Research in Canada
*Extracts and Enterprise*Alison Li

19 The Ontario Cancer Institute
Successes and Reverses at Sherbourne Street
E.A. McCulloch

20 Island Doctor
John Mackieson and Medicine in Nineteenth-Century Prince Edward Island
David A.E. Shephard

21 The Struggle to Serve
A History of the Moncton Hospital, 1895 to 1953
W.G. Godfrey

22 An Element of Hope
Radium and the Response to Cancer in Canada, 1900–1940
Charles Hayter

23 Labour in the Laboratory
Medical Laboratory Workers in the Maritimes, 1900–1950
Peter L. Twohig

24 Rockefeller Foundation Funding and Medical Education in Toronto, Montreal, and Halifax
Marianne P. Fedunkiw

25 Push!
The Struggle for Midwifery in Ontario
Ivy Lynn Bourgeault

26 Mental Health and Canadian Society
Historical Perspectives
Edited by James Moran and David Wright

27 SARS in Context
Memory, History, and Policy
Edited by Jacalyn Duffin and Arthur Sweetman

28 Lyndhurst
Canada's First Rehabilitation Centre for People with Spinal Cord Injuries, 1945–1998
Geoffrey Reaume

29 J. Wendell Macleod
Saskatchewan's "Red Dean"
Louis Horlick

30 Who Killed the Queen?
The Story of a Community Hospital and How to Fix Public Health Care
Holly Dressel

31 Healing the World's Children
Interdisciplinary Perspectives on Health in the Twentieth Century
Edited by Cynthia Comacchio, Janet Golden, and George Weisz

32 A Surgeon in the Army of the Potomac
Francis M. Wafer
Edited by Cheryl A. Wells

33 A Sadly Troubled History
The Meanings of Suicide in the Modern Age
John Weaver

34 SARS Unmasked
Risk Communication of Pandemics and Influenza in Canada
Michael G. Tyshenko with assistance from Cathy Patterson

35 Tuberculosis Then and Now
Perspectives on the History of an Infectious Disease
Edited by Flurin Condrau and Michael Worboys

36 Caregiving on the Periphery
Historical Perspectives on Nursing and Midwifery in Canada
Edited by Myra Rutherdale

37 Infection of the Innocents
Wet Nurses, Infants, and Syphilis in France, 1780–1900
Joan Sherwood

38 The Fluorspar Mines of Newfoundland
Their History and the Epidemic of Radiation Lung Cancer
John Martin

39 Small Matters
Canadian Children in Sickness and Health, 1900–1940
Mona Gleason

40 Sorrows of a Century
Interpreting Suicide in New Zealand, 1900–2000
John C. Weaver

41 The Black Doctors of Colonial Lima
Science, Race, and Writing in Colonial and Early Republican Peru
José R. Jouve Martín

42 Bodily Subjects
Essays on Gender and Health, 1800–2000
Edited by Tracy Penny Light, Barbara Brookes, and Wendy Mitchinson

43 Expelling the Plague
The Health Office and the Implementation of Quarantine in Dubrovnik, 1377–1533
Zlata Blažina Tomić and Vesna Blažina

44 Telling the Flesh
Life Writing, Citizenship and the Body in the Letters to Samuel Auguste Tissot
Sonja Boon

45 Mobilizing Mercy
A History of the Canadian Red Cross
Sarah Glassford

46 The Invisible Injured
Psychological Trauma in the Canadian Military from the First World War to Afghanistan
Adam Montgomery

47 Carving a Niche
The Medical Profession in Mexico, 1800–1870
Luz María Hernández Sáenz

48 Psychedelic Prophets
The Letters of Aldous Huxley and Humphry Osmond
Edited by Cynthia Carson Bisbee, Paul Bisbee, Erika Dyck, Patrick Farrell, James Sexton, and James W. Spisak

49 The Grenfell Medical Mission and American Support in Newfoundland and Labrador, 1890s–1940s
Edited by Jennifer J. Connor and Katherine Side

50 Broken
Institutions, Families, and the Construction of Intellectual Disability
Madeline C. Burghardt

51 Strange Trips
Science, Culture, and the Regulation of Drugs
Lucas Richert

52 A New Field in Mind
A History of Interdisciplinarity in the Early Brain Sciences
Frank W. Stahnisch

53 An Ambulance on Safari
The ANC and the Making of a Health Department in Exile
Melissa Diane Armstrong

54 Challenging Choices
Canada's Population Control in the 1970s
Erika Dyck and Maureen Lux

55 Foreign Practices
Immigrant Doctors and the History of Canadian Medicare
Sasha Mullally and David Wright

56 Ethnopsychiatry
Henri F. Ellenberger
Edited by Emmanuel Delille
Translated by Jonathan Kaplansky

57 In the Public Good
Eugenics and Law in Ontario
C. Elizabeth Koester

58 Transforming Medical Education
Historical Case Studies of Teaching, Learning, and Belonging in Medicine
Edited by Delia Gavrus and Susan Lamb

59 Patterns of Plague
Changing Ideas about Plague in England and France, 1348–1750
Lori Jones

Patterns of Plague

Changing Ideas about Plague in England and France, 1348–1750

LORI JONES

McGill-Queen's University Press
Montreal & Kingston • London • Chicago

ISBN 978-0-2280-1079-1 (cloth)
ISBN 978-0-2280-1080-7 (paper)
ISBN 978-0-2280-1298-6 (ePDF)
ISBN 978-0-2280-1299-3 (ePUB)

Legal deposit second quarter 2022
Bibliothèque nationale du Québec

Printed in Canada on acid-free paper that is 100% ancient forest free (100% post-consumer recycled), processed chlorine free

This book was published with the generous assistance of a Book Subvention Award from the Medieval Academy of America.

This book has been published with the help of a grant from the Canadian Federation for the Humanities and Social Sciences, through the Awards to Scholarly Publications Program, using funds provided by the Social Sciences and Humanities Research Council of Canada.

Funded by the Government of Canada | Financé par le gouvernement du Canada | Canada | Canada Council for the Arts | Conseil des arts du Canada

We acknowledge the support of the Canada Council for the Arts.

Nous remercions le Conseil des arts du Canada de son soutien.

Library and Archives Canada Cataloguing in Publication

Title: Patterns of plague: changing ideas about plague in England and France, 1348–1750 / Lori Jones.

Names: Jones, Lori (Medical historian), author.

Series: McGill-Queen's/Associated Medical Services studies in the history of medicine, health, and society; 59.

Description: Series statement: McGill-Queen's/Associated Medical Services studies in the history of medicine, health, and society; 59 | Includes bibliographical references and index.

Identifiers: Canadiana (print) 20220150060 | Canadiana (ebook) 20220150311 | ISBN 9780228010791 (cloth) | ISBN 9780228010807 (paper) | ISBN 9780228012986 (ePDF) | ISBN 9780228012993 (ePUB)

Subjects: LCSH: Plague—England—History. | LCSH: Plague—England—Epidemiology—History. | LCSH: Medical literature—England—History and criticism. | LCSH: Plague—France—History. | LCSH: Plague—France—Epidemiology—History. | LCSH: Medical literature—France—History and criticism. | LCSH: Plague in literature.

Classification: LCC RC178.G7 J66 2022 | DDC 616.9/23200942—dc23

This book was typeset by Marquis Interscript in 10.5/13 Sabon.

I dedicate this book to the many plague studies friends I have made over the past decade or so. Their constant encouragement and enthusiasm have made this work not only possible, but also a reality.

Contents

Figures xiii

Acknowledgments xvii

A Note on Transcription and Translation xxi

Introduction: Writing Plague 3

1 Creating the Plague Tract 23

2 Producing the Plague Tract: From Author to Stationer, from Manuscript to Print 53

3 Setting Plague in Time: From Never Before to Now, from the Past to the Present 114

4 Seeing Plague in Space: From Elsewhere to Everywhere, from Here to There 161

5 Imagining the Oriental Plague: From Us to Them, from Fearsome Disease to Turkish Threat 215

Conclusion: Rewriting Patterns of Plague 241

Notes 251

Bibliography 319

Index 369

Figures

1.1 Doctor lancing a plague bubo. Frontispiece in Hans Folz, *Item ein fast köstlicher spruch von der pestilencz un[d] anfenglich von den zeiche[n] die ein künfftige pestilencz beteuten* (Nuremburg: Hans Folz, 1482). Reproduced with the permission of Bayerische Staatsbibliothek, Shelfmark Rar., 185. 38

1.2 The Port of Marseille during the Plague of 1720. Etching by Jacques Rigaud after Michel Serre, Wellcome Collection. 50

2.1 Generic woodcut of a doctor examining a urine flask. Title page in Atila, *Traictie tresutile contre la peste* (Paris: Gaspard Philippe, c. 1505–10). Reproduced with the permission of BnF, département Réserve des livres rares, RES-YE-1352. 98

2.2 First page of anonymized French plague tract. (Johannes Jacobi), *Remède très utile contre fièvre pestilencieuse* (Lyon: unnamed publisher, 1501). Reproduced with the permission of BnF, département Réserve des livres rares, RES-TE30-13. 99

2.3 Ornamental title page. Thomas Paynel, *A Moche Profitable Treatise Against the Pestilence* (London, Thomas Berthelet, 1534). 100

2.4 Late sixteenth-century anonymous copy of John of Burgundy's plague tract. Author's own photograph, reproduced with the permission of the Wellcome Collection, Western MS 674, f. 31. 101

2.5 Illustrated folio from Lady Margaret Beaufort's Latin copy of "Bishop of Arusiens" (Johannes Jacobi) plague tract, c. 1485–1509. Reproduced with the permission of the Fitzwilliam Museum, Cambridge, MS 261, f. 1r. 102
2.6 Illustrated folio from Lady Margaret Beaufort's copy of John of Burgundy's plague tract, c. 1485–1509. Reproduced with the permission of the Fitzwilliam Museum, Cambridge, MS 261, f. 23v. 103
2.7 Illustrated folio from King Charles V's copy of John of Burgundy's plague tract, c. 1371, showing a miniature of a robed physician sitting at a writing desk. Reproduced with the permission of BnF, NAF 4516, f. 97r. 104
2.8 Illustrated folio from King Charles V's copy of the Paris Medical Faculty's plague tract, c. 1373, showing a miniature of a seated king being instructed by three robed physicians. Reproduced with the permission of BnF, Français MS 12323, f. 135v. 105
2.9 Fifteenth-century copy of a Hebrew translation by Benjamin bar Isaac of Carcassonne of John of Burgundy's plague tract, c. 1399. Reproduced with the permission of BnF, Hébreu MS 1191, f. 141v. 106
2.10 Sample of sites where manuscript copies of John of Burgundy's plague tract were produced in England. Produced by the author. 107
2.11 First page of French plague tract. Anonymous, *Souverain remede co[n]tre Lepidimye bosse et maulvais aer* (Lyon: Martin Havard, c. 1505–07). Reproduced with the permission of BnF, département Réserve des livres rares, RESP-T-95. 108
2.12 Location of printers of plague tracts in France. Produced by the author. 109
2.13 Commercial and personal relationships between London printers of *The Mirror or Glasse of Helthe*, c. 1520s–80, which contains Thomas Moulton's adaptation of John of Burgundy's plague tract. Produced by the author. 110
2.14 Page 1 from François Ranchin, *Opuscules, ou Traictés divers et curieux en medecine* (Lyon: Pierre Ravavd, 1640). BIU Santé (Paris), Cote: 33587. 111

2.15 Fifteenth-century Phlebotomy Man with buboes in a versified version of John of Burgundy's plague tract. Reproduced with the permission of the British Library Board, BL Egerton MS 1624, f. 216v. 112
2.16 "The Manner of Dissecting the Pestilentiall Body," frontispiece. George Thomson, *Loimotomia, or the Pest Anatomized* (London: Nath. Crouch, 1666), the Wellcome Collection. 113
3.1 Detail of plague broadsheet comprising nine scenes relating to the 1665 outbreak in London, John Dunstall, 1666. Reproduced with the permission of the Museum of London. 144
3.2 London plague statistics for 12–19 September 1665, from John Graunt, *London's Dreadful Visitation: Or, a Collection of all the Bills of Mortality for this Present Year* (London: E. Cotes, 1665), L3, the Wellcome Collection. 145
4.1 Visscher's "View of London." Panoramic View of London, looking across London Bridge from Southwark, 1616. Reproduced with the permission of Bodleian Libraries, University of Oxford, Douce Prints a. 53 (2). 177
4.2 Cities and regions specifically named in French plague tracts. Produced by the author. 182
5.1 Napoleon Bonaparte visiting plague-stricken soldiers at Jaffa in 1799. Engraving by François Pigeot after Antoine-Jean Gros, 1804, the Wellcome Collection. 217
5.2 View of Constantinople from Asia. Engraving by C. Duflos in Jean-Antoine Guer, *Moeurs et usages des Turcs, leur religion, leur gouvernement civil, militaire et politique* (Paris: Coustelier, 1746), volume 1, no page. Reproduced with the permission of BnF, département Réserve des livres rares, J–338. 225
5.3 A Turkish funeral, from the frieze *Ces Moeurs et fachons de faire de Turcz*. Woodcut after Pieter Coecke van Aelst, 1553, the Metropolitan Museum of Art. 225

Acknowledgments

This book marks the culmination of years of research, as well as many years of support and encouragement. My previous career in international health and development had already generated a curiosity, or rather a fascination, with infectious diseases, and so moving into plague studies seemed to be a natural progression when I returned to university to do my PhD in history. Once I started down that road, I was quickly accepted into an international plague studies network. I will be forever grateful for the ways in which I – and my work – were welcomed, encouraged, inspired, aided, and promoted by such a generous group of scholars.

I would like to express my gratitude to my supervisor at the University of Ottawa, Kouky Fianu. After supervising my Master's thesis, which I had decided to do before taking on the greater challenge of a PhD, Kouky let me convince her to take me on as her first PhD student. She proved to be especially adept at finding in my early work many of the tiny threads that, once picked at with some diligence and duly unravelled, revealed the extent of the complex tapestry of themes that run through plague tracts. *Viva il filo rosso*! She constantly challenged me to make my case more convincing and to be bolder, encouraging me to blend traditional English and French historiographical approaches and to work comparatively. The members of my dissertation review committee – Richard Connors, Heather Murray, Sylvie Perrier, and Colin Jones – each offered substantive and very insightful feedback that helped me to improve my dissertation and, ultimately, turn it into this book. I would also like to thank Toby Gelfand, who did so much to introduce me to the history of medicine field, and Laurence Eldredge and Peter Murray

Jones, who graciously acted as my academic hosts during a three-month research trip to the United Kingdom in 2015; both also assisted me with some transcriptions and have remained friends.

I have benefitted tremendously from the sage guidance and longtime warm friendship of Ann Carmichael and Nükhet Varlık, both of whom generously offered detailed comments, suggestions, corrections, and encouragement throughout the long process of this study. They both read drafts of the book from start to end and, along with my dear friend Gillian Neale who did the same, offered much constructive criticism and advice. This book is so much better than it might have been without their engagement and input. Monica Green has been a much-appreciated cheerleader and inexhaustible source of both wisdom and information.

I would also like to acknowledge several colleagues and friends whose support and inspiration have been instrumental. Alpo Honkapohja has become my co-conspirator on all things John of Burgundy; our ongoing research and writing collaborations will, I hope, continue into the future. Susan Einbinder kindly answered my many questions about – and corrected my errors regarding – Jewish tracts and plague writers; she also generously took the time to translate a few tracts for me. Nahyan Fancy and Justin Stearns helpfully explained the intricacies of Islamicate tracts to me. Several others deserve special mention for their ongoing assistance and encouragement: Winston Black, Elma Brenner, Kristin Bourassa, Angie Fehr Costain, Delia Gavrus, Craig Ham, Nichola Harris, Vepe Percival, Heather Plewes, Kari Anne Rand, Brenda Smith, and of course "the Butler," who was a huge help while I spent many hours staring at manuscripts, old printed books, and the computer screen.

The support of numerous institutions has been critical. I am grateful for the generous funding that I received from the University of Ottawa, the Social Sciences and Humanities Research Council of Canada, the Ontario government, the Medieval Academy of America, the Richard III Society, and the Wellcome Collection. The Medieval Academy of America also provided a generous Book Subvention Award to support this publication. Kind assistance was provided by the librarians and staff members at all of the libraries that I visited and/or used virtually during the course of this research: University of Ottawa (particularly the ILL and history specialist teams), Yale Medical Historical Library; the Bodleian Library; Balliol College and St John's College Libraries (University of Oxford); the Cambridge University Library; Corpus

Christie College, Emmanuel College, Gonville & Caius College, Jesus College, Magdalene College, and Trinity College Libraries (Cambridge University); the Fitzwilliam Museum; the British Library; the Library at Wellcome Collection; the Royal College of Physicians; the Royal College of Surgeons; the Society of Antiquaries of London; the John Rylands Library and the University of Manchester Library; Lincoln Cathedral Manuscripts and Wren Libraries; the Palace Green Library (Durham Cathedral); the University of Aberdeen; the University of Glasgow; the National Library of Wales/Llyfrgell Genedlaethol Cymru; the Bibliothèque nationale de France; and the Koninklijke Bibliotheek van België/ Bibliothèque royale de Belgique. I am also grateful for the assistance I received to procure the images that I have included in this book.

I also benefitted from the many comments, questions, and suggestions provided by the audiences at conferences over the years: the Canadian Society for the History of Medicine; the American Association for the History of Medicine; the Canadian Society of Medievalists; la Société des études médiévales du Québec; Society for the History of Authorship, Reading, and Publishing; the International Congress on Medieval Studies; the International Medieval Congress; Medicine, Environment and Health in the Eastern Mediterranean World; A History of the Medical Book at the Huntington Library; Asclepius, the Paintbrush, and the Pen; and the Carleton/University of Ottawa Medieval and Renaissance Society. Showcasing my research through the *Ottoman History* and *Experiencing Epidemics* podcasts was made possible by the kind invitation of Chris Gratien, Nir Shafir, and Ian Hathaway.

I owe the warmest thanks to the editorial, production, and marketing teams at McGill-Queen's University Press, most especially to Kyla Madden, senior editor, who took an interest in this work long before it was much more than some loosely constructed thoughts on paper. Others on the team – including but not limited to Elli Stylianou, Alyssa Favreau, Jennifer Roberts, Filomena Falocco, Mia Renaud, Kathleen Fraser, and Susan Glickman – have all been a pleasure to work with. I am also grateful for the insightful and thoughtful comments provided by the anonymous reviewers; their suggestions and recommendations have improved the quality of this book.

Finally, I thank my family, which supported me throughout this process even if they never quite understood why I went back to school late in life and whatever made me interested in plague. And my dogs, who remind me every day of the important things in life.

A Note on Transcription and Translation

Research for this book draws upon a combination of unedited and edited manuscript and printed texts. Where possible, I have cited from the original unedited sources rather than from more recent editions. I have made my own translations, except where noted. In my transcriptions, I have largely respected the orthography of the authors and printers, in both English and French. I have preserved original spelling (including that of people's names, even when they differ within a text or from one version of a text to another), capitalization, punctuation marks, letter substitution (y/i and y/þ), common orthographic abbreviations and usages (such as y^t and y^e for þat and þe, &c, ß, and ȝ), accents (or lack thereof), and italics, with a few exceptions. I have substituted "s" for the long "ſ" and corrected letter substitutions i/j and u/v to modern usage. I have also expanded word abbreviations (other than those noted above) inside square brackets, omitted both paragraph marks and markers of word divisions, and removed the extra spaces in early modern French punctuation. Unless indicated otherwise, all italics in the quotations are in the original text. I have used contemporary place names rather than their present-day equivalent (for example, Constantinople instead of Istanbul).

PATTERNS OF PLAGUE

INTRODUCTION

Writing Plague

It was about the Beginning of *September* 1664, that I, among the Rest of my Neighbours, heard in ordinary Discourse, that the Plague was return'd again in *Holland*; for it had been very violent there, and particularly at *Amsterdam* and *Roterdam*, in the Year 1663. whether *they say*, it was brought, some said from *Italy*, others from the *Levant* among some Goods, which were brought home by their Turkey Fleet; others said it was brought from *Candia*; others from *Cyprus*. It matter'd not, from whence it came; but all agreed, it was come into *Holland* again.

"H.F.," London, 1665/1722[1]

PATTERNS OF PLAGUE

So begins Daniel Defoe's fictional account of plague in London, set during the great epidemic of 1665. Defoe wrote the book in 1720–21 and saw it published in March 1722, as fear of the deadly disease gripped the imagination of Londoners alarmed by the recent outbreak in Marseille. Defoe's narrator, H.F., recalls in detail how the disease arrived at "the Beginning of *December* 1664, when two Men, said to be French-men, died of the Plague in *Long Acre*."[2] The outbreak was initially confined to "that End of the Town" and appeared to subside after the first deaths; it erupted once again, however, and spread across the entire city. People's "terrible Apprehensions" about the disease were well founded, reflecting both painful memories of past outbreaks and rumours of horrific epidemics raging abroad.

Drawing on the city's official Bills of Mortality, his own observations, and numerous circulating stories, H.F. traces plague's movement across London. He compares its severity to outbreaks in previous decades, recounts weekly mortality statistics as the disease progresses from one parish to another, and ruminates on the path it must have followed from country to country. Increasingly dismayed by the desolation he witnesses while walking the near-empty streets of a city stricken by both disease and terror, H.F. vividly describes the social, religious, economic, and urban dislocation that plague has wrought. It is, he writes, "impossible to say any Thing that is able to give a true Idea of it to those who did not see it, other than this; that it was indeed *very*, *very*, *very* dreadful."[3]

H.F. contends that plague is a scourge that has arisen largely from natural causes: noxious effluvia emitting from the breath, sweat, and open sores of the infected. He reflects on, and then rejects, contemporary theories of infection related to fermentation, putrefaction, and generation, whereby minute organisms – "invisible Creatures" he incredulously calls them – carry the disease from one person to another. Despite his numerous references to divine judgment, H.F. is contemptuous of some people's claim that plague was "an immediate Stroke from Heaven, without the Agency of Means"; such beliefs he considers to be little more than "the Effect of manifest Ignorance and Enthusiasm."[4] Even so, he relates his decision to stay in the diseased city to God's will. While his religious beliefs bring him comfort in the face of so much death, he acknowledges that his brother considers such foolish "Intimation from Heaven" to be no better than the apparent "Presumption [of predestination] of the *Turks* and *Mahometans* in *Asia* and in other Places" that causes them to die from plague in much greater numbers than Europeans and Christians.[5]

Although H.F. shows considerable disdain for the remedies and advice that London's quack doctors offer his fellow citizens, Defoe actually drew quite heavily from contemporary plague tracts – medical treatises about the disease – to write his book. Tract authors of his day, including the English physicians Philip Rose, Richard Mead, and Richard Blackmore, and the French physicians François Chicoyneau, Jean-Baptiste-Nicolas Boyer, and Jean-Baptiste Goiffon, responded directly to the outbreak that spread across Provence. Among the respectable doctors to whom H.F. refers in the immediate context of London's 1665 outbreak is Nathaniel Hodges, himself a notable plague tract author. As descendants of a centuries-old genre of medical writing built on the even older "regimens of health" tradition that provided general health and daily living advice, these physicians' treatises were at once contemporary and timeless, reflecting an intricate weaving of current and longstanding thinking about the causes of and suitable treatments for plague. As widely circulating medical texts, they informed Defoe's – and thus his narrator's – meditations on the nature of the disease. As I argue in this book, these texts likely also influenced and reflected contemporary ideas – as well as our own ideas today – about plague's movements through history and across geographies, its association with foreigners, and its natural locus in particular foreign places.

Plague tracts first emerged as a unique genre of medical literature in response to the massive epidemic that historians call the Black Death (1346–53), the beginning of the multi-century Second Plague Pandemic that affected Eurasia and North (and likely Sub-Saharan) Africa. Despite their familiarity with many sicknesses, fevers, and incapacitating or debilitating conditions, mid-fourteenth-century Europeans seemed completely unacquainted with this widespread disease and its rapid course of illness, high levels of mortality, and unusual signs and symptoms. Although recurrences of the First Plague Pandemic (approximately mid-sixth to mid-eighth centuries) had given rise to long-lasting liturgical responses in the Christian Church, to the establishment of plague intercessors such as St Sebastian, and to some now well-known descriptive accounts, contemporary medical writing about the pandemic did not make it into the medieval medical canon.[6] Furthermore, late medieval European physicians and scholars could make no direct link between the two great pandemics because the sheer breadth and scale of the earlier one was not evident until centuries later. As eyewitnesses to the Black Death, *this* plague was to them both novel and terrifying, unlike any disease then known or written about.[7]

Even so, as soon as plague appeared in the Mediterranean region in 1348, physicians believed that the epidemic's timing and physical characteristics could be logically explained and rationally treated. They trusted this even though the disease's signs, symptoms, and progression – both through people's bodies and across kingdoms and empires – did not fit neatly within traditional medical classifications. Confidence in their ability to characterize and treat the disease was manifested in their plague treatises.

To a large extent, these treatises were formulaic in structure and layout, presenting medical theories and practices in three distinct sections: causes and signs of the disease, recommendations for preventing infection through personal and environmental prophylaxis, and remedial therapies for those who fell ill. Several of the earliest writers produced their texts before plague had even arrived in their cities, and thus also drew on what they were hearing from others to frame their opinions. As devastating outbreaks recurred frequently over the following centuries, these treatises circulated in large numbers throughout Europe and the Middle East. Although plague never again affected so many different places at the same time, peoples' fear that the Black Death could recur generated an "epidemiological narrative" in which the disease increasingly became a touchstone of communal memories and of literary output throughout early modern Eurasia.[8] Alongside a broad range of other types of plague writing, including sermons and prayers, broadsheets, pamphlets, prose, and poems, the treatises' long-term popularity was maintained by the medical optimism and familiar remedies they offered.[9]

One of the fascinating elements of the genre is that although many authors claim to provide something new, the texts' core contents and structure remained relatively static. The same basic medical explanations and advice are repeated across the centuries, although adjustments are evident here and there. The therapeutic recommendations that H.F. scoffs at in the mid-seventeenth century (or that Defoe himself disdained in the early eighteenth) are not that different from those offered in the mid-fourteenth. Even the more religious interpretation of the disease in the sixteenth and early seventeenth centuries, and the emergence of new (and often radical) medical theories and practices between the sixteenth and eighteenth centuries, had little impact on the tracts' formulaic structure and contents. With this longstanding uniformity in mind, the scholarly consensus – much like H.F.'s apparent scorn – has been that plague treatises not only offered unhelpful medical advice at the time but also lack originality and value as primary sources for today's historians. This is the medico-historical aspect of writing about plague to which we have become accustomed: apparent evidence of conventionality, repetition, and conservatism in late medieval and early modern medical thinking and practice. As I show here in a multi-century comparative study of English and French plague tracts, however, there is much more to the writing and reading of plague than is usually assumed. By focusing on their narrative features, by teasing out the often subtle hints in them, and by following the threads of ideas that evolve, I lift plague tracts from the source-dustbin and restore them to their rightful place as valuable historical documents.

Admittedly, the seemingly unchanging advice is puzzling, since the societies that produced and used these treatises changed considerably between the Black Death and the Plague of Provence. They also varied from each other and had different experiences with the disease.

Certainly, by the eighteenth century, treatise authors in both England and France held quite dissimilar views of the world, faced different socio-political problems, and perceived the place of plague in ways that were markedly unlike those of their predecessors in the 1340s and 1350s. Although each wrote about the disease caused by *Yersinia pestis*, local familiarities and epidemiological experiences would not have been exactly the same from one place or time to another: the plague pathogen interacted with different hosts in different ecological contexts, causing the disease itself to manifest "a wide spectrum of variation over space and time."[10] While at times perceived as a universal disease, plague was experienced locally, and no two geographical experiences would have been identical. Even so, as the last major outbreak in Western Europe erupted in Marseille in 1720, a common medical tradition meant that the largely formulaic contents of printed plague tracts differed less from their earlier manuscript counterparts or from one kingdom or city to another than one might expect.

I provide a long view of plague writing over two national histories by "listen[ing] to local voices (in historical sources)" and by examining the tracts for what else, besides medical practices, they can reveal about the societies and times in which they were produced.[11] I focus on treatises generated or circulating in England and France between the mid-fourteenth and mid-eighteenth centuries, and my main interest here is the construction and evolution of ideas about plague's historical timelines, its geographical origins, its causal sources, and its trajectories of spread. Together, these changing ideas point to shifting conceptual narratives not just of the disease, but also of how different actors in different times and places viewed the world around them. How long has this disease been among us, and from where (and from whom) did it come are the key queries that drove my rereading of these historical sources.

Just as importantly, I examine whose perspectives drove the writing and publication of these tracts. Comparing treatises from two different societies allows locally-specific experiences and understandings to be isolated. Many excellent studies of plague tracts have expanded our knowledge of the genre, but this type of comparative study is lacking. Tracing these experiences and understandings across four centuries through a combined historical-geographical lens likewise brings to the foreground wider arcs of material and intellectual change. What I seek to offer here, then, is the construction of a subtle history of changing attitudes about plague sensitively attuned to time and place.

I use a diachronic analysis to re-explore contemporary understanding of epidemic disease and its broader spatiotemporal and sociocultural features. The addition of a series of short synchronic analyses offers a deeper exploration of the backstories of some of the individual treatises and allows illustrative examples to shine through. Ultimately, focusing on the changing discourses about plague in these texts increases our understanding about the broader contents and purposes of these treatises and reclaims their historical merit. I do not address every single tract produced in England and France between 1348 and 1750, but by utilizing a sample of some two hundred tracts, I hope to illuminate the significant value these sources bring to our understanding of the place of plague in past societies.

By the early eighteenth century, plague in England (which became part of Great Britain in 1707 following union with Scotland) seems to have been firmly consigned to the past. Or at least that is how it has been seen since the eighteenth century. Plague is largely absent from official records after the great epidemic of 1665–66, except for minor outbreaks in smaller towns and a few scattered deaths attributed to the disease in London's Bills of Mortality up to 1679. The official record conflicts with recent epidemiological work, though, which demonstrates that the autumnal mortality spike associated with plague continued around London until the late 1720s.[12] Plague also remained a hot topic in London newspapers throughout the latter half of the seventeenth century and into the eighteenth, as stories about outbreaks near and far appeared regularly. The threat that these foreign epidemics posed to English ventures overseas, and even to the public at large should an infected ship arrive in English ports, ensured that journalists and newspaper sellers had a ready readership for stories about plague.[13] The disease was thus still in the minds of English men and women, just not in official mortality statistics.

In France, too, the number and extent of official records of plague outbreaks declined considerably during the second half of the seventeenth century, before the disease returned with force in the early 1720s. This was not the end: plague outbreaks continued in France every single year until at least 1770.[14] Elsewhere in Eastern and Southern Europe, in Russia, and across the Ottoman Empire, they lasted even longer, always threatening that the disease would return to England and France through trade, travel, or some other means. This discrepancy between official records and epidemiological realities helps to explain why plague tracts remained popular in both kingdoms long after the French government had applied a military cordon around the Marseille hinterlands, like a tourniquet to an infected body part, and stopped the 1720–22 outbreak from spreading any further.[15]

Before the Marseille outbreak, political leaders and tract writers alike in both kingdoms agreed that plague was not a native disease; ignoring centuries of local recurrences and tracing its arrival from elsewhere, they recast it as a foreign import. No longer seeing the disease simply as a punishment from God, as the consequence of malevolent celestial events, or as the natural emanation from swamps and urban garbage heaps, they turned their gaze to the bodies and geographical spaces of others. The subtle deletion of a once-grand cosmological and providential framework for explaining plague, and the shift from locally-generated to foreign-spawned sources of disease, has been easy to miss in the treatises because for centuries they otherwise replicated fundamentally similar advice and curative strategies. In missing this shift, we have also failed to notice the critical impact that the assumption of plague's foreign locus has long had on modern plague historiography and epidemiology, two disciplines that have been engaged in a continuous dialogue across centuries.[16] We must then ask ourselves what other changes in and around these treatises we have missed.

By uncovering the value of plague tracts in tracing multiple levels of intellectual change and permanence across late medieval and early modern societies, I offer a new evaluation of their role in the production and dissemination of local knowledge about plague and the disease's place in contemporary history and geography. In short, I argue that continuous and diverse small changes in the tracts' production and contents together comprise a set of non-trivial differences, and that by paying closer attention to something other than their standard medical framework we begin to see these texts as reflections of significant intellectual and cultural innovation.

The very form (material, language, layout, illustrative features) of plague tracts also differed from place to place, from one copy or edition to another, and from one production process to another. The publication of each treatise was thus "a crystallization of social practices" that influenced its content and its form, as well as its target audience; each treatise is, in turn, a reflection of its local context.[17] The treatises' historical value in these two senses – as representatives of multiple yet simultaneous changes across time and as reflections or symptoms of time- and location-specific social practices – has long deserved more attention. Other medical works, such as health regimens, had similarly long and broad histories.[18] Few such sources, though, were repeatedly reworked and republished to respond to current events while maintaining a core of traditional content.

PLAGUE TRACTS AS SOURCES OF INFORMATION ... ABOUT SOMETHING ELSE

To provide better resolution of the many and continuous changes that appeared in plague tracts, I reconsider the place of English and French treatises in the cultural history of medicine, demonstrating how they contribute to "the making of meaning" about the world, about society, and about human bodies.[19] By emphasizing the importance of how meaning is constantly remade through the genre, I engage at different points with intellectual history, social history, literary history, the history of ideas, and the history of the book. My purpose in doing so is to interact with the texts as they were written and produced, to read them closely through the intentions of their producers. I look for both explicit and implicit references to ideas about plague's history and its geography, and then interpret those references in the context of what is known about their producers' lives, eras, and locations.

The research underlying this book was predicated on three intertwined methodological hypotheses. First, that plague treatises as material objects were the unique products of specific agents at particular times, evolving in format, content, and even purpose across long expanses of time and broad ranges of space. Interrogating the social circumstances of a treatise's production can open more of its contents to comparative analysis and demonstrate how these texts moved and transformed – textually, materially, and physically. Scribes, illuminators, printers, stationers, and booksellers all played a role in producing them, not just their original authors. Heavily gilded and illuminated manuscript copies demonstrate the appeal of certain tracts to wealthy (and often well-educated) patrons; treatises that circulated only in plainly written manuscripts served a decidedly more utilitarian purpose. Some plague treatises made the transition to print, while others ceased circulating in new copies once the medium of print gained traction. A relatively small number appeared in both manuscript and print, sometimes circulating in both formats at the same time, but most did not. One might wonder what made some treatises more appealing than others to high-status owners, to printers, or to readers in general.

Paying attention to the non-textual aspects of plague treatises – meaning their material production, including size, illustrations, marginalia, distribution, and so on – also reveals evidence of the value given to different works at different points in time. Likewise, printers who dressed up, edited, or otherwise made an older text seem new participated in the important cultural reconstruction of the genre in the early modern era. Their role needs to be better elucidated. The old-style Gothic typography used on the title page of H.F.'s purported "never made publick before" eyewitness observations, for example, gave his account, or rather Defoe's, a specific kind of historical and perhaps even medical credence: this, the title page suggests, is an accurate rendition of a past event whose contents are both authoritative and informative. Stationers, printers, and booksellers helped generate demand for particular texts and, especially in the early days of print, determined which works made the transition from manuscript to print and which did not. How much the various players in the print industry influenced the longevity and reformulation of plague tracts in England and France deserves more attention that it has received.

Second, even when they borrowed heavily from (or openly plagiarized) their predecessors and contemporaries, plague tract producers betray their time and place. Ideas about plague's historical and geographical origins, for example, were cultural constructions that responded to, and thus changed in line with, what was generally known about the world as well as local socio-political concerns. In many treatises, the finer points of the authors' thinking about plague as a historical, geographical, or socio-cultural phenomenon is laid out either in a preface or note to readers, or so intricately woven into the medical discussion – almost as asides – that they are easy to miss. Reading both the prefaces and the main texts together and accepting that the former were not merely marketing tools allows us to take an *emic* approach that offers critical insights into the authors' mind-sets, times, and places of writing and thus to the social, religious, or political milieu in which their tracts appeared.[20] It also highlights what is unique about each one.

Third, the various concepts that impinge upon and emerge from the plague tracts – space, place, geography, cartography, nature, history-writing, local knowledge, religion, and even disease itself – were in a state of flux throughout the late medieval and early modern eras. We should not be surprised, then, that these texts reflect the tensions of an age that did not "reflect a single coherent cosmology or scheme of classification, but [was] made up out of the debris of many different systems of thought."[21] I show here that using a multidisciplinary methodology that integrates various intellectual traditions and historiographies, that simultaneously explores these works as texts, as objects, and as knowledge, and that blends micro- and macrohistorical methods is necessary to contextualize the production of individual tracts. When they are set within their larger historical contexts and analyzed as textual and material objects, it becomes impossible to see plague treatises simply as medical texts. Instead, they become "cultural artefacts in their own right and not simply as sources of information about something else, not even their apparent referent, plague."[22] Examining the tracts in this light allows the following questions to be asked: What does a close examination of the treatises' material contexts *and* contents reveal about the ways in which they simultaneously captured tradition and novelty? How did their producers shape different representations of plague? Did discontinuities in portrayals of plague's origins and place in society contribute to some tracts' long lives as much as, or even rather than, their continuities in health care advice?

The volume and nature of social, cultural, and intellectual information that can be gleaned from plague tracts by taking a longer cross-cultural perspective that includes both manuscript and print is astounding. Perceptible shifts in their style and content begin already in the later fourteenth and fifteenth centuries. More concrete changes can be linked to broader social and cultural processes such as the humanist movement (circa late fifteenth to mid-seventeenth centuries), which generated a transformation in and mutual integration of various types of learning and knowledge (including historical, geographical, and medical) throughout Western Europe. Humanist medical learning and writing and its "turn to history" relied to a large extent on the new availability of transcriptions and translations of ancient documents that provided wider access to and knowledge about events like disease outbreaks that had occurred in the distant past and in distant places. This, in turn, fostered a new focus on detailing the geographic progression of the disease, on providing daily chronologies of local outbreaks, on making comparative references to previous outbreaks, and on using literary narrative over traditional styles of medical writing.[23] These changes, however, did not happen everywhere simultaneously, or to the same degree.

The humanist movement also played a significant role in upending how people understood their history and its relationship to the present, including experience with plague. Increased access to historical manuscripts following the flight of *émigrés* from Constantinople around the time that the Ottomans captured the city in 1453 engendered a new awareness among Western European scholars that the Black Death of their past was not, in fact, as unique a historical episode as they had thought. Greater knowledge of the past and recognition of present economic and social problems combined to create a sense of longer-term historical change according to which plague was increasingly seen as both a product and symptom of disorder.[24] Especially after the later fifteenth century, changing patterns of social hierarchies, commercial and intellectual exchange, political and religious alliances, and travel and exploration also reshaped and altered the spaces within which people lived their lives. Together, these spatial-perceptual alterations fostered new conceptions of "the Other" and influenced ideas about the places from which epidemic diseases like plague arose.

Recognizing that plague had a longer history and wider geography than previously thought may be one of the most striking shifts that took place within treatises over the *longue durée*. Weakened acceptance of traditional wisdom and the concurrent rise of a more observation- and evidence-based system of knowledge generation also changed the ways in which medical writers approached plague. Authors incorporated new styles of writing, new methods of enquiry, and newly available information about plague's longer history and broader geographical reach into the treatises beginning in the last quarter of the sixteenth century in Italy, France, England, and elsewhere.

At the same time, contemporary discussions of plague were increasingly and more intimately bound up not only with attempts to understand both what the disease was and where it had originated, but also with reactions to other types of perceived societal threat. These included unhealthy (and particularly urban) landscapes, the poverty-stricken underclasses, other diseases such as "the French pox," and religious and political enemies. Embedded in these reactions were new ways of thinking about and understanding the world. Distinct from theories about the disease's ostensible religious or medical cause, though, the question of where plague originated illuminates how encounters with almost four centuries of recurrent outbreaks influenced contemporary understanding about the historical links between epidemics, the specific types of places and spaces that generated disease, and the shifting boundaries between diseased and non-diseased times and places (and peoples). It also highlights the ways in which changing geopolitical concerns played an integral role in shaping these discussions of plague's origins in textual sources that otherwise focused largely on disease treatment and prevention.

These observations raise a number of additional questions that I touch on throughout this book: How did authors, copyists, and (later) printers of plague treatises portray their particular moment in time and place in relation to plague outbreaks elsewhere? What particular views of plague enjoyed the widest circulation or followed the broadest itineraries?[25] What were the natural channels and spaces of circulation, for both the tracts and plague knowledge more generally? How and why did these channels change over time? Identifying changing portrayals of plague's temporal and geographical nature proves to be especially revealing of the ways that access to new information and the evolution of new ways of thinking about the world influenced understanding of disease. The particularities of individual tracts show that they were intimately tied not only to the geographical and historical contexts in which people encountered the disease, but also to the information and knowledge current at the time and place of composition.

Periodic outbreaks of plague over hundreds of years helped to maintain the popularity of the plague tract genre. However, to ensure that particular texts remained (or became) relevant, *au courant*, and demanded by different types of readers, successive authors, copyists, and compilers also had to respond to several layers of transformation, in addition to fears about the disease itself. The Protestant Reformation and Catholic Counter-Reformation, together with the English Civil War and Interregnum and the French Wars of Religion, brought about great upheavals in religion and political structure. The shift from medieval scholasticism to Renaissance humanism, empiricism, and natural philosophy reflected intellectual and cultural movements. The invention of the printing press had profound impacts on communications technology. Experimentation, chemical therapies, new theories of disease causation, challenges to traditional authority, and conflicts between physicians, surgeons, and apothecaries all marked new approaches to medical theory and practice. Administrative responses to plague likewise evolved over time, as did the impact of geopolitical alliances and rivalries on them. The approach that I have adopted allows these various forces to emerge as subtle yet often significant influences on plague tract contents.

Comparing tracts across the span of several centuries and from two politically and culturally intertwined yet separate kingdoms like England and France provides a much richer analysis than would be possible with a narrower focus. Examining discussions of plague's origins or its geography at only one particular moment reveals little about how cumulative and increasingly localized encounters with the disease continuously reshaped people's ideas. I thus investigate not only tracts that responded to the early, universally experienced phase of the Second Pandemic – that is, the Black Death – but also those produced in the context of the longer, later stage of regional and local outbreaks until the middle decades of the eighteenth century.

Contemporary political and geographical boundaries shifted multiple times across the centuries. For simplicity, I have considered Burgundy, Provence, Languedoc, and Avignon as regions of France, while occasional references are made to Scotland and Wales in the case of England. This is not meant to blur significant differences within the two kingdoms: Montpellier, for example, was much more of a Mediterranean cultural, linguistic, and intellectual crossroads than it was a reflection of the royalist Île-de-France, while medieval Normandy, Picardy, and Gascony all had closer commercial and political ties to England than they did to Provence or to Lorraine. Regularly at war and constantly competing with each other, the ruling and aristocratic families in the two kingdoms nevertheless intermarried and shared many common cultural interests. English monarchs established a hereditary claim to the French throne in the 1340s, and continued that claim (often through warfare) until 1801, while the monarchical overlordship of significant regions of France shifted between the two kingdoms according to the vagaries of war. By the mid-seventeenth century, scientific competition between England and France, and between the different providers of health care in each kingdom, was fierce, as was the rivalry between the traditionalist and Catholic Paris Faculty of Medicine and the more Protestant- and innovation-tolerant University of Montpellier. All of these rivalries and competitions were played out through plague treatises.

I have drawn from a corpus of more than two hundred individual treatises, as well as some fifty additional contemporary texts that discuss particular outbreaks. Of the plague tracts that I consulted, more than 70 per cent were either noteworthy for their materiality and/or contained some reference to plague's history or geography. The remaining treatises focused entirely on traditional remedial or curative therapies. Numerous treatises exist in multiple versions, and I consulted as many of these variants as possible for comparative purposes. I also consulted almost twice as many printed French treatises as English ones; this reflects France's larger population and its more prolific manuscript and print production.

THE DISEASE CALLED PLAGUE

Experiences with plague transformed societies so deeply, across such wide expanses of history and geography, that it ultimately gained sufficient cultural weight to become *the* quintessential metaphor of disease, catastrophe, and disorder. Plague treatises offered people one way to understand that disease. While this book steps away from the medical interpretation of epidemic disease, it is important to recognize that the Black Death – which contemporaries called the Great Mortality or the Great Pestilence (*generalis mortalitas hominum* or *magna pestis*) – was neither the world's first encounter, nor its first catastrophic confrontation with *Yersinia pestis*, the pathogen that causes plague. Palaeogenetic evidence documents the existence of the disease in central and northern Eurasia as early as the Late Neolithic and Bronze Age (c.3000–1800 BCE).[26] Better known are the three multi-century pandemics that spread across continents and swept away large numbers of people. The First Pandemic, whose first major outbreak is known as the Justinianic Plague (or the Plague of Justinian) of 541–42 CE, ravaged a wide area from Persia to the Mediterranean to Ireland. It then continued through localized outbreaks until the mid-eighth century. The first widespread epidemic of the Second Pandemic is known as the Black Death of 1346–53; that pandemic then continued in recurrent (regional and localized) waves for several centuries across Eurasia, North Africa and, the evidence now suggests, sub-Saharan Africa. Although plague largely disappeared from Western and Central Europe by the early eighteenth century – the last great outbreaks in the West occurred in London in 1665, in Central and Northern Europe in 1708–13, and in Provence in 1720–22 – sporadic and often severe epidemics persisted in Southern and Eastern Europe for another century. Plague also continued to devastate North Africa and the Russian and Ottoman Empires throughout the eighteenth and nineteenth centuries. After erupting forcefully in China's Yunnan Province in the 1850s, the Third Pandemic spread globally from Hong Kong at the end of the nineteenth century by steamship, reaching the

Americas for the first time.[27] Plague continues to affect human populations in Central and East Asia, Africa, and the southwestern United States to this day.

The three-pandemic chronology is problematic, however, both epidemiologically and historiographically, because of its human focus and its Eurocentricity. Plague certainly caused massive human mortality in the past, but it is not normally a human disease. Rather, it is an ecologically complex disease caused by *Y. pestis*, a single-celled coccobacillus bacterium that occurs naturally among many species of wild ground-burrowing rodents, such as rats, marmots, gerbils, shrews, chipmunks, jirds, jerboas, prairie dogs, deer mice, voles, and ground squirrels. It is spread by their fleas (and sometimes ticks). Other animals can also carry it, including rabbits, goats, sheep, camels, cats, as well as predators such as coyotes, bobcats, and possibly some species of bird. The possible role of human lice in transmitting the disease is also being investigated. Which species act as *Y. pestis*'s host varies by location, meaning that different species act as host in different areas of the globe. Diverse local ecologies, environments, and climates, in turn, can generate altered epidemiological manifestations of the disease – and even variant strains of the bacterium itself as it moves into and adapts to new local conditions.[28]

Y. pestis typically affects certain animals (its natural wild rodent hosts) in particular regions of the world without causing high mortality (in other words, it is enzootic). When it moves into new local reservoirs (host animals and their environments), the bacterium can cycle between rodent burrows and move into new species (and their predators), sometimes killing entire populations yet surviving in a high enough number of rodent nests or burrows to continue its enzootic cycle.[29] In most instances, sylvatic (wild) disease outbreaks are neither visible to, nor do they jump into, humans. In other cases, though, high rodent mortality causes the fleas to seek other hosts, and human activity facilitates spillover into human populations. Localized epidemics, or near-global pandemics, can result. Although we call these three widespread human mortalities *pandemics*, then, they are really *panzootics*, since they were sustained by the bacterium moving through various animal populations.

Distinct strains of *Y. pestis* can circulate simultaneously, each intimately tied to a particular host species and topography. It takes just one strain moving out of its natural host into humans, and then spreading across and through human populations, to create an epidemic or even a pandemic. Further evolution often happens as the bacterium continues to move into new geographies and hosts as the pandemic itself spreads.[30] Different strains of *Y. pestis* are thus associated with each of the pandemics, as well as with different outbreaks within the same pandemic. The lifespans of various strains are not, however, neatly encapsulated within the chronological boundaries assigned to the pandemics themselves. Since some strains survived past the chronological bounds of the major pandemic periods, the beginning of a new pandemic does not mean that the old strains had died out. Eighteenth- and nineteenth-century epidemics linked to the Second Pandemic, for example, continued in the Russian and Ottoman Empires (and around the Adriatic Sea) *after* outbreaks related to the Third Pandemic had already begun in southeast China, as early as the seventeenth or eighteenth centuries. Some strains associated with the Second Pandemic are still active today.

Assuming that plague emerged suddenly and catastrophically close to Europe, circulated there in recurrent outbreaks and then completely disappeared only to reappear centuries later, also ignores its ongoing presence elsewhere, its "'in-between' outbreaks."[31] Current knowledge about the existence and impact of plague outside Europe before the Third Pandemic remains fragmentary and somewhat disconnected, and it is only now starting to be put together to reframe the pandemic narrative. We simply don't know enough yet about what was happening with plague, rodents, and humans beyond Europe in the centuries between the First and Second Pandemics.

In humans, bubonic plague is typically acquired by fleabite, although body lice and human fleas may also play a role in its spread. Fever, vomiting, and distinctively painful and malodorous buboes or swellings in the lymph nodes of the groin, armpit, and/or neck are the most common characteristics of the disease. Blisters or skin discolourations can also appear. The case fatality rate ranges between 40 and 70 per cent if the victim is left untreated, with most deaths occurring about eight days after infection. Pneumonic plague spreads not through fleabite, but rather through the aerosolized droplets of coughing and sneezing. Its signs and symptoms include chest pain, breathing difficulty, and the coughing-up of blood. Septicaemic plague results when a person's bloodstream becomes infected with the *Y. pestis* bacillus (i.e., bacteremia), causing sepsis (a potentially life-threatening condition that occurs when the body's response to an infection damages its own tissues). The bacterium can also enter the body through a gastroenteric or pharyngeal route (by eating infected animal meat).[32] While the bubonic form of plague is now relatively easily treatable with antibiotics, the pneumonic and septicaemic forms remain highly fatal to this day, gastroenteric and pharyngeal only somewhat less so.

The long-accepted (but now rather inadequate) rat-flea-human causal chain of human plague infection stems from the microscopic identification of the plague bacillus by Alexandre Yersin and Kitasato Shibasaburō in Hong Kong in 1894, and the establishment a few years later of the rat and the flea as the bacillus's primary host and vector, respectively. Twentieth-century scholars' understanding of the pathogen and the disease that it caused subsequently relied on observations and conclusions made by scientists in Hong Kong and (slightly later) by the Indian Plague Commission. Yet there were obvious disconnects between medieval and early modern plague experiences in Europe, North Africa, and the Middle East – as recorded by contemporaries – and those made by direct scientific observation in turn-of-the-century East and South Asia. These disconnects included apparent discrepancies in the disease's virulence and seasonality, the rapidity of its spread, the apparent absence (or rather, lack of mention) of rats in many Black Death-affected regions, and even some of the signs and symptoms. Based on these discrepancies, decades of acrimonious debate about whether the Black Death was in fact plague – the disease caused by *Y. pestis* – or some other disease marked late twentieth-century scholarship. A number of other diseases were offered as the real culprits of the Black Death. Since the late 1990s, however, independent international teams of microbiologists working in separate laboratories have confirmed the presence of *Y. pestis* in ancient DNA (aDNA) taken from skeletal remains found in plague gravesites across Europe. Although other diseases were undoubtedly also present at various times and places, the scientific evidence has proven that plague did play a significant role in the high mortalities seen during the pandemics.[33] How and why it behaved differently from more modern outbreaks has yet to be fully explained, but local ecologies, settlement, communication, and trade patterns all likely played a role.

Another point of debate has been whether each new outbreak of plague in Europe, like the great epidemics that initially sparked the pandemics, arrived from elsewhere. The most recent historical thinking and scientific evidence points instead to the establishment and long-term maintenance of local sylvatic reservoirs in Europe itself, during both the First and Second Pandemics. The long-accepted role of the Ottoman Empire as Europe's infector has likewise been challenged. Historical and archaeological work has also reaffirmed the widespread presence of black rats (*Rattus rattus*, the assumed primary carriers of *Y. pestis*) in Europe's Roman era and high and late Middle Ages; the rats' potentially key role in all of the plague pandemics – alongside other wild rodent species – thus can no longer be dismissed.[34] In short, many of the points of argument that underlay longstanding debates about the nature of past plagues are just now being settled or reoriented.

A driving force behind the resolution of these debates has been scientific advancement.[35] Where DNA samples of *Y. pestis* are available, genetics allows us to identify which strain of the bacterium is responsible (and therefore which outbreaks are biologically related). Where aDNA samples can be acquired, palaeogenetics can take us further, identifying which modern and historical outbreaks are related, as well as which seemingly disparate epidemics in the past were biologically connected to each other. Recent and ongoing palaeogenetic discoveries are, in fact, fine-tuning our understanding of individual strains of *Y. pestis*, their relationships to each other, and, sometimes, their movements across both space and time. Current genetic research suggests, for example, that the diversity and antiquity of *Y. pestis* strains in the Tian Shan mountains (along the border region of modern-day Kyrgyzstan, Kazakhstan, and China) make it plausible that the origins of all highly virulent *Y. pestis* strains lie there, even those that later erupted into pandemics elsewhere.[36] Strains long predating the First and Second Pandemics are still found there today.

Some time between the late twelfth and mid-thirteenth centuries, an abrupt polytomy (divergence) occurred in the Tian Shan region that sparked four new branches in the bacterium's lineage.[37] Branches 1 and 2 focalized in long-term reservoirs in Europe, Central Asia, and East Africa, while Branches 3 and 4 moved into Central China, Mongolia, and Siberia. Of the four branches, only Branch 1 has spread *globally* in humans.[38] It may have first established itself locally near the Caucasus Mountains or the Volga River basin before the Black Death.[39] During or shortly after that great epidemic wave, it then split into two sub-branches, each with its own lineage. One of these sub-branches is now extinct, but likely caused most of the plague outbreaks in Europe. The other sub-branch gave rise to the strain related to the *pestis secunda* – the second major wave of Second Pandemic outbreaks around the late 1350s–60s. Retrieved, thus far, from only a few burial sites, that particular strain likely died out in Europe, but the larger sub-branch from which it emerged did survive outside of Europe and eventually generated the Third Pandemic. Yet Branch 1 did not circulate in isolation during the Second Pandemic, and it was not the only one to cause high mortality: during the later Central European and Ottoman Empire outbreaks, for example, epidemics in the Baltics stemmed from a Branch 1 strain and the Ottoman outbreaks from a Branch 2 strain.

Advances in other scientific fields are also contributing to a better historical understanding of plague. Climate science, for example, is revealing the environmental conditions that may have ushered in the First and Second Pandemics, since each appears to have followed new and inherently unstable climatic regimes (in particular, periods of cooling and increased rainfall). Archaeological findings are clarifying the maintenance versus adaptation of burial practices during epidemic episodes (mass graves being an anomaly, not the norm), societal coping mechanisms, and plague selectivity (the latter through pre-existing health status among plague victims and survivors). Immunological studies are revealing complex biological responses to syndemics, which are simultaneous or consecutive outbreaks of multiple diseases, that may help to explain some of the differences observed in how plague manifested across communities. All of these advances, in turn, are fostering new questions to be asked of the documentary evidence.[40]

Physicians contemporary to the Black Death did not, of course, have the benefit of microscopic analysis, climate science, or archaeology to inform their understanding. Nor did their theoretical conceptions of human illness leave room to consider the possibility that rodent-borne pathogens had moved into new environments and crossed the species boundary to infect human bodies, transmitted by ever-present fleas.[41] Instead, to explain this strange and highly lethal disease that had apparently arrived with little warning (aside from its rapid and inexorable progression from east to west, south to north) and that took little heed of its victims' social status, gender, or age, they drew on what they witnessed, blended it with longstanding medical tradition, and offered their thoughts and advice to those who would listen.

Those efforts to explain plague are where this book begins. After summarizing the development and evolution of the plague tract genre, chapter 1 turns to the tracts' medical contents. It describes the thinking behind, and changes in, plague medicine from 1348 to the 1750s, as well as the various socio-cultural factors that influenced how plague was considered from a medical perspective. Chapter 2 then compares and contrasts the places and socio-material conditions of plague tract production in England and France, demonstrating the interwoven nature of intellectual life and materiality alongside the business of publishing and the cooperative nature of production that involved authors, copyists, translators, illuminators, printers, stationers, and consumers. Chapters 3 through 5 examine how thinking about and understanding of the historical and geographical origins of plague both varied between England and France and evolved as political, religious, economic, intellectual, medical, and even publication circumstances changed. Chapter 3 explores the ways in which tract writers used historical referents or precedents to explain plague, and the ways in which these references differed across the medieval-early modern divide and between the two kingdoms. It also establishes the early construction of a historical-epidemiological approach that set plague's origins into a temporal context and allowed it to be historicized as a unique disease. Chapter 4 demonstrates that the spaces tract authors saw as plague-occupied or plague-generating were not entirely dependent on medical norms but rather reflected a constant recalibration of ideas about contagiousness alongside more immediate concerns with urban poverty, religious conflict, and geopolitics. The importance of the location of tract production reappears here too, since the different geographical structures of the English and French printing industries significantly affected whose perspectives were published and publicized. Chapter 5 takes these analyses into the seventeenth and eighteenth centuries, illustrating how place and time interacted to create an understanding of plague as inherently foreign. The chapter also addresses the historical revisionism of the seventeenth century and its near simultaneous consolidation with contemporary geopolitical concerns and perceived success in European healthscaping. Together, these reconstructions of plague marked the beginning of what is now called "epidemiological orientalism," the blatant assignment of Europe's ills – including plague – to the Turks.[42] Despite the many changes that had occurred in the interim, English and French tract writers ended where they began: fearing and pathologizing what might come to them from the East.

I

Creating the Plague Tract

Just like the people in Paris, we and many others feared the corruption on account its nearness.

Pierre de Damouzy, Reims, 1348[1]

RECOGNIZING A NEW DISEASE THREAT

As the earliest known French plague tract writer, Pierre de Damouzy offers a logical place to begin a discussion of the genre's development in the context of the Black Death and its subsequent evolution in France and England. He also provides a starting point to explore contemporary medical perceptions of the disease and the ways in which treatise writers adapted traditional theory to make sense of the apparently new (and later, recurrent) epidemiological threat.

By early 1348, frightening stories had reached Reims about the inexplicable and devastating mortality that was affecting regions to the south and east. In his tract, Damouzy – former regent master in Paris's Faculty of Medicine, physician to Marguerite de France (countess consort of Flanders), prebendary and later canon at Reims – reflected on people's growing fear and anxiety as the deadly *pestilencia* moved ever closer. Most of the neighbouring region was subject to southerly winds carrying the disease; it was only a matter of time before Reims itself would fall victim. Already, Damouzy noted, some places a little further away were showing signs of other pestilential fevers – "*variole et morbilli*" – that were considered to presage the arrival of this new pestilence.[2]

Since he had not yet seen plague with his own eyes, Damouzy forbore from trying to explain it. Instead, he drew heavily from the medical canon to situate the approaching epidemic within accepted knowledge: the works of Aristotle, Hippocrates, Galen, Ptolemy, Haly

Abbas, Avicenna, and Bernard de Gordon all loom large in Damouzy's writing. Foremost in his discussion of the cause of the *epydimia* was corrupted or putrefied air that had been rendered perilous by the combined action of celestial activities and hot and humid winds from the south. Unseasonable weather played its role too: fetid mists and menacing rains that never fell had made the regular *maladies de printemps* especially bad and served retrospectively as warning signs. Damouzy likewise drew from the canonical authors to offer accepted prophylactic remedies focused on purgation, the use of aromatic fumitories, and phlebotomy (the longstanding practice of opening a vein to draw blood in order to remove excessive or unhealthy humours). Alongside these recommendations, he advised his readers to be moderate in their eating, drinking, and exercise, and to avoid bathing and sexual indulgence. He also offered a longstanding therapy from al-Rāzī that, together with good governance, he said would "be a sufficient remedy for resisting" the epidemic; he expected it to work since it had always done so successfully in the past.[3]

Despite Damouzy's optimism, medieval physicians faced bitter and often satirical commentary about their apparent inability – and hence that of traditional medical theory and practice – to halt the epidemic. As Giovanni Boccaccio noted in his mid-fourteenth-century novella *Decameron*, for example, "it seemed that all the advice of physicians and all the power of medicine were profitless and unavailing. Perhaps the nature of the illness was such that it allowed no remedy; or perhaps those people who were treating the illness ... being ignorant of its causes, were not prescribing the appropriate cure."[4] Even so, the disease's arrival provoked several physicians to write about it in a way that contributed to the development of a new genre of medical literature: the plague tract.

The importance of this development should not be overlooked: plague tracts, at least in the Christian European tradition, both belonged to an expanding corpus of health-advice literature and over time became a new genre in their own right. By addressing disease causation, prevention, and treatment together, the treatises in many ways blended two existing genres of medical text: *consilia* and *regimina sanitatis*. *Consilia* – formalized case studies – were diagnostic and treatment/curative texts written by a physician for an identified patient, typically a high-status client, and usually for a specific condition or ailment. Sometimes they included prophylactic advice to prevent the recurrence of the condition being treated. Often turned into case notes, *consilia* also served as teaching tools for medical education; a number of them circulated more widely, but usually only after the advice had been excerpted in such a way as to be applicable to a wider audience.

The *regimina sanitatis* or "regimen of health" belonged to a long tradition that blended advice with Hippocratic dietetic medicine to guide readers about the best ways to conserve or regulate health (of both the body politic and the human body). In its oldest medical sense, the Greek *dietetic* referred primarily to appropriate food intake but also accounted for the broader set of Galenic non-naturals (food and drink, sleep and wakefulness, exercise and rest, passions and emotions, air, and excretion) whose management was necessary for ensuring healthy physical, mental, and spiritual lifestyles. This tradition flourished in the early Islamic world, and medieval European regimens of health emerged from dietetic doctrines translated from Arabic into Latin after the eleventh century. In both cultural traditions, the regimens addressed the actions that one could take to avoid corruption and maintain a healthy equilibrium. While inherently heterogeneous in their aims, intended audiences, and attention given to individual non-naturals, taken together these regimens extended the concept of *dietetics* to encapsulate not only health maintenance but also disease prevention and therapy. Some were composed in European vernaculars as early as the thirteenth century, and this had significant implications for the regimens' longer-term influence: while they were especially popular among the wealthy elite, regimens of health also appealed to educated, non-Latinate audiences that sought medical and lifestyle guidance in their own languages. Since they were meant to provide preventive rather than curative advice, regimens offered neither explanations of the causes of illness (either specific or in general), nor therapies to cure the ill.[5]

Plague tracts brought these two forms of medical writing together, allowing physicians to organize their work into three distinct sections: etiology (cause), prophylaxis (prevention), and remedial therapy. In this way, the writers not only disseminated their ideas about what was causing plague, but also offered advice to readers about preventing the disease through personal and environmental maintenance and how to treat and cure those who became ill. The tracts worked and circulated alongside a larger body of contemporary plague writing, including prayers, sermons, laments, poems, and pamphlets of various kinds, but in the European Christian context served a distinctly medical, rather than spiritual, purpose. In fact, one of the features of Christian plague tracts that sets them apart from their Islamic counterparts, at least in the fourteenth century and most of the fifteenth, is their lack of reference to the disease's religious implications.[6]

Plague tracts also stood apart from the medical *consilia* and regimens on which they were based in that many of their authors claimed to write for the benefit of the general public so that people could, ostensibly at least, care for themselves when they could not access or afford the services of a doctor. As the physician John of Burgundy wrote c. 1365: "I intend, with God's help, to set out more clearly in this schedule the prevention and cure of these illnesses, so that hardly anyone should have to resort to a physician but even simple folk can be their own physician, preserver, ruler and guide."[7] Rather than writing for individual patients or other physicians, as had been the norm with case-based medical *consilia* that were not meant to have any lay or public function, most plague tracts targeted, or at least claimed to target, the "common man, woman, and child." Unlike the popular and relatively generic regimens of health, they responded to public fear about the wide proliferation of a specific disease. Some of the texts reflected their authors' own experience with the disease, while others appeared in anticipation of it.

Jacme d'Agramont, a Catalonian physician, wrote his treatise in 1348 for the councillors and people of Lleida (Lérida), based on reports that he collected about the quickly approaching epidemic. He remarked that if his readers were looking for theoretical explanations or pharmaceutical recipes, they should consult a learned physician; providing such information was not the goal of his treatise.[8] Gentile da Foligno, a physician working in Perugia and Padua in 1348, wrote several treatises, each for a different audience, which reflected his experiences with the practical problems of combating plague. Abū Dja'far Ahmad ibn 'Ali ibn Muhammad ibn Khātima Al-Ansari (better known as Ibn Khātimah), a Muslim author in Almería (Andalusia), based his 1349 treatise on a combination of personal experience treating plague victims and the knowledge of others. Damouzy's prevention-focused tract, prepared as plague approached Reims, was much like the one issued a few months later by the Paris Medical Faculty, itself written at the behest of France's King Philip VI; Damouzy may well have written his tract at the Medical Faculty's request, the latter using it to complete its own work. The Jewish physician Abraham Caslari of Besalú (Catalonia) wrote a tract in 1349 after the disease had spread through his region and moved on; in contrast to many of the others, his work was clearly intended for readers learned in both medicine and highly technical Hebrew.[9] A few of these early authors, including Agramont, Caslari, and Foligno, died from plague not long after writing their tracts.

Complicating any attempt to identify a definitive genre in these early tracts is the fact that they vary considerably in length: some are short and concise (one to five pages), while others provide extended and often detailed discussions of the meaning and nature of the disease – alongside other narrative – that run to hundreds of pages. Regardless of length and level of detail, however, in the Christian and Jewish European contexts their contents are largely formulaic. The first part elaborates on the causes and prognostic signs of plague and is typically grounded in traditional theoretical and/or astrological frameworks. The second part provides guidance on how the disease might be avoided, focusing primarily on maintaining the six non-naturals and keeping a clean home environment. The third part offers a range of therapies, both prophylactic and curative, including herbals, cordials, plasters, and phlebotomy. The texts are based on traditional Galenic principles and draw heavily from the eleventh-century medical canon of the Islamicate natural philosopher Avicenna (Ibn Sīnā), as well as other traditional and authoritative sources.[10] By the early modern era, the style of the tracts change: they become longer, more narrative, and often include a religious component. Still organized around the three-part medical core, many of the later treatises offer stories about local outbreaks, engage the reader in medical debates, or consider plague in a broader social context.

Most of the earliest Christian plague tract authors, meaning those who wrote their treatises between 1348 and 1350, were well-esteemed, university-educated physicians; some held university chairs or other high-status medical positions in the papal and royal courts or in large towns. Not surprisingly, they primarily composed their treatises in urban centres of learning and/or in major universities, including Bologna, Perugia, Montpellier, Paris, and Lleida. In an era when university medical training was highly regarded, these authors' treatises carried significant intellectual weight. Non-Christian writers of the earliest tracts included Islamicate scholars in Andalusia and Syria such as Ibn al-Khaṭīb, Ibn Khātimah, al-Shaqūrī, and Shams ad-Dīn adh-Dhahabī, as well as Abraham Caslari, a Jewish physician practicing in Girona and Besalú. These men absorbed the university medical curriculum via translation, personal relationships, and/or personalized study, but were not part of the formal university system.[11] Many authors named themselves in their treatises, although a few remained anonymous. Some, like Agramont, Foligno, Khātimah, and Caslari, wrote as individuals; other authors, such as the Faculty of Medicine in Paris, wrote as a collective.

The professional and popular utility of plague treatises is evident from their quick proliferation and uptake. At least twenty-four, and likely closer to thirty, different texts appeared between 1348 and 1350 alone.[12] By the later fourteenth and fifteenth centuries, hundreds of treatises (originals and copies or adaptations of originals) circulated throughout Europe, North Africa, and the Middle East, responding to recurrent outbreaks. While the first authors wrote primarily in scholarly Latin, Arabic, or Hebrew, with only a very few like Jacme d'Agramont writing in the vernacular, by the later fifteenth century the majority of plague tracts circulated in the vernacular (English, French, Italian, Spanish, Catalan, Flemish, German, Ottoman Turkish, and so on). By then, production had also moved beyond academic settings and into other urban centres, attesting to the importance of these works as reflections of both universal experience and local concerns. The cadre of authors likewise expanded relatively quickly beyond those with university training to include surgeons, apothecaries, clergy, political administrators, and other generalist or specialized writers and translators in the Christian and Hebrew traditions as well as historians, jurists, and ḥadīth scholars in the Islamicate tradition.[13] This broadening of authorship indicates, in turn, that as plague came to represent a socio-political phenomenon rather than simply a medical or religious one, a wider range of writers felt drawn circulate their ideas about it. Plague tracts addressed medical professionals and scholars as well as a varied audience that included wealthy patrons and other literate readers. Many of the treatises explicitly include preventive and curative recipes for both the rich and the poor, in order to assist not only practitioners but also literate caretakers or patients who could use such advice directly.

Some plague treatises circulated as individual texts written into medical books, while others were copied into composite manuscripts and miscellanies. With the advent of printing, the tracts continued to circulate alone as well as appearing within larger compendia, including surgical books, hygiene manuals, almanacs, and a variety of other works. Most of the earliest printed treatises had circulated first as manuscripts; after the mid-fifteenth century, printers selected the most popular ones and republished them in the new format for wider audiences. Printed tracts then contributed to a growing and broader corpus of writing on plague that became increasingly moralistic (in the face of the Reformation and Counter Reformation), more literary (as the disease was increasingly drawn upon as a cultural metaphor in literature, theatre, and song), and ultimately more newsworthy (in the sense of outbreaks being tracked and discussed in newspapers beginning in the seventeenth century).[14]

Plague treatises were widely translated, adapted, and disseminated into the nineteenth century, their popularity maintained by recurrent outbreaks of a disease that continued to generate fear along with high levels of mortality. Texts on other specific conditions, sets of symptoms, or diseases – such as ague, various fevers, the pox (*morbus gallicus*, now known as syphilis), scrofula (king's evil), epilepsy (falling sickness or falling evil), and leprosy – as well as texts that addressed topics such as midwifery and children's illnesses were also common throughout the late medieval and early modern eras. Treatises on plague, however, proliferated to a level that in some years exceeded the combined production of medical books on all other types of diseases or conditions. Plague was, then, the disease that required sustained textual attention, and the disease that ultimately came to represent the ills of contemporary society.

RESPONDING TO A NEW DISEASE THREAT

Plague Tract Medicine: Tradition Reigns

> I have been asked by my friends to write something about the cause of this general pestilence … And they asked that after explaining the cause I should discuss appropriate remedies, drawing on my own opinions and medical advice.
>
> Geoffrey de Meaux, Oxford, 1349[15]

Extensive studies of plague medicine have concluded that the uniformity of the treatises' arrangement and, to a large extent their contents, points to the evolution of a genre of medical writing that was, at least initially, predicated more on extensive borrowing and copying than on developing innovative theories or sharing locally-specific information.[16] By combining authoritative medical knowledge and theory (that is, scholastic humoralism) with practical experience, the treatises responded to both professional and public concerns about the disease. Many authors integrated their personal experiences and observations into the tracts, both to bolster their own credibility and authority and to make their works more appealing by appearing useful, pragmatic, and based on actual success.[17] For the most part, though, they simply built on the maxim that a healthy person enjoyed balanced humours, lived moderately, attained mental, physical, and spiritual equilibrium, and avoided the conditions that caused illness. Like all medicine of the time, plague medicine was predicated on the understanding that disease or ill health was the result of an imbalance in a person's four humours (blood, black bile, yellow bile, and phlegm) and their respective qualities (hot, cold, wet, and dry). Humoral balance, in turn, could be negatively impacted by mismanagement of the non-naturals, as well as by contra-naturals (pathological conditions). Since one of a physician's key roles was to maintain and promote the health of his patients, not just to prevent disease, a successful medical practice entailed developing expertise in rectifying humoral imbalances alongside administering drugs and knowing when surgery was necessary.[18]

Whatever the origins and impulse for plague treatises, before 1400 the genre and its contents were well established. Even so, experience with plague challenged medical thinking that was more attuned to dealing with individuals or, at most, localized groups of people, and that typically explained disease as the result of imbalanced humours, complexions, or poor habits. This was what Galenic medicine had taught: illness was caused by a blend of external and internal factors, but was manifested individually because each person's constitution was different. French physician and astrologer Geoffrey de Meaux noted in 1349 that he had been asked to write about the disease, "showing its natural cause, and why it affected so many countries, and why it affected some countries more than others, and why within those countries it affected some cities and towns more than others, and why in one town it affected one street, and even one house, more than another, and why it affected nobles and gentry less than other people, and how long it will last."[19] In other words, for most tract writers this disease was not behaving in the same way as other, more familiar diseases did.[20] As such, existing explanations needed to be reworked to clarify how this widespread, high-mortality disease had been generated and spread.[21]

Medieval physicians typically pointed to two sets of causes for plague. Thirteenth-century Christian scholastic philosophy dictated that even though God ruled everything on earth (that is, was the prime cause), natural laws could also be understood as secondary causes. As a result, although plague was ultimately generated by a supernatural power, it was also part of a natural order that encompassed causes both remote and universal, and near, particular, and terrestrial. In direct contrast to both religiously oriented discussions and their Islamic tract-writing counterparts, Christian treatise writers rarely invoked divine causes before the late fifteenth century.[22]

Universal and remote causes embodied either natural or supernatural agents, such as adverse astrological conjunctions and earthquakes that affected many people in geographically distant places. The conjunction of Saturn, Jupiter, and Mars, in 1345 – and the devastating earthquake on 25 January 1348 centred in the eastern Alpine Friuli-Venezia Giulia region of modern Italy (but felt as far away as Strasbourg, Milan, Pisa, and Regensburg) – were repeatedly invoked as having sparked the pandemic because they had produced evil vapours capable of corrupting the air that were then spread widely by the wind. A subsequent earthquake in the Apennine Mountains eighteen months later bolstered the belief among some writers that earthquakes might be to blame.[23] Particular or near causes, for their part, included environmental factors such as stagnant bodies of water, unburied corpses, damp enclosed spaces, human and animal waste, or industrial by-products – essentially anything that gave rise to a foul odour. Paradoxically, one wonders if the foul-smelling industrial byproducts included effluents from the very processes that were used to produce parchment, paper, and ink for books like the plague treatises themselves.

In any case, the key to the generation of plague was the altered air that, when breathed in, was drawn to the heart where it corrupted a person's "lyfle spyrytes."[24] Tract writers also noted human-specific factors that facilitated the disease's entry into the body. These helped to explain why only some people in a community became sick and died, or why some communities were affected and others were not, even though everyone breathed the same air. Physicians made recourse especially to variations in individual humoral balances, which rendered some people more susceptible than others to the infected air. John of Burgundy, for example, analogized that just as fire could only burn in material that was combustible, so too could pestilential air only cause infection in those people in which the corrupted air "fynde mater of ye body redy to receyve corupcion."[25] Others, like Abraham Caslari, rejected cosmological and altered air explanations; in his assessment (based on personal experience with the disease), the fevers were "humoral-pestilential, not a universal pestilence."[26] Thus Caslari argued that only immediate causes should be considered: poor diet was known to corrupt people's humours, but celestial changes had no diagnostic value.

Most physicians distinguished between major and minor levels of plague transmission. The former entailed transmission of the disease from place to place, while the latter represented human-to-human transmission, which itself could occur by three different modes: breath, skin perspiration, or gaze. They recognized that close proximity to persons sick with plague increased one's own chances of becoming ill. As Guy de Chauliac wrote in 1363, the disease was so contagious that people could catch it from each other through a glance alone.[27] Theories suggesting that disease could be transmitted through air corrupted and putrefied by malign astrological conjunctions or earthquakes and other terrestrial features – which supported longstanding ideas of miasma, an unseen poisonous vapour containing particles of decomposed matter that caused disease when it entered people's bodies and upset their humoral balances – and/or by contagion were thus longstanding and not seen to be contrary. They were, instead, successive stages of the disease's dissemination along a broad spectrum of possibilities.[28] Tract authors argued both that corrupted air had infected the bodies of the ill and that the plague-infected returned the corruption to the air and infected others through their breath or gaze.[29] A small number of early authors, including Jacme d'Agramont and Alphonso de Cordoba, also raised the spectre of malicious human agency in generating and spreading the disease.[30]

As Pierre de Damouzy had done, many of the later fourteenth-century tract authors noted a variety of signs that seemed to precede or foretell the arrival of plague: extreme or unseasonable temperatures and weather, severe winds and rains (or lack thereof), and even the sudden appearance of frogs, reptiles, or insects out of the ground. Physicians' suggested preventive measures were complex and multivariate as a result, and aimed at identifying places that were or could be protected from infected air, at correcting or purifying the infected air, at keeping the body resistant to infection, and at avoiding contact with infected people.[31] These approaches to disease management had been, with minor cultural and geographic differences, common since the time of the Ancient Greeks. Now they had to be made to fit plague.

Yet this disease differed from what physicians had read about in their medical books, and a few recognized that what they saw conflicted with their medical training.[32] Some contemporary lay descriptions of the Black Death (and of later outbreaks) are sufficiently graphic to give us a sense of what the disease might have looked like to those who lived through the pandemic. The Piacenzan notary Gabriele de' Mussis, for example, decided "to set ... out in writing" the four stages of the disease's progress through people's bodies so that the "symptoms of this pestilential disease" could "be made plain to all."[33] It began with "chilly stiffness" and a "tingling sensation" that he likened to being pricked by the points of arrows, perhaps as a nod to Christian iconography of the martyrdom of St Sebastian that showed the plague saint embedded with arrows. Mussis described the next stage of the disease as a "fearsome attack which took the form of an extremely hard, solid boil." In some people, the boil emerged in the armpit, in others it developed in the groin. In all cases, it then led to an "acute and putrid fever" and severe headaches. Finally, it "gave rise to an intolerable stench ... [and] vomiting of blood" and additional swellings elsewhere on the body. "Behold the swellings," he advised, for these were "warning signs sent by God." Other writers, like Giovanni Boccaccio and English chronicler Geoffrey le Baker, described plague in much the same way, noting a progression of bodily signs and symptoms.

There are, however, few such graphic descriptions in the Black Death-era medical texts. Even if they mentioned abscesses in the armpit or the groin, many of the earliest tract writers did not describe the signs of plague in any detailed way. In 1348, the physician Jacme d'Agramont noted that the "pestilence and mortality ... is accompanied by very terrible symptoms," yet his description of them was rather laconic and detached: fevers, abscesses, "smallpox or measles, and ... worms [or loss of] memory."[34] Damouzy likewise pointed to a variety of non-evocative signs and symptoms that he associated with putrid fever, such as stinking sweat and breath, pustules, and intestinal pain. Others indicated that the disease's onset included a range of signs: fever, fainting and weakness, sweating, spasms, confusion and anxiety, ulcers, difficulty breathing, vomiting, diarrhoea, pain, and haemorrhaging. Worms sometimes accompanied these symptoms, while a black tongue and glandular swelling also appeared in some victims.

By the 1370s, a few writers in Montpellier believed that they had to come to terms with the physical signs of plague; here, more than anywhere else in the fourteenth century, physicians attempted to assimilate what they were observing to traditional medical theory. They did so by explaining the emergence of buboes in terms of humoral pathology. An excess of humours in the brain would generate a swelling behind the ear, they said; an overabundance in the liver would cause a bubo in the groin; and a surplus in the heart would give rise to one in the armpit. Even so, they provided little actual description of the swellings or other signs, other than to vaguely link excessive humours to "buboes, erysipelas, carbuncles, and other different kinds of abscesses."[35] Writing some decades later, the papal physician Raymond Chalin de Vinario linked three separate outbreaks of the disease (1348, 1378, and 1382) by referring both to their common cosmological causes and their similar signs, these being large abscesses, fever, worms, and black spots.[36] Traditional medical authorities had, of course, addressed painful apostemes or swellings, fevers, and stinking putrid matter, but not in the catastrophic and dramatic form that physicians and other medical practitioners now witnessed in their patients, their families, and sometimes themselves. It was only as plague became a recurrent phenomenon that descriptions of its physical signs became more graphic, first in German and Italian texts from the fifteenth century and later in French and English ones. Local norms related to the acceptance and integration of personal observation (the appearance of ill bodies being one of these) into medical texts thus guided the content of plague treatises in a particular direction that we do not see in generic, pre-existing health-advice treatises.[37]

Even when they did not describe or even mention the main signs of plague, some of the tracts included therapies or cures that address the buboes in one way or another. Gentile da Foligno, for example, recommended scarifying, cauterizing, or cupping the apostemes to attract and evacuate the poisonous matter collected in them, and then covering them with plasters to dissolve the accumulated pus. More often, physicians recommended phlebotomy. Phlebotomy served both as a preventive measure – to ensure a healthy humoral balance that would protect against disease – and as a curative measure, with bleeding in this case allowing plague poison to be safely removed from the body. Which vein was most suitable for bloodletting typically depended on the condition being treated: the cephalic vein was often opened for conditions above the neck, while the basilic or hepatic vein was preferred for conditions below the neck. The median or cardiac vein was also frequently used; in practice, each vein in the body was associated with specific illnesses and opened as appropriate. Key to the proper practice of bloodletting were the concepts of "derivation," or the letting of blood from a vein close to the affected body part, and "revulsion," or the letting of blood from the furthest possible vein. Each method was predicated on careful diagnostics and indications of particular illnesses.[38]

Tract authors listed the veins suitable for bleeding, depending on whether the bloodletting was for prophylactic or therapeutic purposes and, if the latter, on the bubo's location. Writing around 1365, John of Burgundy noted that the pestilential sores erupted in the emunctories or purging spots of the body's three main organs: in the "arm-holis," in the groin, or under the ears. As such, the best veins were the cardiac, saphena, and cephalica, respectively. Like his contemporaries, he advised that special care should be taken to let blood only on the same side of the body as the bubo itself, because otherwise the uninfected blood would be removed rather than the poisoned blood; furthermore, the plague poison itself would be drawn across the body and thus infect the heart: "ther is two harmes: oon, if thow bleede on that other side, the goode bloode and cleene in thi side nat corrupt nat venymed shal be drawen out of, and the evil bloode shal dwel stil ther. And than the body is fiebler for defaute of goode bloode … and the harme is more, for than the bloode that is venymed shal passe overthwert the herte and venymeth it and hastith a man to his endynge."[39]

The key was not just knowing which vein to bleed, but also the timeframe within which to do it. It was important to be bled as soon as one felt the "prickyng of bloode or flakeryng" that indicated infection, and especially within one to six hours, since (as a later version of John's tract states) "lettinge blood in tyme is a specyall meanes of cure."[40] Waiting too long, by contrast, would cause mortal danger: if "ther passe xxiiij houres the matier than is gadred and harded and wil nat passe out of the veyne if it be striken." Some tract authors argued that bleeding after obvious symptoms had appeared was simply too dangerous and should be avoided.

Phlebotomy was not the only therapy that physicians suggested as both prophylaxis and cure. In addition to recommending a prevention-based regimen that focused on avoiding certain foods (especially non-sour fruits and red meats because of their corrupting influences on the body) and too much bathing, sex, and sweating (because these activities opened the pores to infection), tract authors also included a wide variety of aromatic or medicinal therapies meant to both protect against infection and act as cleansers. Since the infected air was the most immediate problem, correcting or changing it was of paramount importance. Many tract authors encouraged their readers to flee infected areas or, if they could not, to stay in their homes after making them more salutary. The geographical implications of this advice are discussed below in chapter 4 (where to locate one's home, which windows to leave open, and so on), but encompassed in this advice was aromatic fumigation. If stench propagated unhealthy air, then sweet or pleasant-smelling air was by extension healthy: burning aromatic woods, spices, and herbs was a protective measure against infection meant to cleanse both rooms and people's bodies. Suitable woods included juniper, cypress, oak, pine, sandalwood, wormwood, willow, poplar, and fig; among the best herbs and plants were aloe, mugwort, marjoram, oregano, rosemary, saffron, lavender, violets, water lilies, roses, and laurel. Other recommended substances included ambergris, camphor, frankincense, myrrh, musk, and mastic. Separate options existed for the rich and the poor, and also for the winter and summer months. Some scents could be sprinkled on the hands and face, rinsed or chewed in the mouth where appropriate, or carried around in pomanders.[41] Homes could likewise by sanitized with vinegar mixed with aromatic rosewater or something similar.

Like phlebotomy, the purpose of many plague medicines was either to prevent infection in the first place or to purge the body of humours that had become corrupted by the infected air. Foods such as vinegar, garlic, onion, and sour or acidic fruits were frequently recommended because they both preserved health and were believed to help cure plague. Herbs such as fennel, rue, borage, bugloss, angelica, and blessed thistle were also promoted. Tormentil, dittany, pimpernel, and scabious were prescribed regularly for their ability to help patients avoid infection. Simple medicines prepared from natural clay (such as Armenian bolus and *terra sigillata*) were anti-inflammatory and anti-diarrheal. Composite medicines blended multiple ingredients and were typically prescribed in the form of electuaries (paste), syrups and juleps (sweet drinks), powders, or pills. The Paris Medical Faculty, for example, recommended pills containing aloe, myrrh, and saffron, as did John of Burgundy, who stated "pillule rosarum [made of aloe, saffron, and fumitory syrup] bien woundirly excelent of preservacioun ... and he that usiþ this governaunce may be preserved from the ... corrupcioun of the aire."[42] These pills acted as a laxative, but were also believed to prevent the development of buboes. John, like many of his contemporaries, also recommended theriac, which was one of the most commonly prescribed compound medicines for both prevention and therapy. Popular among the ancient Greeks and used as a universal antidote against poisons and ills of all kinds, it appeared in a variety of recipes, sometimes comprising up to eighty different ingredients, including a heavy dose of opium.[43] Finally, cordials were meant to strengthen the heart, brain, and liver. Some authors recommended wearing or even ingesting precious stones such as emeralds, sapphires, rubies, and amethysts to counter the effects of poisoned air. By suggesting a variety of local or abundant substances and a few exotic, costly ones, tract writers hoped to allay patient fears.

On the whole, there was little substantive change in plague medicine for centuries. Even as tract writers grappled ever more boldly with the reality of personal experiences that seemed to contradict, or at least not accord with, what they had learned from their books, medical practices and remedies alike typically remained confined within the traditional canon. Whatever their preferred therapy, the authors' empirical interpolations became key components of plague treatises amongst a growing popular readership: references to everyday knowledge and familiar medicines met readers' desire for texts that provided useful explanations and recommendations.

Providing evidence of successful first-hand experience also bolstered the perceived value of some writers' therapies (see figure 1.1). The papal physician Guy de Chauliac suggested that he had survived the plague epidemic of the early 1360s when his own "external apostemes were brought to a head with figs and cooked onions mixed with yeast and butter; then they were opened and treated as ulcers. The tumors were cupped, scarified, and cauterised."[44] Alongside recommendations for pills, bloodletting, and purifying the air, Chauliac offered a recipe for an electuary of his own making, drawn "from the teachings of Master Arnald of Villanova [c. 1240–1311] and of the masters of Montpellier and Paris." Some decades later, Blasius of Barcelona claimed to have survived plague by having his buboes cut open and evacuated, as recommended by Albucasis and Avicenna. Both men had, in other words, survived plague by relying on traditional treatment practices offered up as something not just new but also personally verified.

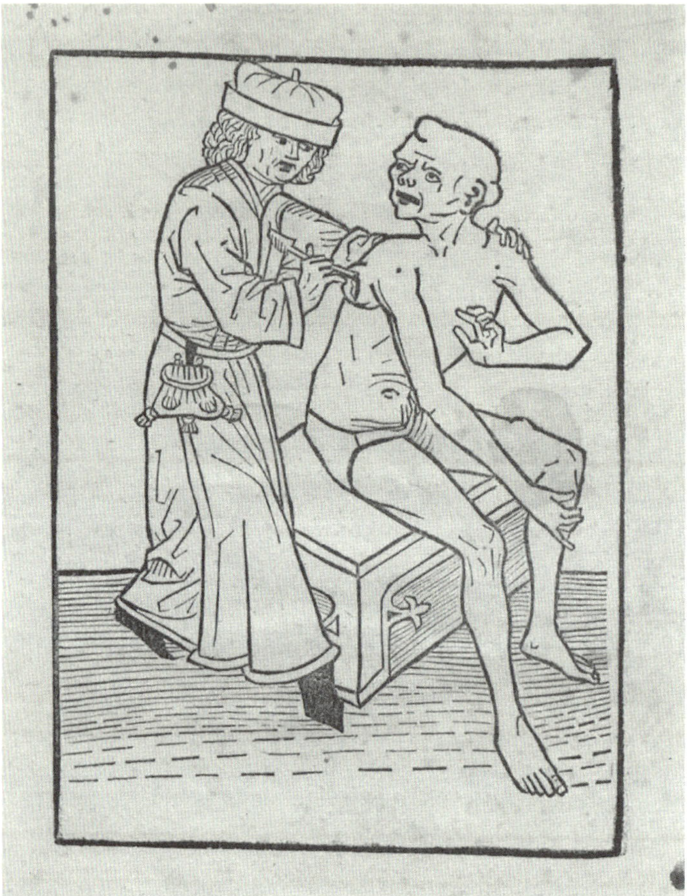

1.1 Doctor lancing a plague bubo, frontispiece in Hans Folz, *Item ein fast köstlicher spruch von der pestilencz un[d] anfenglich von den zeiche[n] die ein künfftige pestilencz beteuten*, 1482.

More than a century later, tract writers continued to emphasize the tried-and-true value of their proffered remedies. Sébastien Colin, a physician from Fontenay perhaps best known for his polemic attacks on apothecaries as medical imposters and deceitful traders, claimed in 1566 that his therapies against plague were authentic because they had been "first written in the Syriac language by Rhazes, interpreted in Greek by Alexandre Traillian and newly translated from Greek into French" by himself.[45] Somewhat less controversially, Parisian physician Pierre Drouet claimed to "have had conference with the best learned Phisitions both in England, Germanie, and many other places" from whom he learned secrets that enabled him to "cure many kindes of diseases. Amonge all which secrets I have gathered together manye rare and verie effectuall remedies ... against the infectious Pestilence."[46] For the most part, these purportedly "rare" remedies were little different from those recommended by Drouet's much earlier predecessors: avoid infected places; air out and sprinkle sweet water throughout the home; burn a variety of aromatic woods and herbs; apply liniments comprised of wax, camphor, saffron; and use ointments made of roses, violets, cinnamon, cloves, lavender, agarwood, and numerous other ingredients. Perhaps Drouet's primary effort, like that of many of his contemporaries, was simply to reassure readers about the efficacy of traditional medicine. Doing so also created the illusion that the unchanging medical advice being offered in plague treatises was better than any alternative. But, as a closer look at Drouet's tract shows, other types of therapy were by this point pushing strongly against traditional Hippocratic and Galenic theory.

Plague Tract Medicine: Tradition Falters

Surely in this one point God wonderfullye declareth his providence, when he teacheth us to applye strong and deadlye poysons.

Pierre Drouet, Paris, 1576[47]

By the sixteenth century, in addition to repeating traditional plague therapies and citing classical authorities, Pierre Drouet and many of his contemporaries also offered more eclectic preventives. In doing so, they followed the Swiss physician Paracelsus (Philippe Aureolus Theophrastus Bombastus von Hohenheim) and the Flemish chemist/physician Jan van Helmont, both of whom countered traditional humoral theories and offered in their place chemical, mechanical, and corpuscular explanations of the body and of the world.[48] Yet, in some cases, these alternatives were packaged and presented not as novel therapies, but rather as part of longstanding (or at least trustworthy) tradition. Drouet contended, for example, that "if a hole be made in a hasyll nut, and the kernel be pulled forth with a pin, and the place fylled up againe with common quicksilver, and hanged about the neck, it preserveth a man wonderfully from the pestilence."[49] This, he learned, had saved the life of the French King Henri II (r. 1547–59) during a siege in Germany. Other chemical and natural therapies meant to drive away plague poison included electuaries made with arsenic, oils containing viper or scorpion venom, ointments of vitriol (sulphuric acid), and antimony-based vomitories. Some of these chemical therapies had long histories in ancient medicine, as Drouet was quick to point out: "as *Galen* sheweth" was a phrase he repeated numerous times.[50]

At first, both Paracelsianism and Helmontism appealed primarily to religious dissenters and political reformers in the sixteenth and seventeenth centuries. Medicine in this era was being pulled in multiple directions: intellectual, religious, and political. Some English writers incorporated these new medical-chemical theories – and the heated debates that they generated –into the tracts they wrote in response to London's great outbreak in 1665.[51] George Thomson, for example, was a keen proponent of the new chemical medicine and accused his Galenic opponents of being "fugitive physicians ... false Impeachers ... [and] a company of grand talkative Imposters" whose efforts against plague brought only "evil effects" because of their opposition to "Fundamental Truths" and their belief in "Dogmatical Fancy."[52] Thomson argued that plague was a contagious, venomous gas that, once in the body, acted as a "Domestick Enemy we carry about us, ready to betray us."[53] To combat this enemy, Thomson proposed measures that were decidedly chemical, rather than herbal or lifestyle-oriented: sulphur, tartar, salt, and so on. Tracts like Thomson's evidently served purposes and addressed audiences in ways that differed radically from the formulaic passages of earlier centuries.

In France, such ideas were initially equated with heresy and greeted with suspicion, but were nevertheless adopted into a theoretical system of medicine that tended to blend the new ideas with the old.[54] Several sixteenth-century writers, including royal physician Oger Ferrier, Bordeaux physician Pierre Pichot, and Pierre André, a surgeon in Poitiers, advocated the use of alternative remedies such as sulphuric acid, mercury, and antimony as plague therapies. In 1629, Pierre-Jean Fabre, a physician in the southern French town of Castelnaudary, recommended chemical medicines as the antidote to the poison of plague. These included arsenic, antimony, sulphur, mercury, saltpetre, and coal, and were to be used alongside the more commonplace herbal remedies promoted by others.[55] Other tract writers, though, like the Nîmois physician and legal expert Jean Suau, opposed alchemical medicine altogether, castigating "spagyrist imposture and [its] many abuses to medicine, surgery, and pharmacy."[56] As in England, the debate about the respective value of traditional versus new medicine was carried out, in part, through the pages of plague treatises.

At the same time, a new empiricism based on clinical observation and inductive reasoning served as a counterpoint to Galenism and its emphasis on deductive epistemology.[57] Early modern treatises dealt more openly with non-traditional medical theory and novel remedies than had their late medieval counterparts, and this in turn makes evident a kind of discontinuity in plague medicine.[58] The wonderful flexibility of the plague treatise becomes most apparent in this era, masked by its stodgy rhetorical framework.

Another shift from Galenic medicine came from the religious turn that many tracts took after the late fifteenth century. Medical, astrological, and religious approaches to addressing plague were not completely distinct even in the mid-fourteenth century, with secular medical practices operating alongside and in conjunction with religious healing. Although they sometimes acknowledged that divine punishment was the highest cause of plague, fourteenth- and fifteenth-century tract writers generally did not engage directly with the discussions of humankind's sinfulness or the wicked state of Christendom that filled contemporary religious writings about plague. Such thinking may have been implicit, but was rarely stated explicitly.[59] However, descriptions of plague's causes shifted in a significant subset of tracts produced in the decades leading up to the religious upheaval of the sixteenth century. This was due, in part, to the greater number of clerics and other religious writers who began writing plague treatises and the likelihood that they were responding to both a different perspective on what caused the disease and a different publication environment. The integration of increasingly religious rhetoric is discernable even among physicians and other medical writers, especially during the Reformation and Counter-Reformation, as these writers were motivated by their own convictions – or possibly by the increasing popularity of religious writing – to add moralistic content to treatises that otherwise maintained their medical focus. Certainly, religious writing on plague surged, especially during the sixteenth and seventeenth centuries: rising literacy rates and the technology of print enabled the publication and dissemination of a far greater number of prayers, sermons, and lay religious responses than had been possible during the manuscript era. In the Protestant context, Scripture became the touchstone of religious writing about plague, even in medical tracts, while Catholic writers placed much emphasis on the disruption plague wrought on the possibility of a good death.

Already by the 1470s, an adaptation of John of Burgundy's tract by English Dominican friar Thomas Multon emphasized the primacy of divine retribution for human sinfulness to understand plague etiology and incorporated long extrapolations from the Bible, such as the narrative of 2 Kings 24.[60] This type of commentary, and indeed this same biblical passage, had been commonplace in sermons and moral texts since the Black Death, but its appearance in otherwise medically-oriented plague tracts – and especially its incorporation into a tract whose original version had contained no reference to God, sin, or divine retribution – represents a definitive change in both tone and content. Multon's tract made the transition to print before 1530, and in that format acquired an even stronger moralizing tone.[61] Religious content became a regular feature in European plague treatises in the early sixteenth century, part of the much larger effusion of devotional writing more generally. This is perhaps most noticeable in German-speaking lands, where university-trained reforming physicians attempted to encourage piety on the pages of their tracts by employing "Protestant rhetoric on medical and spiritual issues, even repeating Martin Luther's statements."[62]

Religious tracts in England and France often replicated the format, structure, and style of plague treatises, using much of the same explanatory, descriptive, and remedial language as their medical counterparts. In some cases they incorporated medical authority, not to support it but rather to dismiss or debate it in favour of causes and therapies that were more spiritual in nature. "Plague, properly speaking," the French priest Estienne Ydeley argued in the 1580s, "is a rod of God sent on earth, and on the iniquity of the world, to punish sinners, and to admonish them to leave their evil life behind and to return to our Savior and Redeemer Jesus Christ."[63] Ydeley, who acted as chaplain to plague victims in Besançon, offered a treatise that, like its medical counterparts, discussed the causes of the disease, how to preserve the healthy, and how to treat the ill. To him, though, "the plague is not a disease, but a rod of God." He placed significant emphasis on maintaining the cleanliness of body, soul, and living spaces as part of one's duty towards God, but refrained from offering preservatives and other medicines against plague. Instead, he prayed that "all who find themselves tainted by the disease of plague will have recourse to spiritual medicine."[64] He did not eschew the herbal therapies found in the medical tracts altogether; they just took second place to spiritual advice and were promoted as being more curative – applied to buboes they would aid in physical healing – than preventive.

This turn to religion in plague tracts has already received scholarly attention.[65] Moralistic tracts had wider and broader circulation during the religious turmoil of the sixteenth and seventeenth centuries than did tracts less able to reflect or engage with contemporary social (rather than just medical/health) concerns. The degree to which tracts like Multon's and Ydeley's situated the origins of plague within a religious framework rather than in a medical one thus "contributed to [a] cultural construction of epidemic disease" that differed significantly from that of earlier eras.[66]

Although relatively numerous, the solely religious plague tracts typically authored by clerics or other writers remained in the minority in both England and France.[67] It is, perhaps, more useful to consider them in the broader context of religious writing (and speech) about plague, rather than simply in opposition to medical writing. Certainly, preachers considered medical issues; in one such case, during an outbreak in London in 1603, a public debate took place in their pamphlets between Henoch Clapham and James Balmford. Clapham argued that faith alone saved one from plague, while Balmford urged his congregation to believe that plague was contagious.[68] Yet what set the religious tracts apart from their more clearly medical counterparts was their emphasis not on people's bodily health but rather, in the French context, on "the violence done to the community of saints and the disruption of religious ritual" and, in the English, on the need for redemption and salvation.[69] They were less focused on providing advice for environmental and personal prophylaxis than on countering and mitigating individual and community sin and restoring the Christian community.

Sixteenth-century physicians, surgeons, and other medical writers who invoked religion in their tracts typically presented a blend of spiritual and physical health explanations, treatments, and preventive recommendations. Some argued, often through the addition of an entire subsection of religious rhetoric and proselytizing, that plague resulted from divine wrath. They included moralizing commentary and called for prayer and penance, but then offered more traditional medical explanations and treatments. The mid-sixteenth-century Aberdeen physician Gilbert Skene, for example, wrote that the first and principal cause of plague was contagion blown onto earth as the "scurge and punischment of the maist just God."[70] The primary means of preventing the disease was thus returning to God and pacifying his wrath. Yet Skene also recognized the traditional medical causes of plague (even lamenting that it would be "difficill and tediouse" to list all of them) and offered a long list of remedies and therapies that were much the same as those found in tracts with no religious content. Even alchemically oriented writers like the French surgeon Pierre André listed "rods and chastisements" from God first among the causes of plague; none of the many chemical remedies he offered would work without God's permission.[71] In communities torn apart by religious factionalism, writers and readers might well have needed religious comfort and consolation in addition to medical advice.

In some cases, the injection of religious content into plague treatises reflected the tensions of the era, and a more nuanced reading of their contents reveals an ideological agenda suggesting that the Christian community had become plagued by heretical beliefs. Much of the existing scholarship on England has focused on religious reformers; here, "the [human] body and its diseases functioned as a nexus for fraught sixteenth- and seventeenth-century discursive battles ... led by Protestant reformers intent on restoring 'health' to, and for, the 'common wealth'" and who were "convinced of endemic spiritual, moral and social 'disease' under Roman Catholicism."[72]

Yet English Catholics felt the same way about their Protestant neighbours. Physician (and later advisor to Queen Mary I) Thomas Phayer, for example, could have been referring to Lutherans in his mid-sixteenth-century warning that "the venemous air [of plague] itself is not half so vehement to infect, as is the conversacion or breath of them that are infected already."[73] His recommendation to "every chrysten man, that is in doute of thys dysease to cure first the fever pestylencial of hys soule" might likewise have been meant to highlight the spiritual danger posed by reformist ideas. Phayer's tract was not an original piece of work; rather, it was an adaptation of a French treatise written before 1520. It is important to read these suggestions about the Lutheran infection as a religious interpolation into a text that had much less to say on the matter and that certainly did not carry this connotation when originally produced. The tract's author, the Angers professor of medicine Nicolas Houssemaine, had noted simply that "breath or venomous vapours" could infect an entire region.[74] The idea that plague could be spread by breath appeared in the earliest tracts and relied on Galenic tradition. Phayer thus extrapolated from Houssemaine's work, turning the latter's medical idea about how plague was spread through breath into an argument that people who rebelled against traditional religion brought plague upon their communities by speaking of – that is breathing out – their heretical beliefs. Later in the century, an unidentified Protestant author revised Thomas Multon's (Catholic) adaptation of John of Burgundy's tract yet again, laying the blame for plague squarely at the feet of "the governors of the churche of God and the expounders of the word and law of God [who] doe transgrethe and swarve from ther dutie."[75] This speaks to a strong sense of the roles and responsibilities that those who led, governed, and spoke for the English Protestant Church – that is, the "the churche and law of God" rather than the Catholic church of Multon's day – were expected to fulfill. And yet, in both Phayer's tract and the anonymous revision of Multon's work, the medical therapies remain intact, much as they do in similar tracts from France.

While religious literature continued to flourish in seventeenth-century England, especially during plague outbreaks, tract writers tended, for the most part, to turn away from religious discussion. It can be difficult to see what was actually changing within plague tracts at this time, because the word "plague" was harnessed to political and religious purposes. There were no large outbreaks in London during the period that included the Civil War (1642–51), the Interregnum (1649–60), and the Restoration (1660). There was a small outbreak in London in 1641 that prompted the publication of a few remedial and religious tracts. The civil war spread small local outbreaks rather widely, as large armies moved across the kingdom and into people's homes. Some of these, such as the ones in Barnstaple and Oxford in 1644, led to accusations of heresy and lax morality by writers of one religious denomination against their opponents, each blaming the other for generating plague. The surge in Puritanism tied to the Civil War also bolstered divine and providential interpretations of plague, and several editions of religious tracts admonishing the "plague of schism" and the "plague of civil war" appeared in the 1640s and early 1650s.[76] Religious tracts mimicking plague treatises also maintained the emphasis on sin as the cause of disease, regardless of which side of the civil war their authors supported. In 1644, for example, royalist Church of England clergyman Lionel Gatford wrote that "The *Plague* of the *Soule* is the originall or principall cause of the *plague* of the *body*. And therefore without all dispute the best and surest, if not the onely course for avoiding or expelling the *Plague* of the *body*, is to avoid or expell the *Plague* of the *soule*. No disease, say *Physitians*, can be taken away, unlesse the cause be taken away; and the cause being removed, say the *Naturalists,* the effect removes with it; and the onely way that the *Scriptures* prescribe to get quit of any judgement, is first to get quit of Sinne."[77]

Yet references to these interwoven religious and political upheavals were rarely included in medically focused tracts. Increasingly after the Restoration of King Charles II in 1660 – a political and social event that had a significant impact on English medicine – religious and medical explanations of disease separated once again, with tracts dedicated to the one less often invoking the other.[78] In fact, an increasing number of English writers rejected, often very openly, divine explanations of plague and the religious content of plague tracts decline significantly. In the early 1670s, Nathaniel Hodges felt that in discussing the possible causes of plague he had at the very least to acknowledge the role of God, lest he "incur the Suspicion of Atheism."[79] Fifty years later, John Quincy, who translated Hodges's tract from Latin into English, went much further in railing against religious writers of any sort who "either out of Ignorance in other Causes, or out of an affected Devotion, thought it their Interest to come in to this Opinion, and pretend to do greater Cures by certain religious Performances, and their Intercession with Heaven, than was in the Power of Medicine, of which they knew but very little."[80]

In France too, a burst of religious factionalism enters a small subset of plague tracts in the sixteenth century, driven in large part by the decades long Wars of Religion (c. 1559–1629) and buoyed by the proliferation of polemic invective produced by both sides of the religious divide. While religious writers tended to speak directly to divine wrath as the cause of the disease, several tract authors – most notably Claude de Rubys (1577), Nicolas de Nancel (1581), François de Courcelles (1595), and Jean Grillot (1629) – referred instead to religious enemies whom they blamed for the spread of plague. I discuss this religious enemy angle in more detail in chapter 4, but would note here that, as in England, the religious content of French plague tracts largely fell away after the wars ended. Early eighteenth-century writers like François Ranchin, chancellor of Montpellier's Faculty of Medicine, might still have noted that "plague is recognized as a scourge of God" and discussed the work done by churchmen to forestall an epidemic, but they reverted to the medical approach of their pre-Reformation predecessors.[81]

Plague Tract Medicine, Tradition Revised

Other circumstances were to contribute to the increase in mortality in Marseille: surprise, *the lack of experience of the doctors and surgeons*, and the operative causes that were present there in particular.

Pierre Baux, Nîmes, 1722[82]

Many aspects of Western medicine had changed by the early eighteenth century. Paracelsus had taught that diseases were specific entities, not simply the result of imbalanced humours; they thus required specific (usually chemical) treatments. Experiences with "new" diseases of the early modern era, like syphilis (*morbus gallicus*, or the French pox), had reinforced this view, and Girolamo Fracastoro's conclusion that some diseases were spread through miniscule "fomites" or seeds of the contagion became more widely accepted (but also hotly debated).[83] Andreas Vesalius's sixteenth-century anatomical works had fostered a new sense of the human body and how it functioned, leading to a significant growth in anatomy-through-dissection studies. William Harvey's trials with and detailed descriptions of blood circulation had confirmed the work of earlier experimenters; although initially rejected, Harvey's ideas were, like those of Paracelsus, Vesalius, and Fracastoro, ultimately incorporated in one form or another into the medical canon. An ongoing series of (often competitive) experiments by members of London's Royal Society, France's *Académie royale des sciences,* and Italy's *l'Accademia nazionale dei Lincèi* (among many others) likewise led to advancements. Reading the medical treatments in early modern plague tracts, though, one might not readily notice these developments.

What one does notice, however, is a further turn towards observation and experience over book learning alone.[84] The Parisian physician Pierre Drouet recalled a plague outbreak in Lyon during which he had seen "men fell downe dead to the grounde, eve[n] as they were going in the streets."[85] He claimed that his knowledge about plague had been gained through a combination of first-hand experience, a prodigious review of Hippocrates and Galen, deep questions posed by his patron, and studying treatments with famous medical men. Francis Herring, a Fellow of the College of Physicians in London, had his treatise – "First published for the behoofe of the City of *London*, in the last visitation, 1603" – duly reprinted in 1625 with updates based on what he had observed and learned about the disease during the earlier outbreak.[86] George Thomson, a physician and pamphleteer, dedicated part of his work in 1666 to revealing the truth he had uncovered through dissecting one of his patients who had died during the London outbreak. Thomson looked back upon his twenty years of experience treating plague victims, and the three times he had contracted the disease himself, to disparage other physicians' treatments. In these cases and many others, the writer claimed to have developed a better understanding of plague through his own direct experience.

In some ways, these testimonials are not so different from those made by tract authors in the later fourteenth century; they too claimed to have gained knowledge of plague through experience. John of Burgundy was clear about the need to rely on the accumulated wisdom of those who had actually lived through the disease and treated its victims. Raymond Chalin de Vinario stated at the outset of his treatise that he had read the works of modern doctors, especially those in Paris, Montpellier, and Avignon, and augmented their most useful knowledge with his own observations. By the sixteenth and seventeenth centuries, however, earlier authorities no longer seemed to matter, their scholastic approaches largely ignored if not disdained. Instead, in paying tribute to accumulated wisdom, early modern authors turned to more recent experts: Jean Fracastoro, Jean Fernel, Paracelsus, Marsilio Ficino, and Montanus, among others. As Thomas Thayre noted, it was necessary to consult "the best learned Physitions *in this age*," alongside one's own observations.[87]

The third-generation London physician Stephen Bradwell, who studied at Cambridge but did not complete his degree, offered in his two plague tracts knowledge he had acquired "both by *Reading* & *Experience*."[88] His first tract, published in 1625, was "Collected out of the best authors, mixed with auncient experience, and moulded into a new and most plaine method." Bradwell wrote in that first edition that he "may not take upon me to cure the Sicke, because I meddle not with the Sicknesse (for to practise on the *Plague* now, would prove a plague to my Practise hereafter)."[89] He did take it upon himself to treat the ill, however, and realized that he had much to learn. By 1636, when his second tract appeared, he claimed that there were very few physicians still alive who, like himself, had remained in the city and gained "experience of the last great Sicknesse." Because he had stayed and treated patients against his original intention – and had spent much time since then learning as much as he could about the disease "out of the Choycest Authors" – Bradwell argued that he was now especially well placed to "prescribe a course of *Physicke*, such as both my much reading, and also my manifest Experience in the last great *Visitation*, have preferred to my best approbation."[90]

Often vociferous debates about whether plague was spread by miasma or contagion – two poles on the transmission spectrum that had been significantly less controversial centuries earlier – marked another clear difference between the eighteenth-century plague tracts and those of the mid-fourteenth century. The later treatises found plague transmission to be less straightforward: these debates, as well as the variety of theories from which they emerged, caused one early eighteenth-century tract writer to exclaim "'Twould take an Age to recite the many Guesses made concerning the Causes of [plague]; for as each Age has had a Philosophy peculiar to itself, so their Reasonings have been brought down to a Congruity therewith."[91] So too did phlebotomy become a contested method of prevention (and, in some cases, cure). In most other ways, though, the medical contents of the treatises were, if not the same, at least not entirely unlike those of earlier centuries.[92] This may be due to the fact that by the time plague broke out again in Marseille in 1720 (see figure 1.2), the disease seemed to be on the wane in Western Europe. Most of the medical men who wrote tracts during that outbreak had had much less direct experience with it than their predecessors, and so had to rely on old knowledge. This time, though, it was knowledge from the sixteenth and seventeenth centuries that counted, not the experiences of fourteenth- and fifteenth-century physicians.

Sent to Marseille to report on the state of the outbreak in October 1720, Monsieur D.M. Pons, a physician in Montpellier's Faculty of Medicine, quickly realized that his book learning was insufficient. He lamented that his understanding of the disease was based solely on tradition and presumption, learned from "professors [who] had never actually seen the plague."[93] Pons was surprised to see that the city was afflicted with "the true Plague, described by all the Authors who have written about it."[94] He experimented with various remedies, ultimately relying on remedial therapies long recommended by his predecessors in their plague tracts. He acknowledged that some of his ideas might appear to be extraordinary, not only because they were to some extent new, but also because they directly contradicted what he had learned at university. Other French plague tracts of the early 1720s likewise focused almost exclusively on the authors' personal observations

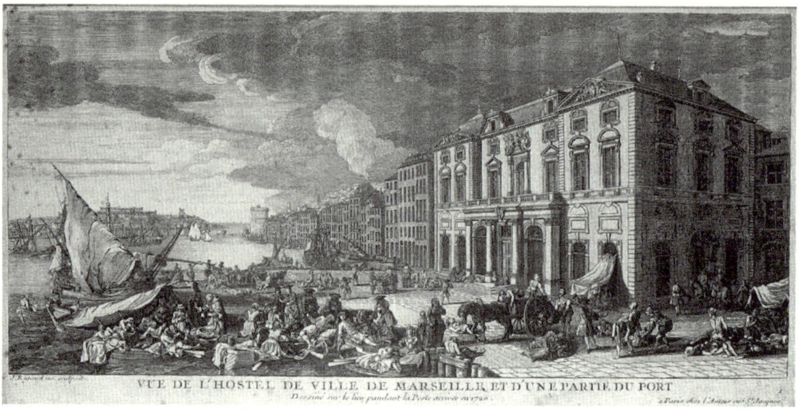
VUE DE L'HOSTEL DE VILLE DE MARSEILLE, ET D'UNE PARTIE DU PORT

1.2 The Port of Marseille During the Plague of 1720, etching by Jacques Rigaud after Michel Serre.

about, encounters with, and reflections on the Marseille outbreak. Treating a large number of infected people daily over a short period of time and "opening and dissecting many cadavers" offered them, as François Chicoyneau, François Verny, and Jean Soulier noted, a unique opportunity to test their formal medical learning against "a certain number of evident and incontestable facts" of a real-life disease outbreak.[95] What this contrast made clear to them was that the high mortality in Marseille could be traced, at least in part, to physicians' and surgeons' lack of experience with and insufficient training for a disease that had caught them all by surprise. They were, in Pierre Baux's words, "*novices dans ce fait.*"[96]

Unlike Pons and his colleagues, eighteenth-century English tract writers had no opportunity to test either their education or their assumptions: the outbreak did not reach London. But this did not stop them from engaging in a heated debate about the relative merits of Richard Mead's idea that plague spread through infected trade goods against theories that Richard Brookes contended were "Founded upon the Experience of those who were Practitioners when [plague last] raged."[97] As another writer, Joseph Browne, argued the "most learned Physicians of [earlier] Times" had actually observed plague first hand and could therefore speak with more authority on the subject than modern physicians who had no experience.[98] According to most eighteenth-century English writers, traditional ideas should not be dismissed quite so readily. As Brookes passionately stated: "Whoever writes with any tolerable Success upon the *Plague*, must found his Opinions upon the Observations and Experience of his Predecessors; for they alone are able to inform us of the different Fortune of a various Practice ... However specious or conclusive the Reasonings of some may be, yet they satisfy us no farther than they have *Experience* for their *Foundation*."[99] It was clear to many that the observations and experiences of their predecessors mattered more than book learning for truthful discussions about plague. Indeed, one of the hallmarks of the eighteenth-century tracts is this reliance on clinical observation, direct or indirect, as an enduring component of cross-temporal learning. Theories of what caused plague, by contrast, continued to be a source of significant debate, even if the remedies to treat the disease would have looked surprisingly familiar to tract writers of the fourteenth century.[100]

CONCLUSION

Across the larger Mediterranean world, plague tracts emerged as a new form of medical literature and advice in response to the Black Death. Blending the format and structure of existing genres and incorporating traditional medical theory and practice alongside novel observations, experiments, and authorities, the treatises enjoyed enduring popularity for centuries. Their ultimately widespread authorship, their quick vernacularization, and their reflection of religious difference and adaptation to cultural change meant that the tracts could speak to divergent audiences while maintaining a largely formulaic structure and offering familiar advice that underpinned medical practice in Christian, Jewish, and Islamic communities alike.

The first serious studies of these texts in the early twentieth century generated a succession of catalogues, partial transcriptions, and editions from modern-day Germany, Italy, France, Spain, and the British Isles.[101] Since then, further transcriptions and significant analytical studies have cast a wider net, producing invaluable information about the specific contents, authorship, and dissemination of individual treatises and of targetted subsets of the genre.[102] Many of these investigations have examined particular aspects of plague medicine and medical change across time. Nevertheless, even where change has been identified – some of it quite radical and groundbreaking – the broader scholarship has tended to accept that "long-favoured texts" were simply republished during multiple outbreaks, that "novelty [was] rare," and that even eighteenth-century tracts were "uncontroversial and traditional ... [simply] summaris[ing] old ideas and old remedies."[103]

If the medical contents of plague tracts largely remained if not consistent then at least consistently traditional, we might be excused for thinking that they remained so in their entirety. As the next chapters show, however, we do a disservice to these sources if we simply stop at their formulaic contents without looking deeper into what else they reveal about how thinking about plague changed over time. Over the many centuries of the Second Pandemic, they are full of small changes, unique commentaries, and locally relevant non-medical discourses. Taken together, these variations point to significant cultural and transformations beyond the tracts' medical contents. Approaching the treatises as individual productions through which to view non-medical change, and doing so in a comparative fashion, thus highlights the tapestry of information that is embedded in plague tracts. The first point of departure is to examine more closely who produced these texts, and where and how they did so.

2

Producing the Plague Tract

From Author to Stationer, from Manuscript to Print

There was a pestilence in Montpellier and I could not avoid the community because I went from house to house to cure the poor sick … My colleagues were incredulous that I kept my life.

Johannes Jacobi, Montpellier, c. 1357–74[1]

PLAGUE TRACTS AS INTELLECTUAL AND MATERIAL CULTURAL OBJECTS

Not long after the second wave of plague passed through his city, Johannes Jacobi (also known as Jean Jacme) reflected on the role that he had played in aiding the sick and dying, especially the poor. While the wealthier members of the city could flee the advancing disease, and indeed were often advised to do so, those without the means to escape were left to fend for themselves. Despite widespread public condemnation of physicians, whether for their inability to cure the disease or for their cowardly refusal to stay and treat the ill, not all of them chose to run away. Jacobi was an important man in the city: professor of medicine, between 1364 and his death in 1384 a chancellor at the Montpellier Faculty of Medicine, personal physician to the Duke of Anjou, and occasional physician to Avignon popes (Urban V, Gregory XI, and Clement VII) and King Charles V. Yet he was among those who stayed and risked their own lives in an effort to save others.[2] For protection, he likely followed the advice he offered to other physicians: stand far away from the patient, keep your head facing the door or window, and make sure that the windows remain open to the north and east. When he wrote about this experience, Jacobi used the relatively new plague tract format to structure his ideas and recommendations.

In addition to his illustrious medical and teaching career, Johannes Jacobi authored several well-known medical texts. The practice compendium *Secretarium practica medicine,* written at the request of King Charles V, offered a head-to-toe discussion of diseases and other ailments. Other works included a treatise on fevers and a practical text on kidney and bladder stones intended for other doctors and students. He also seems to have translated several medical treatises from Arabic into Catalan.[3] But the most copied and thus most influential of his written works was the plague tract. Like others of its genre, it discusses the causes and signs of plague, recommends preventative measures, and offers therapeutic treatments. In writing the tract, Jacobi clearly drew on his own experience: not only did he stay behind in Montpellier to treat the sick during an outbreak, but he may have contracted the disease himself, surviving only with some difficulty.

Jacobi's tract survives in several different manuscript versions. The first appeared in verse, possibly as early as 1357, and was read aloud to the clergy in the diocese of Montpellier. Jacobi later rewrote the tract, first in French prose and then in Latin prose, possibly in the 1360s or 70s.[4] Another shorter tract, entitled *Preservatio pestilentie secundum magistrum Johanem Jacobi*, appears to have been copied down in 1371 by Pierre Chartreis, a Genovese scribe and later a canon. Chartreis may have studied medicine under Jacobi and this version of the tract could be his recording of notes taken during one of Jacobi's lectures.[5] Unlike the longer tract – which follows the typical cause, prevention, and treatment format – Chartreis's text focuses more heavily on prophylaxis and remedy. If it was copied from one of Jacobi's lectures, it likely reflects those therapeutic aspects of the disease that Chartreis found most interesting or useful for his own needs.

Jacobi's Latin prose tract survives in about forty manuscript copies, mostly unadorned and simple productions. Although it was popular on the Continent, only four fifteenth-century Latin copies of the tract are known in England. Through the later fifteenth century and well into the sixteenth, this treatise continued to circulate widely. By this time, though, it was circulating in print, in multiple languages, and, most importantly, under someone else's name.

Unpacking the specific contexts and conditions of an individual tract's production and reproduction enables us to step back and look more closely at these works as objects, as examples of material as well as intellectual culture.[6] Authors, copyists, translators, illuminators, and later printers – and alongside all, consumers – each played a tangible role in the creation and recreation of the treatises and the knowledge within them. At the same time, each treatise is itself a product that marks the coming together "of a unique community of producers and consumers, a community of which the [treatise] it produces will be, strictly speaking, the only instantiation and record."[7] Here, I explore who produced these treatises and where and how they did so, revealing in the process their uniqueness and their ties to particular places and times.

The intellectual and physical production of plague treatises was not uniform in England and France. French authors produced some of the very first, in 1348–50, and continued to be prolific in their output thereafter. By contrast, despite authoring other famous medical works, Englishmen mostly offered only translations of a very small number of Continental treatises for at least two hundred years. The same few tracts circulated in England in manuscript and then in print until the last decades of the sixteenth century. Even though English-authored tracts started to appear in greater numbers in the later 1500s, French production continued to far outweigh English into the eighteenth century.

In both kingdoms, plague tracts appeared not just as simple, unadorned texts copied into small manuscripts, but also as ornate, gilded, and professionally illuminated editions destined for royal readers. The earliest printed tracts were reproductions of popular treatises still circulating in manuscript, but the greater variety of French manuscripts continued into print. The small size, tight interconnectedness, and London-based concentration of England's print industry also influenced that kingdom's tract production and content in other ways, not only limiting which treatises appeared on the market but also ensuring that their content and format attracted readers specifically in that city. France's larger and more dispersed publishing industry – a reflection of its much greater population and regionalized demography – meant that more authors had the opportunity to write about their experiences with local outbreaks. This presented a wider range of voices than was possible in England.

All of this points to the significant influence that location played on plague tracts.[8] The format, time, and place of a tract's production left its mark on both its contents and its physical materiality. Whether it was an original manuscript from a fourteenth-century university faculty in Paris, a handwritten copy made for the occupants of a fifteenth-century manor in the North Riding of Yorkshire, an adaptation from manuscript into print by a stationer in London, or a physician's draft meant to go directly to print in eighteenth-century Béziers, each treatise contains within itself "both geographical and historical coordinates … [and] individuality."[9] Each responded to a particular outbreak, a particular set of fears, and a particular moment in history.

Like many other kinds of books, plague treatises were mobile.[10] The ideas and beliefs within them were largely, albeit not universally, accepted throughout Europe, yet as individual tracts travelled from one place to another, their contents were sometimes adapted or revised to respond to local concerns. Translators both helped existing works to circulate in a new language and offered a "unique and creative transformation of the source text into a new … environment," whereby "local equivalents [were inserted into the text in the place of] the settings, customs, religious practices, and so forth of the original."[11]

Scholarship tracing the work of specific scribes reveals their role in the circulation and localization of many kinds of popular texts.[12] Identifying traceable changes in a certain genre or text's material form, practical function, or literary presentation as it transitioned from manuscript to print and was updated and modernized has also been fruitful.[13] While much has been done to identify the outputs of individual authors, scribes, editors, translators, and printers, studies of specific texts or groups of texts often neglect to trace all those people whose combined time, effort, and intellectual contributions might have been crucial to these books. I have attempted to close that gap by digging deeper into the production processes of plague tracts.

Work on the creation and dissemination of knowledge about the natural world in the early modern era has clearly established that the question of *who* did the actual printing (and reprinting) of books was as important to their success as the identity of their purported authors. Just as vital was the relationship between early printers and their circle of contacts, including those who provided the manuscripts from which printed versions were made.[14] It was through the agency of printers and stationers that later plague treatises reached their audiences; the decisions that these men and women made determined how these tracts looked, how the material contained within them was presented, and their availability and affordability. Like manuscript producers before them, printers oversaw editorial changes such as additions, cuts, and the reorganization of existing texts, including works that were more than one hundred years old. This enabled them to regularly reissue editions that were, in effect, new books that contained modern messages and advice, and that sometimes had new authors.[15] The indispensable agencies of authors, copyists, translators, stationers, and printers were thus inextricable components of any plague treatise's manufacture and, by extension, of its very character.

The choices that producers made about a tract's appearance – the presence or absence of illustrations and ornamentation, the size, the quality of parchment or paper, the script or typeface used, and so on – also reflected both the specific conditions of its publication and its expected readership. Different formats and styles enabled manuscript texts, for example, to serve a variety of separate yet overlapping functions: informative, reflective, and performative.[16] Richly elaborated presentation copies held different meanings than workaday versions of the same text. Early printed tracts closely resembled their manuscript counterparts, or at least the plainer and more ordinary copies, suggesting that they too targetted a particular kind of audience. The fonts they used likewise indicated the literacy levels of their expected readers.

Unpacking the production processes of plague treatises and who was involved in them, then showing how those processes evolved over time and place, can tell us about contemporary societies and cultures as well as about the generation, organization, and consumption of knowledge. For otherwise formulaic and outwardly generic plague tracts, these variable aspects of their production – the location, the players involved, the physical formats utilized, and their mobility – had very real implications for their longevity. And, as I explore in later chapters, the who, when, how, and where of tracts' production also influenced how they discussed the locations that plague occupied. Such aspects of production, in turn, made individual tracts especially relevant, or irrelevant, to particular audiences at particular times.

Returning to Johannes Jacobi's tract, we can see some of these considerations in play. Following its wide popularity in manuscript, this text became the first plague tract printed in both France and England. Around 1476, the Lyonnais printer Guillaume le Roy published the French version, with Jacobi's authorship intact: *Regime de lepidimie*. Le Roy was born in Liège and, under the patronage of Barthélémy Buyer, established the first printing press in Lyon in 1472–73 after being trained by German printers in Venice. He is credited with being the first European printer to specialise in vernacular books, and printed the first book in the French language, Jacobus Voragine's *La légende dorée*, in 1476. He also printed a French edition of Guy de Chauliac's surgical manual.[17] Jacobi's French treatise did not circulate beyond le Roy's single edition, although Gaspard Philippe, who later became the first printer in Bordeaux, published an adaptation of it around 1505; here, Jacobi's name is curiously replaced by a fictitious one: a Greek named Atila[18] (see figure 2.1). This tract also appeared in just one edition. No Latin treatise was printed in Jacobi's name.

This does not mean that Jacobi's popular Latin tract did not appear in print. In Paris around 1480, Ulrich Gering, who had established the first press in France, produced an adapted and abridged edition.[19] However, Gering not only removed Jacobi's name as author, but added a colophon (statement at the end of a book) that attributed the treatise to someone else entirely: "Kamiti, Bishop of the city of Arusiens in the Kingdom of Denmark, expert professor in medicine."[20] Early twentieth-century scholarship suggested that this was an unintentional error. Although numerous scholars have attempted to identify the mysterious Danish bishop, more recent arguments posit that the Parisian printer, "on the lookout for new material to supply to an ever-increasing demand" in an era of recurrent outbreaks, was likely more calculating in appropriating the text and saw this as an opportunity to put what looked like a new work into the marketplace.[21]

The majority of other incunables (books printed before 1500) of this Latin treatise were copied almost verbatim from Gering's adaptation. Antoine Denidel produced at least two further editions in Paris (in 1498 and c. 1500). Multiple Latin editions printed in Antwerp, Leipzig, Cologne, Nürnberg, and Freiburg note the author variously as Kamitus, Kamintus, Kamiutus, Kanutus, or Ramitti. Translations in Dutch, German, and Portuguese attributed to Kamiti also appeared before 1500.

Within a few years of printing the Latin Kamiti treatise, either Gering or one of his subsequent partners (Johannes Higman) produced a new edition in French translation. In this version, Kamiti is no longer the purported author; instead, the remedies contained in the work were simply "approved by many doctors in medicine."[22] In dropping the Kamiti attribution from the French edition, Gering sought to publish yet another tract for a different audience. Between 1490 and 1520, that unattributed French version was reprinted in Paris at least seven more times by five different printers (Antoine Caillaut, Estienne Jehannot, Jacques Nyverd, Guichard Soquand, and Jean de Pré), with slightly variant titles (see figure 2.2).

The Latin copies of the Kamiti tract and Le Roy's earlier French treatise correctly attributed to Jacobi were all printed in quarto; the French Kamiti translation appeared only in octavo, similar to almanacs and remedy books that were meant to be easily portable. Both its content and its style were designed to appeal to a more middling audience than the larger works meant to attract higher status readers to the relatively new medium of print.

In London, William de Machlinia thrice printed an English translation of the Latin tract in 1485 that attributed its authorship to "the most expert Doctour in phisike Bisshop of Arusiens in the realme of Denmark," without naming Kamiti specifically.[23] It is possible that King Henry VII supported the tract's English translation and triple printing to counter a dual crisis: concerns about his legitimacy as king and the first outbreak of the sweating sickness.[24] The treatise may have become known to Henry or members of his court during their exile on the Continent. Although it was originally written to address plague and not the new disease that England faced, Henry's encouragement and/or patronization of its publication was largely a political imperative to "contest the notion that the Sweating Sickness was a divine rebuke" to his kingship and "to counteract ominous political gossip and to provide an authorised, if still unofficial response to the epidemic."[25] Whatever Henry's involvement or motivation, the printed tract proved to be popular in England as well: five further editions or versions appeared by 1536: Wynkyn de Worde printed two (London, c. 1509 and c. 1511), while Jan van Doesborch (Antwerp, c. 1520), Thomas Berthelet (London, 1534), and Thomas Gybson (London, 1536) printed one each. All but one were printed in quarto. Fifteenth- and sixteenth-century manuscript copies of this "Bisshop of Arusiens" tract also appeared, in Latin and in English, all post-dating and thus copied from the printed version.[26]

The edition of Jacobi's tract that Berthelet printed is worth looking at in a little more detail. In 1534, Thomas Paynel – Austin friar and canon at Merton Abbey in Surrey, religious diplomat, chaplain to England's King Henry VIII, and translator – added the plague treatise to his growing list of published books. The title page acknowledges that Paynel had translated the text into English, but neither the prefatory comments nor the contents indicate the text's original source. Instead, the reader is advised that it is Paynel who is offering "certayne profitable thynges for the co[m]mon weale, and agaynst pestilence."[27] Throughout the tract, Paynel used the first person pronoun "I" to take ownership of the proffered explanations and advice: "I intende," "I wyll ordinatly wryte," "To this question I aunswere and say," "I wolde counseyll them," "I had experience," and so on. Even though English versions of the tract had already been printed multiple times, Paynel (or, more likely Berthelet) decided that the treatise was no longer widely known, and that a newer version would be useful. Paynel thus translated it anew, likely from one of the French editions (since he mentions neither Kamiti nor the Bisshop of Arusiens), claiming that he had done so for the profitable benefit of the English "common weale."[28] He also removed his exemplar's prologue. In its place, he proclaimed his own humility, noting that due to his "poore lernynge" he was willing to be corrected by "auncyente maysters and doctours."

Paynel was a well-known humanist translator and focused on providing non-Latinate readers with moral guidance, including both religious texts and practical instruction related to medical and household problems. Aside from the plague treatise, his early medical works included two translations from Latin: the medieval *Regimen sanitatis Salerni* in 1528, and Ulrich von Hutten's contemporary treatise, *De guaiaci medicina* (into *De morbo gallico*, or On the French Disease) in 1533. Both books were successful enough to appear in new editions over subsequent decades.

Generating book sales benefited both author (here, Paynel) and printer, and Paynel's translation may have been done at the behest of his printer, Berthelet.[29] From 1530 to 1547, Berthelet was the king's printer and bookbinder, responsible for printing royal statutes and proclamations, as well as other works that the king and his council deemed important for broad dissemination. The King's Printer operated under rules, privileges, and legal and political principles that were independent of those of London's Stationers' Company. Berthelet thus held considerable status and authority in London, and anyone reading works that he printed "would have understood that the text was doing official service."[30] He was prolific: in addition to official texts and statutes, Berthelet printed more than 252 titles, including all of the works written by the humanist diplomat and scholar Sir Thomas Elyot, various religious tracts, and a number of learned legal treatises.[31]

Berthelet had also printed all of Paynel's earlier translations, and the two enjoyed a beneficial working relationship: Paynel's books provided good economic returns. In the preface to his translation *De morbo gallico*, Paynel reflected on this close collaboration between translator and printer, noting that that book had resulted directly from him "being at London to talke with" Berthelet about his previous work, the *Regimen sanitatis*: "And thus in talkynge of one boke and of an other, he [Berthelet] came forthe and sayde: that if I wolde take so moche peyne as to translate into Inglysshe the boke that is intitled *De medicina guaiací, et morbo gallico* wryten by that great clerke of Almayne Ulrich Hutten knyght, I shulde, sayd he, do a verye good dede."[32] Paynel's translations thus simultaneously served economic, humanist, and charitable impulses, while Berthelet as printer assigned them a sense of officiality.

A similar motivation likely spurred Berthelet's decision to suggest retranslating and reprinting the plague treatise. He certainly would have recognized the profitability of earlier editions of the treatise, given both its economic returns and the remedial benefits that it offered. In light of the epidemics that continued to trouble London in the early sixteenth century – sweating sickness in 1528 and plague in 1529–30 – there were incentives to produce a modernized version of a popular text.[33] The most recent English edition had been printed a decade and a half earlier, in 1520. The only other printed plague tract then in wide circulation was Thomas Multon's late fifteenth-century translation and adaptation of a different mid-fourteenth-century treatise, one written by John of Burgundy; it too might have seemed out of date.[34] Multon's treatise – with the author's name now spelled "Moulton" – had already gone through at least two print editions in recent years, and it was a reasonable bet that English readers would eagerly purchase another tract to give them guidance against a recurrent and deadly disease.

Berthelet printed the treatise using a small black-letter type, described as being "of the form known as Secretary, and of a body between Small Pica and Long Primer."[35] Despite Berthelet's status, this typography likely signalled that the book targeted people with basic or functional reading skills rather than more highly educated readers who could understand Roman typefaces. Black-letter was, for example, the type commonly used in primers, almanacs, public documents and proclamations, and plague orders.[36] Berthelet used the same (or similar) font in several other medical texts meant for a wide audience, including Paynel's translations of *De morbo Gallico* and the *Regimen sanitatis Salerni.* The tract's small and portable octavo size suggested that it was meant for ready and regular use, rather than to be occasionally consulted like the larger quarto-sized *Regimen.* An architectural border topped with a cherub's head graced the title page. Both the title and

Paynel's name appeared as a text block set within the bounds of an intricately decorated monument that resembled a triumphal arch or epitaph (see figure 2.3). Since printers used their title pages both to define the status of a book and as visual marketing tools, an elaborately decorated title page implied that the text carried weight and authority, even if it was meant for rudimentary readers.[37] This style of title page was much more common in Italy than it was in England. Berthelet used similar architectural borders on many of his works, and doing so both visually distinguished his productions from those of his competitors and signalled the particular importance of his work.

Berthelet seems to have miscalculated the tract's profitability, however: unlike Paynel's other medical translations (and unlike Elyot's oft-reprinted *The Castel of Helth*), the plague treatise proved to be less appealing to purchasers than anticipated. Only one edition appeared in print, while a newly updated version of the Jacobi treatise materialized just two years later, in 1536, under the auspices of another (unnamed) translator and a different printer (Thomas Gybson).[38] Perhaps it was Paynel's (and thus Berthelet's) decision to stick with a straight translation rather than alter the older French text so that it addressed England's current political and religious concerns that rendered the work less marketable.[39] Despite the authoritative appearance of Paynel/Berthelet's treatise and its association with a respected translator and a highly regarded printer, and even despite the tract's long and broad circulation in its earlier forms and formats, this work could not and did not meet its readers' needs any longer. Simply put, it failed to offer them the interpretation of plague that they had come to expect. Indeed, even Paynel's apparent personalization of the text with numerous self-references was translated directly from the original. Paynel seemingly had nothing new to say about plague and its contemporary impact.

Until it faced competition in the ever-expanding print marketplace that was able to respond more quickly to contemporary tastes, Johannes Jacobi's fourteenth-century plague tract, with and without acknowledgment of his authorship, had a longer and broader shelf life than many of the other treatises produced in France in the early decades of the Second Pandemic. Its dominance was not due to it being the first of the tracts, nor even the one written by the most prestigious author, but because in building on the experiences and ideas offered by a growing corpus, it proved to be the most malleable for later producers.

MANUSCRIPT TRACTS AND THE EARLY TRANSITION TO PRINT

Authors/Copyists/Translators

Written by me Raymond Chalmelli, master of arts and of medicine, and physician to our lord pope.

Raymond Chalin de Vinario, Avignon, 1382[40]

Of the extant plague treatises written anywhere before 1350, at least one quarter were composed in France. Pierre de Damouzy, former regent of the Paris Medical Faculty (1325–28), wrote the first one as plague approached Reims in August 1348. At the request of King Philip VI, the Paris Medical Faculty produced its own work a few months later, in October. Like Damouzy, the members of the Faculty did not have any direct experience with plague when they wrote about it, although the epidemic was already causing high mortality in surrounding regions. The plague tract was their first major scholarly work, and its contents reflect the Faculty's pre-eminent position in astrological science. Several other writers associated with either the Paris Medical Faculty or the renowned Faculty of Medicine at Montpellier, which also attracted scholars from across the Continent, produced treatises during the Black Death: Alfonso de Córdoba, an Andalusian physician (1348); Johannes von Göttingen, a German physician, bishop, and astrologer (1348–49); an anonymous Montpellier author who addressed his text to the University of Paris (1349); and the physician and astrologer Simon of Covino (1350). Another physician and astrologer, Geoffrey de Meaux, produced a treatise in 1349, while Bernard Alberti, a physician in Montpellier, wrote his before 1350. Two additional anonymous treatises may have been written before 1350.[41]

Translators reproduced the Paris Medical Faculty tract in several vernacular languages, making it another of the more widely circulated treatises during the early waves of the Second Pandemic (it survives in at least twenty-five manuscript and print versions). New treatises also appeared in response to subsequent outbreaks. Members of the Montpellier Faculty alone produced about twenty-five separate works before the mid-fifteenth century.[42] Alongside Johannes Jacobi's tract, the most well known and influential treatises (or related texts) that circulated widely over the succeeding centuries are those by the

Montpellier- and Paris-trained papal physician and surgeon Guy de Chauliac (who included discussion of the plague epidemics of 1348 and 1361 in his surgical treatise of 1363, *Chirurgia magna*), and Montpellier Faculty of Medicine's chancellor and court physician Jean de Tournemire (also known as Johannes de Tornamira), who wrote in the 1370s. Both Guy de Chauliac and Jacobi included some reflection on their personal experience of contracting the disease; other authors drew either from their professional observations of plague victims or indirect knowledge gained through discussion. Another papal physician in Avignon, Raymond Chalin de Vinario, wrote of his experience living through four separate waves of plague: 1348, 1361, 1373, and 1382; he prepared his tract following the last of these outbreaks.

Almost all of these early writers in France were associated with seats of authority. Most were affiliated with the universities. The Paris Medical Faculty wrote as a collective, but Jehan le Lièvre was a regent in the same institution and wrote his own tract before 1418. Tournemire, Jacobi, Valescus de Taranta (1401), Michel Boeti (<1421), and Jacobus Angeli (<1450) were all affiliated with the University of Montpellier. Tournemire, Jacobi, Chauliac, and Vinario were also tied to the papal court. These men's proclamations about plague and its remedies presented not just a sense of medical authority, but also shades of religious and even political authority. Taranta and Angeli embedded their tracts within larger medical compendia; Taranta's covered practical medicine, while Angeli's encyclopaedic work addressed medicine more broadly. Blasius of Barcelona studied at Toulouse and practiced there as well as in Montpellier and Sicily; he wrote his treatise in 1406 at the request of King Martin of Aragon.[43] Like Guy de Chauliac and Johannes Jacobi, Blasius treated his own plague symptoms and survived to write about the experience. Another fifteenth-century French tract writer was Theobaldi Loüet (Theobaldus Loneti), a physician from Besançon whose tract reflected his experience treating patients during a plague outbreak in Rome in 1424.

Jewish physicians living and working in Avignon during and after Black Death also wrote their own plague tracts, the most notable being Isaac ben Todros. In his treatise of 1377, Todros claimed to be opposed to the use of anti-plague pills because they would not transport the medicine to the extremities quickly enough; he nevertheless described in his treatise how his own recipe could successfully be converted into pill form. He also criticized what he had read in some Christian tracts, notably a tendency among the writers (and medical practitioners) to ignore individual patients' circumstances and complexions and to assume a one-size-fits-all approach to explaining and treating the disease.[44]

The late fifteenth-century tracts of the Tournai physician Joannes Spierinck are also notable for their connections to both the French and English kingdoms. In 1480, Spierinck, physician and councillor to Philip the Good (Duke of Burgundy, 1419–67), his son Charles the Bold (Duke of Burgundy, 1467–77), and Charles's wife Margaret of York (sister of English Kings Edward IV and Richard III), wrote a plague regimen for Margaret. This work was likely a response to either an outbreak in 1479 in the Low Countries, where Margaret was then living, or one in England in 1480 during her visit there. Some decades earlier, Spierinck had written a plague regimen addressed to James II, King of Scotland (1436–60).[45]

In contrast to the French tracts penned from 1348 onwards, the earliest treatises produced in England date only to the end of the fourteenth or early fifteenth centuries, decades after the Black Death and the subsequent second, third, and even fourth waves of outbreaks. The vast majority of tracts circulating in England through the late fifteenth century were versions of that written (according to the treatise itself) in 1365 by the Liège-based physician John of Burgundy. This tract survives in more than 130 manuscript copies in multiple versions, a variety of physical appearances – from simple workaday to professionally illuminated – and in several languages (Latin, French, English, Dutch, and Hebrew). Three significant adaptations to the tract were made, most likely the products of English innovation from the turn of the fifteenth century. One, an epistolary version commonly referred to by its opening words (*Dilectissime frater*, or Dear brother), survives in twenty Latin copies, plus two English translations. The second adaptation incorporates material from John of Burgundy's tract along with text from elsewhere; it survives in two English copies.[46] The most commonly attested adaptation, however, is a shortened Middle English version attributed to John of Bordeaux that survives in more than fifty manuscripts.[47]

Manuscript copies of this popular tract continued to appear into the early seventeenth century, long after the treatises of later writers and translators had transitioned to print (see figure 2.4). Upwards of 90 per cent of the extant copies of John of Burgundy's treatise were produced in England; of these, at least three-quarters were in English, the greater part from the fifteenth century. This was, in essence, *the* English plague treatise of the late Middle Ages. Due to its ubiquity, John of Burgundy's work has been considered to be "the parent of a whole host of variants and descendants, and [it therefore] provides a key to much of the [plague tract] literature" in England.[48] Another early English tract writer was John Malverne, physician and rector of St Dunstans in the East (London) around the turn of the fifteenth century.[49] The self-described Dominican friar Thomas Multon wrote another substantially adapted version of John of Burgundy's treatise during the third quarter of the fifteenth century. Multon's tract survives in just one manuscript copy but, as discussed below, it did have a long life in print in the sixteenth century (as "Moulton").[50] The London-based Norman physician Thomas le Forestier penned a tract in 1485, at the beginning of the first outbreak of the English sweating sickness, which closely followed the format and content of contemporary plague tracts. It too survives in only a single manuscript copy.[51] Continental tracts also circulated in limited numbers, including copies and translations of fifteenth-century treatises attributed to Johannes Jacobi, to "Blascus, physician to the King of Aragon" (i.e., Blasius of Barcelona), and to Benedetto Reguardati, physician to the Duke of Milan (Francesco Sforza), the latter printed posthumously in the late 1470s. At least three anonymous tracts appear in fifteenth-century English manuscripts, the "Tractatulus de salute conservanda contra pestilentium," "Breve opusculum de pestilentia," and "In nomine."[52] Others have either not survived or been discovered.

It is puzzling that composition of new plague treatises appeared so late in England, especially since English physicians wrote authoritative and widely circulated texts that focused on the diagnosis and treatment of other illnesses both before and after the Black Death. Why so few appeared during the first century or more of the Second Pandemic has not yet been adequately addressed. I use the term "original" here to mean texts that an author wrote (or, more typically, compiled) himself, rather than translating or adapting someone else's work. Certainly plague tracts were, in most cases, full of widely accepted medical theories and therapeutic recommendations; in that sense, there were few truly original productions after the mid-fourteenth century.[53] Some of the translated/adapted treatises also included small amounts of new content that arguably transformed source texts into something quite different.[54] However, it is important to separate imported and adapted works from those written without direct referents, as they indicate different writing and thinking processes.

Most of the often-copied, often-translated plague treatises of the late English Middle Ages were written before the fifteenth century, and so the initial availability of possible treatise-writers likely mattered. The late creation of medical faculties in England, and their subordination to theological study, meant that there was a comparatively smaller number of English university-trained physicians at the time of the Black Death compared to what one would find on the Continent.[55] By extrapolation, there were fewer English university-based medical writers like those who wrote the earliest plague treatises.[56] Learned medicine in this era was Europe-wide, however, so political boundaries did not hinder the sharing of ideas and information – just as they did not hinder the sharing of disease pathogens. Furthermore, the socio-linguistic region encompassing southern England and northern France ensured a lively interchange of medical information (along with trade goods and other exchanges) across the Channel; some English medical students went to the Continent to learn medicine, and Continental physicians and surgeons served alongside their English counterparts in England's royal courts and noble households.[57]

This does not explain why so few (if any) English medical authors wrote about plague during the Black Death or the epidemics of the following decades, a noticeable absence given English production in other medical subjects. Plague had moved quickly through Western Europe in 1347–48, arriving in England's southern counties by the late summer of 1348. In advance of its arrival, knowledge about the disease was already available, witnessed in numerous papal, episcopal, and royal letters.[58] Yet surviving evidence suggests that no English physicians used the emerging plague tract genre to explain the approaching epidemic or to suggest, in writing, preventative and curative treatments as their French counterparts did. Nor would they do so for almost two hundred years (aside from a few notable exceptions).[59] This points to larger questions about English medical writing, and about English medical writers and their interests and motivations, that deserve more attention than can be given here.

Despite the paucity of tract authors in England, however, we are able to trace in some detail a not insignificant number of tract owners as these manuscripts moved across and through kingdoms and were repeatedly recopied.

Places of Production and Owners

Here begynneth a nobyll tretys made by a right worthy physician named maister John Burdeus agaynes the malady of the pestilence.

Margaret Beaufort's copy of the shorter version of John of Burgundy's tract, London (?), c. 1485–1509[60]

Lady Margaret Beaufort, countess of Richmond and Derby and mother of England's King Henry VII, had a morbid fear of epidemic disease, including plague. Her first husband, Edmund Tudor, had died of plague in November 1456, only a few months before Henry was born. At the time, Margaret was only thirteen years old. Between then and her own death in 1509, she faced numerous epidemic disease outbreaks, including plague, influenza, and the sweating sickness. Especially during the years of Henry's kingship (1485–1509), both plague and sweating sickness were frequent visitors, sometimes concurrently.[61] At least two of her grandchildren died from epidemic diseases – the baby Edmund in 1500, possibly of plague, and Arthur, heir to the throne, in 1502, possibly of sweating sickness. Although she may not have had direct contact with them, several high-ranking members in Henry's service contracted, and some succumbed to, plague or sweating sickness.[62] Recent research indicates that Henry's mother-in-law, Elizabeth Woodville (widow of King Edward IV), also likely died of plague in 1492.[63]

Surrounded by such fearful and deadly epidemic diseases, Margaret did what she could to help herself and others. Through her will, she left funds to keep the manor house at Malton (Cambridgeshire) in good repair "soo that the maister and scolers may resort thidder, and there to tary in tyme of contagious siknes at Cambrige, and xercise their lernyng and studies."[64] She owned a book of hours that contains both an image of St Christopher (a plague saint) and several prayers calling on him to shield her against plague.[65] Some of the numerous anti-plague recipes found in a large medical manuscript owned by the Scope family, which was closely connected to Margaret, may have come from her. At the least, a number of the recipes are repeated, or are very similar to, those found in Margaret's own medical manuscript.[66]

This latter manuscript contains not just anti-plague recipes and prayers, but also two versions of the "Bishop of Arusiens" (Johannes Jacobi) treatise – one in Latin and one in English – and two versions of the John of Burgundy tract, one epistolary version in Latin and the shorter English text attributed to John of Bordeaux (see figures 2.5 and 2.6).[67] Whether it was commissioned by or for Margaret has not yet been determined, but its existence points both to ongoing concern about plague within the highest levels of late medieval society and the value the nobility placed on plague tracts.

Margaret was not the only high-ranking commissioner or owner of a plague tract. The Paris Medical Faculty tract was produced in 1348 at the behest of King Philip VI.[68] His grandson, King Charles V, owned at least two different tracts made in the early 1370s: the first by John of Burgundy and the other by the Paris Medical Faculty (see figures 2.7 and 2.8).[69] English courtiers such as Sir John Paston II also commissioned copies of the John of Burgundy tract along with other medical and alchemical texts.[70]

Other tract owners were somewhat lower on the social scale, yet their ownership of copies of the same tracts trusted by the nobility demonstrates their wide appeal. Pierre Chartreis, a medical student who later became a physician and canon in Montpellier and Geneva, prepared an early Latin copy of Johannes Jacobi's treatise in 1371; the Augustinian Monastery of St Marienwolde, located in Frenswegen, Lower Saxony, owned a manuscript containing Latin copies of Johannes Jacobi and Jean de Tournemire's tracts in the fifteenth century.[71] Two fifteenth-century Latin copies of John of Burgundy's tract can be traced to France: to a Montpellier medical student named Petrus de Oultre c. 1412–22, and to Bauduin Cauwet of Lille, a minor nobleman associated with the fief of Molinel in Lomme c. 1423.[72]

A Hebrew translation of John of Burgundy's tract of 1399 from Carcassonne is also notable. The translator, Benjamin bar Isaac of Carcassonne, began with an interesting reflection on the transmission of medical knowledge across religious boundaries: "When I saw this work closed up among their treasures, tried and verified by respected physicians, I plied all my efforts towards getting it out of their hands in order to translate it from their language into the holy tongue, so that it could bring aid and glory to us and to those who come after us"[73] (see figure 2.9). We do not know yet where Benjamin found his exemplar. It is reasonable to assume that additional copies of these treatises and many others were held in French monasteries and copied by French medical practitioners, clerics, and gentry.

English ownership of plague tracts was just as broad-based. In the mid-fifteenth century, Richard Trewythian, medical practitioner, astrologer, and moneylender in London, owned a copy of the Latin plague tract written by Blasius of Barcelona.[74] John Somerset, physician to Thomas Beaufort (Duke of Exeter) and Humphrey of Lancaster (Duke of Gloucester), owned a manuscript containing a copy of John Malverne's early fifteenth-century "Remedium contra pestilentium." Rouland Brugges, possibly a London lawyer in the late fifteenth-/early sixteenth-century, acquired a manuscript that included a plague tract; he later purchased several printed tracts.[75] A number of miscellanies contain more than one tract, indicating that for their owners, plague was a significant, ongoing concern, regardless of their occupation or social status.

Copies of the John of Burgundy tract can likewise be traced to a wide range of institutional and individual owners in England. The Barber-Surgeons of York, for example, had a copy, as did an archiepiscopal household in Southwell (Nottinghamshire) and several abbeys and priories from southwest England to Scotland.[76] Many individuals spread across the kingdom held copies: a monk in Norwich, a parson in Leicestershire, a minor lord in the North Riding of Yorkshire, a London-based herald and antiquary, and a physician and a barber-surgeon in London.[77] While most copies of this particular treatise appear to have been copied directly by and/or for their owners/users, six more are traceable to commercial production in London and Westminster[78] (see figure 2.10).

By the late Middle Ages, London and Paris were major centres for manuscript production, as many of the people engaged in the trade (scribes, painters and illuminators, parchminers, binders, and stationers), importation, and sale increasingly converged in these cities. Growing literacy rates and the clustering of legal, regal, government, mercantile, and large religious institutions – and the many people employed by them – created a growing demand for manuscript books that made market-oriented copying profitable. In Paris, the presence of schools (eventually to become the University of Paris) and increasing willingness by the aristocratic class to spend money on courtly culture also encouraged the concentration of manuscript producers in that city.[79] Added to this was the sheer size of the two cities, in relative terms, which necessitated a great many parish churches, fraternities, gilds, schools, hospitals, almshouses, local government institutions, and professional networks, all of which relied on books to function.[80] At the same time, the introduction of paper, which was much less expensive than parchment, had made books increasingly affordable for literate but non-aristocratic or clerical readers, such as tradesmen, merchants, and artisans.[81]

Even so, manuscript plague tract copying and ownership were widely diffused in France and England, both geographically and socio-economically. Furthermore, many of the same tracts appealed to readers in both kingdoms. This too should not be surprising. Southern England especially was intimately connected through language, commerce and trade, education, diplomacy, and familial ties to a broad region of north-western Europe, and the English Channel served not as a barrier but as a channel of circulation.[82] In this context, a tract written in Liège, like John of Burgundy's, could move to Paris and to England. Just as plague moved along trade and communication routes, so too did the treatises written to explain and address it. Indeed, high mobility was a key characteristic of many of the manuscript-origin tracts, but this changed significantly when local, printer-enabled production began to dominate after the late fifteenth century. I will examine that change below, but first it is important to briefly consider the material aspects of manuscript plague tracts in the two kingdoms and the initial transition to print.

Materiality and the Transition to Print

> Here begynneth a litel boke the whiche traytied and reherced many gode thinges necessaries for the infirmite & grete sekenesse called Pestilence.
>
> "Bisshop of Arusiens," London, 1485[83]

Manuscript plague tracts appeared in various sizes and formats, each designed to suit its intended audience or users. Some were written on parchment, others appeared on less expensive paper. And, while manuscript medical treatises were not uncommonly illustrated with images of surgical tools and procedures, urine flasks, anatomical diagrams, and the like, images are rare in manuscript plague tracts. The main exception to this rule is a small number of tracts that were prepared for wealthy aristocratic or royal owners. The two tracts owned by France's King Charles V in the early 1370s, for example, are found in richly decorated, folio-sized manuscripts (approximately 235 x 155 millimetres). The physician Gervaise Crestien commissioned both manuscripts for the king and the royal scribe, Raoulet d'Orléans, prepared at least one of them. In addition to many elaborate marginal decorations, the John of Burgundy treatise includes a miniature of a robed physician sitting at a lectern consulting a large manuscript, possibly the treatise itself. The Paris Medical Faculty tract boasts a miniature of a seated king speaking with (or being instructed by) three robed physicians – members of the faculty, perhaps. One of the physicians is in the process of handing a book to the king, again possibly the plague tract (see figures 2.7 and 2.8).[84] In both instances, the physician's importance is highlighted, as is the physician's relationship with the king.

A small number of English copies of John of Burgundy's tract were produced with a similar level of elegance and skill. A small (120 x 80 millimetres) deluxe parchment volume dated to 1449, associated with the physician Thomas Betrisden, contains a copy of the tract that is, like the other texts in the manuscript, decorated with gilt initials and border flowers and vines.[85] The fifteenth-century Guild Book of York's barber-surgeons is full of detailed medical and surgical drawings, as well as heraldic images, portraits of sovereigns, and guild ordinances; this quarto book (275 x 190 millimetres) would have held pride of place in the guild building.[86] Fifteenth-century commercial producers in London or Westminster created at least six variously sized manuscripts containing medical and alchemical texts that included several versions of the John of Burgundy tract, most likely produced as bespoke commissions.[87] Two from the later decades of the fifteenth century are large (240 x 160 millimetres and 241 x 175 millimetres, respectively), lavishly decorated (including with gilt initials), and on vellum (higher-quality parchment often made from calf skin).[88] Although somewhat smaller, at 195 x 145 millimetres, Margaret Beaufort's tracts are also on vellum and professionally illuminated (see figure 2.6). Prepared some time between 1485, when Henry became king, and 1509, when both Margaret and Henry died, the manuscript's decorations include not only flowered borders and coloured initials on gold, but also elements of Margaret's arms and badge – such a portcullis – together with the red dragon and silver greyhound found on Henry's arms.[89] In the early years of the printed book trade, the production of these deluxe manuscripts signalled continued interest not just in plague tracts in general, but in John of Burgundy's tract in particular. In all cases, their ornate production suggests that this tract (in its various versions) was fit for French kings, wealthy English nobles, and successful medical practitioners. But there is, for the most part, little sign of use in them.[90] We might wonder then, what the purpose was of a tract that explained the cause of plague and offered remedial therapies if it was not actually used; perhaps possession of it, and the information it contained, offered some level of comfort all on its own.

Individual treatises may have circulated originally as pamphlets. In both France and England, however, aside from the deluxe versions described above, most extant copies are either contained in medical miscellanies used by university-trained physicians, rural doctors, barber-surgeons, and lay practitioners, or inserted into general miscellanies produced and/or used by clergymen, gentry families, and (later) antiquarians. Most were pocket-sized, at only 90 x 60 millimetres, or only modestly larger (around 200 x 140 millimetres); in both cases, they were portable, intended for regular consultation. What most distinguishes these tracts from those produced for higher-status owners is their lack of decoration and their layout: they were copied onto the available blank spaces in manuscripts, sometimes squeezed onto pages with little internal marking to clearly distinguish them from the texts that preceded or followed, aside from (sometimes) a rubricated (i.e., coloured) title or initial. Other kinds of adornment are rare. The scripts are not always neat and careful; often they are tiny and cramped. Some appear on parchment, but most are on paper. All of this indicates that these treatises were produced neither for presentation nor for sale, but rather for use. Indeed, many do show signs of use, including marginal pointers (manicules) to important paragraphs or remedies and commentary about them.[91]

In the mid-fifteenth century, John Porter, the member of parliament for Worcester, added a copy of the John of Burgundy treatise to the end of his personal composite manuscript that also includes texts on hunting, heraldry, chess, and biblical and culinary matters. A few decades later, Thomas Ponteshyde, a rector of Blystow (Cornwall), prepared a manuscript while he was in Essex in which John of Burgundy's tract follows works on astrology, mathematics, medicines for horses, and a herbal. Monastic scribes working on cartularies (books of charters) or chronicles typically added the treatise to the empty leaves or pages at the end of a section while others compiled miscellanies that were largely medical in nature. Manuscripts prepared within fifteenth-century provincial gentry families, such as the Whartons (Westmorland) or the Thorntons (North Riding of Yorkshire), included plague tracts together with a variety of other medical and culinary recipes, romances, and political and religious texts. Physicians and surgeons, like "Charles Whytte Cittezen and Barboure Cirurgyon of London" and an otherwise anonymous German surgeon in Grenoble, incorporated plague treatises within larger medical miscellanies containing surgical texts, zodiacs, recipes, and regimens. The Montpellier medical student Petrus de Oultre blended a plague tract in among his lecture notes, two columns to a page, with barely a marker to denote where it began and where it ended, aside from a manicule that points to an important passage.[92]

Later, antiquarians sometimes copied plague treatises onto empty leaves in older manuscripts, as the sixteenth-century herald Sir William Dethick did in Sir John Paston's fifteenth-century "Grete Boke," or as Sir Edmund King, physician to King Charles II, did in an old medical manuscript that he had acquired.[93] In these cases, we can sometimes identify the exemplar from which the antiquarian copied and trace the copyist's attempts to modernize, or not, the text's language and terminology. Given the context in which some of these copies were made, they more likely represent the antiquarian's interest in what they called "historical curiosities" than a copying of the tract for actual use. Even at this late date, though, we can find copies of plague tracts being written in manuscript, with revisions and/or new contents added. Two such tracts, one an adaptation of John of Burgundy's tract and the other an adaptation of Thomas Multon's, were copied for use or study by a surgeon, an apprentice surgeon, or perhaps even a cleric who had a special interest in surgery and wound management. Some quite old tracts thus still served their original purpose centuries after they were first written, albeit with some modernization, such as the anonymous author who updated the tracts to reflect a Protestant worldview[94] (see figure 2.4).

These late manuscript copies demonstrate the long-term value that certain tracts continued to hold over time. But manuscript production also continued well beyond the advent of print. Some later sixteenth- and seventeenth-century treatises – like those by the astrological physician Simon Forman (1593 and 1607), Samuel Collins, anatomist and personal physician to King Charles II (c. 1665), English apothecary William Boghurst (1666), and French vicar Alexis Allaire de Lozeillère (c. 1685) – appeared *only* in manuscript, even though in some cases they give the appearance of having been intended for print.[95]

By the 1470s and 1480s, printers played an increasingly dominant role in deciding which treatises were going to be published and which, therefore, became available. In addition to the adaptation of Johannes

Jacobi's plague treatise, which, as noted above, was the first printed in both France and England, Thomas le Forestier's English treatise on the *sudor anglicus* (English sweating sickness) was expanded to include plague and appeared in Latin and French print in the early 1490s.[96] In 1501, the Lyonnais printer Martin Havard published an anonymous tract that he proclaimed had been "composed and approved by many doctors and other great clerks in medicine in Avignon when the great pestilence reigned there"[97] (see figure 2.11). This treatise, he said, contained numerous recipes "very profitable for the conservation of human bodies." By 1520, that tract had been reprinted four times: twice by the Lyonnais printer Claude Nourry and twice in Paris (once by the frères Marnef and once by an unnamed printer).[98] Midway through the treatise is a discussion of anti-plague pills whose formulation is attributed to a "Master Jacques, Jew of Avignon," making it likely that that the tract originally circulated in manuscript.[99]

Through the first two decades of the sixteenth century, the most commonly reprinted French plague tracts were the various versions of just two medieval treatises: Jacobi's fourteenth-century tract and the "Avignon" text. In England as well, the earliest printed and constantly republished tracts were the adapted version of Jacobi's work and Thomas Multon's reworking of John of Burgundy's treatise. All were adapted from manuscript. To continue their accounts, we too should transition to the story of print.

PRINTED TRACTS POST–1500

Authors and Translators

> [N]othing is more necessary nor more desired in the time of dangerous sicknesse and perill of death, then to present unto the person so standing, the meanes to preserve him from the violence of the same, and to restore the sicke from imminent perill of death, unto his former estate of health … [and so] This treatise (gentle reader) I have penned, and present unto thee.
>
> Thomas Thayre, London, 1625[100]

Although his work was unremarkable in terms of the genre, Thomas Thayre was among the first of a small group of English authors who penned their own plague tracts rather than translating Continental sources and adapting them to an English readership. Writing in 1603, Thayre, a self-described (but unrecorded and thus unlicensed) surgeon and medical writer, promised to provide his readers with the "most excellent and approoved remedies ... the true and perfect cure of the pestilence."[101] The second edition of Thayre's treatise appeared in July 1625 during another serious outbreak, just as the number of deaths started to increase significantly. In this later edition, Thayre claimed to be drawing upon his personal experience treating the disease and counselled his readers to use the recommended medicines early, "for delay breedeth danger; and death commonly followeth, and medicine comes too late when nature is overcome by the sicknesse."[102] He asserted that "no man had as yet written any treatise wherein was contayned such speciall and excellent medicines." Of course, other writers claimed that they too offered something new and special, yet they, like Thayre, typically proposed the same blend of spiritual, medicinal, lifestyle, and administrative recommendations that were common to this era. Original production did not necessarily mean original ideas.

For the most part, the adapted versions of Johannes Jacobi and John of Burgundy's works dominated English plague treatise production and circulation well past the mid-sixteenth century. The final English edition of the "Bisshop of Arusiens" version of Jacobi's tract was printed in 1536, but new editions of Thomas Multon's (i.e., Moulton's) wholesale translation and adaptation of John of Burgundy's tract continued to appear until 1580. Other tracts were slowly coming on the market, but they too consisted primarily of translated and (sometimes) adapted Continental treatises. In 1544, Thomas Phayer translated and adapted Nicolas de Houssemaine's French treatise, first printed some two and a half decades earlier. Phayer was a lawyer, member of parliament (1447, and again 1555–59), and licensed physician (he had practiced medicine for twenty years before being formally licenced in 1558). An expanded edition of his large volume of translated medical texts containing the plague treatise appeared in 1553 and became another of the most reprinted English medical books of the sixteenth century.[103] In 1578, the physician Thomas Twyne's *A New Counsell Against the Pestilence* offered a translation of Pierre Drouet's Latin tract of 1572; the following year, the writer Thomas Hill translated an Italian tract by Leonardo Fioravanti that was a decade old.[104]

At the height of a serious outbreak in London in 1603, Thomas Lodge – lawyer turned author turned playwright turned physician – published his first medical text, a plague tract. His objective, he claimed, was to help the poor who had no recourse to greedy professional medical help and so suffered inordinately for lack of self-help knowledge. Lodge also detailed another reason for publishing this work: to re-establish his good credentials. A neighbouring unlicensed practitioner had posted a series of unaddressed advertisements for miracle cures outside of Lodge's business and, while this generated an influx of patients into Lodge's shop seeking those cures, it also overburdened him. Worse, he felt, it "prostitute[d]" his profession to the "base and servile desire of mony," tarnishing his reputation as a serious and honest medical practitioner.[105] To restore that reputation (so that "the world might conceive of me ... that I preferre a common good") and "under a great desire to doe good unto my neighbors," Lodge claimed to have "faithfully gathered out of the most approved Authors" the true explanations of and cures for plague. Furthermore, he stated, all other treatises that were currently available were so "confusedly hudled up, without either forme or Methode" as to be not only useless but also harmful to those who tried to read them. Nowhere in his tract did Lodge mention that all he had really done was to translate and loosely adapt a fifty-year-old treatise written by French physician François Vallériole that he (Lodge) had aquired from Vallériole's son Nicolas. He concealed this by having the work printed under his own name.[106] Among other popular tract authors in translation in the seventeenth century were French surgeon Ambroise Paré and Dutch physicians Isbrand van Diemerbroeck and Paul Barbette.[107]

Not all sixteenth- and early seventeenth-century English treatises were translations, but most of the earliest medical practitioners who wrote original treatises lived during the reign of Elizabeth I.[108] While their contents were similar and typically compiled from existing sources, these writers' tracts were not direct translations of others' work. Overall, though, before the early seventeenth century, the most reprinted English texts were translations and adaptations of treatises from Continental Europe. Indeed, even in the mid-seventeenth century, Richard Smith, secondary of the Poultry Compter (a small prison) in London, found it useful to translate and copy by hand treatises written by sixteenth-century Spanish and German physicians alongside numerous other religious, political, and literary texts related to plague.[109]

It was not really until the plague outbreak of 1578 – and even more so that of 1603 – that English writers responded to local epidemics with their own treatises, a point at which all the Crown's continental possessions were lost, the breach with the Church in Rome was irrevocable, and English printers increasingly stopped reproducing medieval texts. Most authors were still physicians or clergymen, as the earlier translators/adapters had been, but they also worked as apothecaries (William Boghurst, 1666), surgeons (Dale Ingram, 1755), members of parliament (Simon Kellwaye, 1593), poets and career writers (John Quarles, 1665), pamphleteers (George Thomson, 1665), and naturalists and botanists (Richard Bradley, 1721). By the late sixteenth century, discussing plague and its role in society through the tract genre was no longer the purview of medical and clerical writers alone. Writers still followed the formulaic structure and contents, but many added their own perspectives by focusing on aspects of plague causation and prevention that appeared most important (or, alternatively, most ridiculous) to them. Many also addressed contemporary concerns that they linked to the plague outbreaks.

Other than Nathaniel Hodges's Latin *Loimologia* and the English translation of Paul Barbette's Dutch composition, both of which appeared in print in 1672 (Hodges's treatise was a reflection on the 1665 outbreak), no significant medical treatises on plague appeared between the great plague outbreaks in London (1665–66) and Marseille (1720) – an absence that correlates with the declining public awareness of plague. Although outbreaks did not stop in England after 1665, they remained largely unrecorded (or were diagnosed as something else). A few general medical books in the 1690s and early 1700s contained sections on plague alongside discussions of other diseases, and broadsheets providing plague remedies continued to be printed and posted. There was, however, a noticeable lack of tract production over this half century as large, high-mortality outbreaks essentially ceased. Small, localized outbreaks did not instil the same sense of fear that drove treatise production because they typically occurred outside London, and therefore beyond the printing industry's interest.

By contrast, serious continental outbreaks, such as the one in Central and Northern Europe in 1708–13, and more especially in Marseille in 1720, caused significant concern in England and spurred a larger output of plague tracts than any time before: between July 1720 and the end of 1722, more than thirty different treatises appeared in English. Adding in the multiple editions of some tracts, and the reprinting of older treatises (some decades or even a century and a half old) brings the output closer to seventy. Many of the authors, as in earlier outbreaks, were physicians: Philip Rose, John Quincy, George Pye, John Pringle, an unnamed "Physician in York," and so on. An anonymous tract attributed to the seventeenth-century royal physician Charles Scarborough also appeared in 1722. Journalist Daniel Defoe produced a tract entitled *Due Preparations for the Plague, as well for Soul as Body.* Other authors were anonymous: "Well-wisher to the publick," "Explainer," "Philanthropos," "Lover of Mankind," "Mr. Place," and the general "Englishman." Of these later treatises, the work of Dr Richard Mead is particularly interesting, not just for its preventative recommendations that centred on quarantines, *cordons sanitaires* around infected towns, the isolation and removal of suspected cases to plague hospitals, and even the possibility of death penalties for resisters, but also for the fierce debates about contagion to which it gave rise among many other writers.[110] Several English treatises compared Marseille's outbreak with London's epidemic of 1665, and in doing so rehashed the contents of mid-seventeenth-century treatises. A compilation entitled *A Collection of Very Valuable and Scarce Pieces Relating to the Last Plague in the Year 1665,* for example, appeared in 1721 as a reminder of the previous London outbreak. Some eighteenth-century writers deliberately repackaged seventeenth-century opinions and observations, either to refute Mead's contention that plague could be transmitted via imported merchandise or to bolster their own ideas. Still others translated texts that emerged directly out of plague experiences in southern France, presenting them as eyewitness accounts.[111]

In France, we see quite a different pattern emerge. The pace of new treatise production was increasing already before 1500, and between the first quarter of the sixteenth century and the first quarter of the eighteenth, hundreds of new plague texts appeared, primarily in the French language. Some writers, like Jehan Guinter d'Andernach, provided French versions of their own Latin texts to reach broader audiences.[112] However, so many treatises qualify as original French works that it is impossible to describe them all here in equal depth.[113] The stories of many of these authors will, in any event, appear in the chapters that follow.

Many French tract writers were associated with prestigious centres of medical teaching or the court, much like their fourteenth-century predecessors. These included university chancellors, deans of medical faculties, professors, and royal physicians whose tracts were imbued with academic and/or royal status.[114] The majority of authors, in fact, were still university-trained and practicing physicians.[115] As in England, though, and to a much greater extent, after the fifteenth century the occupations of French treatise writers expanded considerably. We find among them royal councillors, civic administrators and royal officials, health commissioners, apothecaries, surgeons, Jesuits and other religious authors, and the like.[116] The early eighteenth-century outbreak across Provence generated a greater upsurge in treatise writing and production than any previous outbreak: almost forty new works appeared between 1720 and 1722 alone. Many of these were written by physicians tasked with treating the sick; they were thus able to provide direct accounts of what they were witnessing and experiencing. Some of their tracts were quickly translated into English and made available for the London market.

One notable difference is that, unlike in England, tracts continued to appear regularly in France throughout the seventeenth century, even during the reign of Louis XIV as the number and severity of plague epidemics fell almost to levels that had led the English to abandon production. Another difference was the tendency of each newly authored French tract to appear in only a single edition after 1500. The adapted-from-manuscript French tracts produced in the early decades of print had each seen multiple editions over the years, while sixteenth-century English tracts issued under the names of Thomas Moulton, Thomas Phayer, and William Bullein went through even more editions (more than twenty, nine, and four, respectively), and over a longer period of time. Yet only six of more than two hundred and fifty French tracts that were first printed after 1500 went through five or more editions; most of these are from the seventeenth century.[117] After the late sixteenth century, only a small number of English tracts went through multiple editions, too; in these cases, an author, like Thomas Thayre or Francis Herring, updated his tract with new information following a subsequent outbreak, or like Richard Bradely and Richard Mead, was well-connected and oft-published anyway.

The decision to publish a second or subsequent edition of a plague tract lay, for the most part, with printers and stationers, not with the authors. This also meant that which tracts saw the broadest circulation, indeed which even got published at all, was a matter of printerly agency, whereby early printed books held the views and opinions of the men who printed them and, by extension, were selected to serve particular interests.[118] In some cases, of course, these interests were primarily economic, as early printers recognized the financial incentive to produce tracts that were already popular in manuscript. We have seen this above in the case of Johannes Jacobi's tract and its transition to print under a new name. How this agency played out in later decades, and how printers and their location affected the publication of plague treatises after the early sixteenth century are the issues to which we next turn.

Printers and Publishers

> This treatise hath pass'd the view and approbation, both of juditious Physitians and Chirurgians, and hath been judged worthy to have a new vesture put upon him, and to be vindicated from the obscurity and darknesse it hath lain involved and eclipsed in this many years.
>
> Gertrude Dawson, London, 1652[119]

With these words, London printer Gertrude Dawson introduced her most recent medical book – a plague tract – to purchasers, apparently having rescued it from decades of neglect. She took advantage of print technology to redress an old manuscript text (that is, put a new vesture on it) and published it "on purpose for the publick good," noting that one of King James I's surgeons had "formally commended it to publick view" many years earlier.[120] The experiences of later surgeons had subsequently "confirmed, strengthened, and approved" its contents, all of which were predicated on "the most excellent" medical authorities, both past and present. It is unclear whether the original manuscript text existed, or whether its alleged link to the early seventeenth-century court of the late King James I was a shrewd marketing ruse on Dawson's part. Regardless, after a single edition in print the tract appears to have run its course.

Like other plague tracts available at the time, Dawson's first sought to explain the nature of the disease, calling it a "pernitious and contagious Fever ... reckoned to be one of the number of those which are called *Epidemia*."[121] After describing the basic signs and symptoms of plague, the tract then lists a range of possible causes and modes of transmission. These fall across a broad miasma-to-contagion spectrum: unnatural heat, flooding, and/or drought; air, food, and water corrupted by a multitude of rotten and stinking odours; and the clothing or other possessions of already-infected persons. Even dogs, cats, pigs, and weasels could be blamed for carrying the infection from one place to another. But, the treatise warned its readers, whatever explanation one accepted, it was truly a just punishment from God for humankind's sinful ways. The first and primary means of preventing the disease was thus prayers and penance. The second was to flee. Only the third was medical, encompassing sound management of the six non-naturals and numerous herbal and alimentary concoctions in liquid, powder, pill, or pomander form. Wearing a venom-resisting sweet bag or quilt over the heart and carrying a nosegay completed the prophylactic regime. A description of the signs of infection – both good (red botches with pus) and evil (black botches without pus) – leads into the tract's final section, which provides numerous cures to rid the infected body of its plague poison: blood-letting (in the correct vein, of course), purging, and ripening the bubo until it bursts.

This tract's contents were very much like all the others that were already available. Why Gertrude Dawson – one of a very small number of female English printers who published a plague tract – went to the trouble of taking a manuscript that was at least decades old and reproducing it in print is an interesting question.[122] She noted in her preface that she had no doubt that the unnamed author had had charitable intentions in writing the treatise and, given the various epidemic dangers that still faced London's residents, she might have felt that it offered useful assistance. The last serious plague outbreak in London had occurred in 1636; there was a smaller outbreak in 1641, and the next was not to appear until 1665. Perhaps the outbreaks of 1650–51 in Bristol, Shrewsbury, and Newcastle, or the epidemics of smallpox, measles, and fevers affecting southeast England influenced her.[123] Or she might just have decided that it was a profitable time to put a new tract on the market, since few had appeared in almost two decades.

Gertrude Dawson was a prolific printer. Among her many publications were other medical works, including an obstetrical treatise, household remedy books for women, a treatise on urine, more preservatives against plague and smallpox, and intellectual treatises written by members of the Royal Society. In 1657, five years after publishing the plague treatise, Dawson printed the first English medical dictionary, entitled *A Physical Dictionary*, for John Garfield, another printer and bookseller of medical titles. Garfield was an apprentice to Hannah Allen, herself a prolific printer of radical Puritan works and a friend of Dawson's. Dawson had printed works for Allen to sell in 1649. Both women were the widows of printers of medical texts and

John Dawson had printed Stephen Bradwell's plague treatise, *A Watch-Man for the Pest*, in 1625. All three still-living printers – Dawson, Garfield, and Allen – had personal connections in the local empiricist medical and apothecary communities.[124]

Most of the books that these printers produced had clearly named authors who actively sought to have their works published and sold; in other cases – as with this anonymous plague tract – the printer used her own voice to assume agency, to identify herself with (but not as) the treatise's possibly long-dead author, and to declare that she was printing the treatise for the public or "common good."[125] The notion or presumption of serving the common good was evident in many late medieval books regardless of where they were published, and manuscript plague tracts (both English and French) often contained proclamations of having been written for the benefit of the common man, woman, and child who had no recourse to a physician. What separates the manuscript treatises from the printed ones is that even when scribes removed markers of authorship during the copying process, they did not typically insert their own name in its place.

Printerly agency, by contrast, emphasized the intellectual and physical labour that went into the production of books. It also served to promote the printer's identity as the book's producer and thus as the provider of the profit that it delivered, often in the place of an otherwise anonymous or unnamed author. Dawson's declaration of having produced the plague tract for the public good demonstrates that this practice endured at least into the mid-seventeenth century. Printers also enacted their agency through other means, such as presenting old works as new ones by obfuscating authorship, or by creating and then meeting market demand for particular texts. Thus, in both England and France, printers were not simply the producers of books others had authored, especially in the early decades of print. Rather, they played an integral role in determining which treatises to print, to whom to attribute them, and what format they took. As well as being the purveyors of mechanical production, printers and stationers directed and acted alongside authors, translators, and editors.

This is evident in Ulrich Gering's late fifteenth-century publication of Johannes Jacobi's tract under the invented authorship of "Kamiti," as discussed above. Here, the very act of inventing a new author for an already widely circulated manuscript – a new author who presented both expert medical and authoritative religious credentials – points to printerly agency and intention. That this agency was implemented in Paris, when the treatise's original author was affiliated with the Faculty of Medicine at Montpellier, may not have been accidental, given ongoing rivalries between the medical faculties in those two cities. The earliest printed and most commonly reprinted plague tracts in both France and England into the first half of the sixteenth century, in fact, were not written by contemporary authors reflecting on their encounters with or understanding of the disease; rather, they were old texts given new life with new authors, new "vesture," sometimes a new language, and new readers. They were, in other words, the products of a small number of printers in Paris, Lyon, and London.

In addition to the "Kamiti" tract and the "Avignon" treatises noted above, the recycling of a third French tract from manuscript to print is worth noting. Between c. 1519 and 1530, the Lyonnais printer Claude Nourry produced five editions of yet another old plague treatise. The same tract had already appeared in print elsewhere: in a 1519 edition from Basel, the Swiss author, humanist, Protestant reformer, and self-proclaimed "doctor of medicine and the seven liberal arts" Joachim von Watt claimed to have translated it from Latin into German.[126] Nourry likely copied his edition from an Italian one that appeared in Venice around the same time, as it, like Nourry's, is attributed not to von Watt but to unnamed doctors from Basel.[127] Von Watt's work is not original either, and seems to have been translated and updated from an older manuscript circulating in southern Germany; both the older version and Von Watt's contain similar images of a phlebotomy man with buboes.[128]

After 1520, a growing number of French printers started to produce plague treatises as more and more original tracts were written; at least two hundred and four individual printers can be identified between the early sixteenth and early eighteenth centuries, but only thirty-two of them printed more than one. Les frères Bruyset in Lyon (1720s), Raymond Colomiez (1620s) and C.G. Le Camus (1720s) in Toulouse, and Philippe Planche in Geneva (1720s) each printed at least three different tracts.[129] The concentration of these multi-production printers in the eighteenth century reflects the upswing in tract production during the Plague of Provence. In short, the practice of printing plague tracts was widespread, both in terms of the number of printing houses involved and, as we will see, their geographic location.

By 1470, printers had set themselves up in Paris, taking advantage of the structures and markets already established for manuscript book production and the university market. But before 1500, print industries of various sizes existed in twenty-one different cities, as well as in various smaller towns. The kingdom's large population could support multiple, vibrant manuscript and print book production centres, and its less formally centralized system of government and commerce demanded it: large cities such as Lyon, Rouen, Orléans, Toulouse, and Marseille acted as regional political, economic, and commercial centres quite separate from Paris.[130]

The real success of provincial printers came during the religious and political conflicts of the sixteenth century. In particular, presses established in Rouen, Orléans, La Rochelle, Montauban, Montpellier, and Nîmes emerged as significant Protestant printing centres, while publishing houses in Reims, Le Mans, and Tours, among other places, focused on producing Catholic works, as well as official mandates and acts.[131] Less than half the plague treatises published in France between 1490 and 1725 were the products of Parisian printers; about 15 per cent came from Lyon, 7 per cent from Toulouse, and 5 per cent from Rouen. Small numbers of works were also printed in other centres, including Troyes, Poitiers, Anvers, Vienne, Douai, Caen, Angers, Bordeaux, Montpellier, and Dijon (see figure 2.12) This decentralized industry ensured that French authors were able to publish their reflections on local (i.e., non-Parisian) outbreaks, and that the treatises echoed the experiences and concerns of writers and producers across the kingdom. Furthermore, French-language treatises were also printed in Amsterdam, Leiden, Lausanne, Geneva, Zurich, Strasbourg, Tübingen, Heidelberg, Cologne, and even in London.

In England, the situation was entirely different. By the mid-sixteenth century, France was the most populous kingdom in Europe and its total population was five times larger than that of England. Its largest cities (Paris, Rouen, Lyon, Orléans, Marseille, and Toulouse) each had at least 50,000 persons, while in England only one city, London, boasted a population over 15,000. It was in London that the English print industry centralized, maintaining for some time the dominance of Continental works and their adaptation to local tastes. By the 1390s, the area around St Paul's Cathedral was a well established book-craft neighbourhood and, within a decade, a single guild (the Stationers Company) united the interests and oversight of all aspects of book production and sale. Over the course of the fifteenth century, this region of London, along Paternoster Row, had become the *de facto* centre of manuscript book production in all of England.[132] Over the last quarter of the fifteenth century, first Westminster and then this area near St Paul's Cathedral came to house England's nascent print industry, ensuring continuity from the commercial manuscript production centre to one dominated by the printing press. In 1557, by which time printers far outnumbered manuscript producers, the Guild of Stationers received a Royal Charter of Incorporation that gave it significant authority to control printing in the kingdom. Outside London, printers established themselves under the patronage of local monastic or university institutions at Westminster, Oxford, St Albans, Tavistock (Devon), Cambridge, Canterbury, York, Ipswich, and Worcester. These were small operations, though, and other than the printing houses established in Oxford, Cambridge, and York, all were ultimately unsuccessful. The Printing Act of 1662 renewed the restriction of printing to London, Oxford, Cambridge, and York, but outside London the number of printers always remained low.[133]

This directly affected the production (and, as I argue in later chapters, the contents) of English plague tracts. First, a geographically concentrated printing industry, accompanied by the slow spread of booksellers outside of London, likely contributed to the continued manuscript copying of the John of Burgundy treatise long after the rise of print: the availability of printed alternatives was perhaps limited outside the city. Second, a printing industry that was both geographically concentrated and tightly interwoven meant that the choice of printed tracts was limited within the city of London as well, at least for the first six or seven decades of print. The "Bisshop of Arusiens" adaptation of Johannes Jacobi's tract was the only one available in print in English until the late 1520s. Then, a new tract came on the market that not only displaced the "Bisshop" tract but also completely dominated the print market for decades thereafter. This was Thomas Multon's adaptation of John of Burgundy's fourteenth-century tract. More than half a century after Multon, printer Robert Wyer incorporated the text into a larger medical miscellany entitled *The Myrour or Glasse of Helthe*. Wyer and ten other printers then republished the work more than twenty times by 1580. Excerpts from the treatise also appear in the seventeenth- century surgical work *The Compleat Bone-Setter*.

London printers and stationers were conservative, preferring "to produce lots of editions of established [manuscript] texts which had already enjoyed success in Latin [or in English] in the fifteenth century rather than [risk profits] with new texts [written] by contemporary authors."[134] The earliest printed English medical books resembled their manuscript counterparts in both content and format, with regimens, recipes, books of secrets, and other household aids being copied directly. Technical medical books for English readers were imported from the Continent until the later sixteenth or early seventeenth century. Significantly new titles started to appear in larger numbers only after the late sixteenth century.[135] The same trend characterized printed plague tracts: the most common treatises for the first century of London printing were either adaptations of medieval manuscripts that had already seen long lives or translations of older (printed) Continental treatises. This both limited the publication of new ideas and ensured that the same messages were repeated.

Moulton's *Myrour or Glass of Helthe* was the most popular medical work of the sixteenth century not only because it responded to English anxieties and concerns, but also because no competition was allowed to enter the market. The repeated reproduction of the same work (in the same medical compendium) reveals links between each of the eleven printers who published at least one edition of this treatise. They were all connected through widow inheritances, marriages, apprentice/successor relationships, business partnerships, or, interestingly, through landing in jail at the same time and place for the same crime (see figure 2.13).[136]

The book's first printer, Robert Wyer, produced the most editions, making subtle textual and /or format and material changes to each new edition before passing his materials, equipment, and printer's device to Thomas Colwell around 1560. In his two editions of the book, Colwell used Wyer's printer's device and type as his own, as did the printer and bookseller Hugh Jackson, who succeeded Colwell and married his widow after the latter's death in 1575. Robert Redman, the second to publish Moulton's treatise, around 1540, is known to have pirated other printers' works, and it is reasonable to think that he did the same with Wyer's plague tract before passing it on through his wife, Elisabeth Pickering, and her successor, William Myddleton.[137] Both Colwell and Jackson apprenticed with William Powell, who succeeded Myddleton after marrying his widow; Colwell and Jackson possibly inherited materials indirectly from Redman and Redman's successors in this way, as well as from Wyer directly. In 1543, Myddleton, Thomas Petyt, and Richard Kele were imprisoned together for almost one month in Poultry Compter, along with five other printers, for allegedly transgressing Privy Council publication rules and publishing unlawful books.[138] Kele's printshop was located on Poultry, not far from the prison; so too was that of John Allde, his apprentice, who was likewise imprisoned in 1568. Petyt, Kele, and John Waley were booksellers as well as printers; along with the printer Robert Toye, they ran neighbouring shops and engaged in several collaborative projects. Petyt and Redman also co-printed at least one English edition of Coverdale's Bible. Petyt, Kele, Toye, Waley, and Myddleton each printed the *Myrour or Glass of Helthe* at least once around 1545–46.

The printer's name, emblem, and/or date of printing is missing from some extant copies of the treatise, making it difficult to trace its passage from one printer to the next. Nevertheless, it is possible to compare changes in layout, spelling, and woodcuts over time. The first page layout in Wyer's 1540 edition, for example, appears in most editions printed after that date, with minor changes only in word breaks and spelling. Redman's sole edition of the book looks almost identical and appeared around this same time, suggesting that it was his possibly pirated copy that most subsequent printers adopted. Redman's wife, Elisabeth Pickering, made a few orthographic changes in her edition, which Myddleton reproduced exactly before producing a second, slightly different version. Kele, Toye, and the unnamed printer who published "for Rychard Jugge" – then a bookseller and later a printer himself – adopted Myddleton's second edition almost wholesale. Waley's three editions are very similar to Myddleton's. Colwell, who inherited Wyer's works, repeated Wyer's c. 1540 layout, spelling, and iconography. Jackson's later edition was likewise much the same, although he added a new title page. Petyt's edition, though, is closer in style to one of Wyer's earlier versions; he also used the same woodcuts that appear in Wyer's work. A "substantial citizen" who educated and freed at least eleven apprentices, and who produced a sizeable number of books, Petyt's "preference for letting others establish a book's vendibility before reprinting" is clear in this case.[139]

In this light, this tract – and the larger miscellany of which it was a part – might be better considered as standard house stock that was passed down (or borrowed) from one printer and bookseller to another than as a work that was reprinted solely because of customer demand. After all, it was printers and booksellers who "enabled the manufacture, promotion and circulation of these written and printed books ... [and] the promulgation of knowledge, news, and authority was business."[140] This treatise was clearly good business.

The period c. 1545–46 saw the greatest production of "Moulton's" tract: nine editions produced by six different printers. It is in this period that the prison connection between Myddleton, Petyt, and Kele, combined with the partnerships that Petyt and Kele enjoyed with the other printers, led to the treatise's greater availability. There was a plague outbreak in London in 1543, and additional outbreaks occurred in other towns between 1543 and 1547 (Reading, Salisbury, Bristol, Exeter, Worcester, Norwich, Lincoln, and Newcastle, among others).[141] Whether any of these outbreaks spurred this sudden outburst of printing is not known. The 1543 outbreak coincided with the printers' time in prison. This was also a period of intense religious, political, and economic uncertainty. The Italian Wars, which England and the Holy Roman Empire fought against France and the Ottoman Empire, had been exorbitantly expensive and resulted in no significant gains. A French invasion of England seemed plausible. A disastrous war with Scotland was ongoing. English coinage was debased. The Third Succession Act of 1543 reinstated Princess Mary, a devout Catholic. The heir apparent, Edward, was still a young boy and Henry VIII's health was poor. The treatise might have served as a way for printers to respond (uncensored) to these troubles. After 1560, only those printers who had inherited the tract directly from Robert Wyer continued to publish it. The treatise excerpts that were incorporated into the surgical manual in the mid-seventeenth century were then printed multiple times by the same printer (Thomas Rooks) for the same bookseller (Nathaniel Crouch).[142]

Similar kinds of connections can be seen in the repeated publishing of the two other English plague tracts most reprinted in the late fifteenth and sixteenth centuries. Of the eight editions of the adapted (that is, "Bisshop of Arusiens") version of Johannes Jacobi's treatise printed between 1485 and 1536, six were the product of three Low Country printers: William de Machlinia, Wynken de Worde, and Jan van Doesborch.[143] Machlinia and Worde were among England's earliest printers, and each enjoyed patronage from the first Tudor monarch; Doesborch collaborated with both Machlinia and Worde to select the English texts that he then published in Antwerp.[144] Five of the nine editions of Thomas Phayer's treatise came from the shop of one man, Edward Whitchurch, who had been arrested along with Myddleton, Petyt, and Kele in 1543 for printing unlawful books. Two other printers of Phayer's work, Abraham Vele and Henry Myddleton, were also linked to the printing of Thomas Moulton's treatise: Vele received a bequest in Thomas Petyt's will and Henry Myddleton was the son of William Myddleton.

Since none of London's printers and stationers printed a new – that is, original – plague tract before the late sixteenth century, unlike their French counterparts, one might reasonably argue that they in effect created, and then supplied, the most popular treatises in the first century of English print. After the 1570s, as more original English plague treatises appeared, and as the English print industry expanded, the number of printers engaged in publishing these works also increased. Few, if any, printers published more than one plague tract, though. Printers might have worked only with particular authors, and there were sufficient printers willing to publish the treatises to offer authors a choice. There was no monopoly on the production of tracts, or in the production of medical titles more broadly. The genre was secularized to the point where many different authors and printers could profit from it. Unlike the earlier, translated treatises, most of the later, original treatises circulated in a single print edition; only a small number lasted in circulation much beyond the epidemic to which they responded. By the seventeenth century, writers, printers, and readers viewed the older treatises as out of date, and most disappeared from printers' stock (although a few, like Phayer's, reappeared again in response to the plague outbreak in Marseille). As plague increasingly became associated with the broader ills of a society wracked by religious and political controversies, newer works purported to address modern concerns, reflected changing socio-economic conditions, and spoke to new issues when and as they arose.

London's concentration of population and treatise producers meant that its urban experiences with and perceptions of the disease were those that appeared in print. Even so, the circulation of books, from author to printer to bookseller to purchaser (and onward to other readers in other places and times) was a critical aspect of the tracts' lives as textual objects. Though they were produced almost entirely in London, one can assume that plague treatises reached readers well beyond that city, carried and distributed by peddlers alongside the more formal bookselling networks, as well as by members of religious orders, merchants, and any other kind of traveller.[145] Historians who have studied these peddler networks do not discuss plague tracts, but it is not difficult to imagine the treatises being distributed in this way, along with almanacs and other small medical books.

It was, in fact, not just ongoing plague outbreaks but also the tracts' small, cheap format that contributed to their increasing popularity in the age of print. Materiality played an important role in their appeal to different kinds of audiences.

The Subtleties of Materiality

I dedicate this book to the living and to posterity. If it is censured by the learned and the curious, I will patiently suffer their judgment and stop my pen, excusing myself upon the prayers of my friends who desired this first part of my Opuscules. If they judge it to be acceptable, I will pursue my plan and will soon provide the second part. The first Treatise on the Plague is only an excerpt, or an abridgement of the larger work that I prepared in Latin.

François Ranchin, Lyon, 1640[146]

In 1640, François Ranchin, professor of medicine in Montpellier and an avid antiquities collector, produced a large medical book that contained a plague treatise as its core. At close to four hundred pages, the tract was, he claimed, just an excerpt of his much longer Latin treatise. A copy of the book held at the Bibliothèque nationale de France is octavo in size and loosely bound in quires (section or collection of pages) inside a (now) worn and torn vellum cover. It is weighty. To guide his readers, Ranchin provided a detailed table of contents, or rather, several tables of contents, since the first breaks the book down into ten simple parts while subsequent tables provide more detail about each section. The text is printed in several different typefaces, each with a separate function: headings, prefaces, chapter summaries, and main text. Atop each section heading sits a woodcut that resembles the upper portion of an ornamental, architectural arch. All chapters begin with an enlarged capital letter set within vines. Other minor ornamentation separates prefaces from the body of each chapter and signals the end of every section. In many respects, Ranchin's book looks like others of its era. It bears little resemblance, however, to the plague tracts of earlier centuries (see figure 2.14).

In the early years of print, the format of plague treatises hardly changed from the workaday versions commonly found in manuscript: they appeared most often on cheap paper with few decorations. At this point, the tracts' black-letter typefaces targeted the functionally literate. They were sold unbound or incorporated into larger medical miscellanies for about two to three pence in England, or about two to three sols in France (in comparison, a building craftsman or labourer in southern England earned approximately six or four pence per day, respectively; in France, the ratio was similar).[147] Their materiality and cost suggest that printed treatises were intended for a new audience: no longer were they the preserve of clerics, physicians, or higher status individuals who had owned manuscript copies. Instead, they were now for the middling sorts – those with enough income to afford their purchase and the ability to read at a basic level. Until the later sixteenth century, English plague treatises appeared in some variant of black-letter type, with headings and main text typically being in the same typeface. As literacy rates increased in England, printers more often used the blend of Roman types that were already common in French books before the mid-sixteenth century, with capital letters signalling titles and subtitles and italics used for prefaces, summaries, and emphases.

The size of printed plague treatises also changed over time, and differed between England and France. In France, the earliest printed treatises – le Roy's Johannes Jacobi tract (1476), the Latin Kamiti treatises (c. 1480–1500), Martin Havard and Claude Nourry's editions of the "Avignon" tract (c. 1505–15), and the first edition of Nourry's "Basle" text (c. 1519) – were in quarto, or approximately 250 by 200 millimetres.[148] All of the Latin tracts continued to be printed in quarto after 1500, their format perhaps meant to appeal to a higher status audience. Learned works like anatomy and surgical texts were also typically printed in quarto or even in the larger folio. Ulrich Gering's French version of the Kamiti treatise, by contrast, appeared in the much smaller octavo. Gering's decision to print the Kamiti tract in French, rather than just in Latin, and in a smaller size, was a calculated decision to target two separate audiences with what was, in essence, the same work in different formats. More than two-thirds of the hundreds of French-language treatises printed between 1500 and the 1750s appeared in octavo size; a further one quarter came in an even smaller pocketsize.

In England, all versions of the "Bisshop of Arusiens" treatise, except for Thomas Paynel's translation of 1534, appeared in quarto. Since this was the only plague treatise printed in the fifteenth century, the earliest English printed works were all quarto-sized. In the sixteenth century, though, most English plague treatises, like all editions of Thomas "Moulton's" tract (c. 1530–80), appeared in the smaller octavo. Thomas Phayer's oft-printed treatise (c. 1543–96) appeared once in quarto, but more often in either octavo or the tiny sextodecimo (approximately 100 x 150 millimetres). In the seventeenth century, medically oriented tracts were printed most often in quarto, while their religious counterparts appeared in octavo. By the eighteenth century, both types of treatises appeared almost exclusively in octavo.

The different sizes clearly set English printing apart from its French counterpart. The size and format "of a book has its own story to tell ... since it reflects the author's and printer's view of the purpose and audience for it."[149] Applying this logic to plague tracts, some must have evoked an audience or purpose that was more important than others, on par with (or just slightly less valued than) academic anatomy and surgery texts, which tended to be produced in quarto or folio formats for more learned readers. Overall, the genre seems to have had, at least in the fifteenth and seventeenth centuries in England, a nobler purpose than textbooks and regimens, which appeared almost exclusively in octavo format for students and household use. If this assessment for English medical print can be extrapolated, it also appears that vernacular treatises held higher value initially, and for a longer period of time, in England than they did in France. As octavo-sized books after the seventeenth century, though, plague treatises in both kingdoms often resembled pamphlets: small, inexpensively produced, roughly stitched, and portable texts used to disseminate medical information, to advertise proprietary medicines, and to communicate medical, religious, and political debates.[150] They had become, in a word, commonplace. Even so, one of the major differences between eighteenth-century printed tracts and their predecessors was their sheer length: some ran to many hundreds of pages, literally being doorstop-sized tomes. This seems to have relegated them anew to a genre geared towards scholars, no longer a specialized version of a generic health-advice book.

Like their manuscript counterparts, few printed tracts were illustrated. Aside from printers' emblems, authors' portraits, simple ornamentation, or decorated initials, less than 10 per cent of vernacular printed treatises contained any kind of illustration. Those images that were included were typically generic woodcuts of physicians at work, humoral temperaments, or astrologists (see figure 2.1). These images were not specific to the tracts, since printers often used the same woodcuts repeatedly in a variety of books. Although printers initially designed illustrations for specific passages in specific texts, they (and their fellow printers) tended to reuse the same woodcuts so many times for decorative purposes that the images ultimately lost their initial meaning.[151] The few images that were used in plague tracts tended to be simple prior to the mid-sixteenth century, but by the later sixteenth and especially the seventeenth centuries became more detailed. This artistic evolution occurred alongside an expansion of plague art more generally, in style, content, and complexity.[152]

Images perhaps designed specifically for inclusion in plague tracts – such as the Saints Roch and Sebastian, the famous plague doctor, or phlebotomy men with buboes (see figure 2.15) – were rarer, appearing in less than fifteen treatises out of the entire French corpus and typically only in a single edition each. Aside from the doctor and the phlebotomy men, plague-specific images were largely religious in nature. Plague saints represented both healing and intercessionary powers against divine wrath, while illustrations of God, avenging angels, and/or devils shooting arrows or swinging scythes at humanity, or pouring poisonous liquids upon it, appeared commonly in miniatures, paintings, and other contemporary media about plague.[153] Not surprisingly, these types of images appeared most often in texts that focused on religious, rather than medical, explanations of plague. And, while earlier manuscript and print versions of the phlebotomy man with buboes implied a medical intention – such as in Claude Nourry's French edition of Joachim von Watt's tract in 1519 – by 1581 Jean Stratius, the printer of Estienne Ydeley's plague treatise, had given the image itself a decidedly more spiritual tone: surrounding the image are the words "the plague is not an illness but a rod of god."[154] Most of Stratius's production was Catholic religious works, and Ydeley's tract downplayed the medical aspects of disease causation and treatment and emphasized divine wrath. The iconic early modern plague doctor, by contrast, was a thoroughly secular figure.

Images are even more rare in printed English treatises. Nowhere do we see an early modern counterpart to the lavishly decorated commercial copies of John of Burgundy's tract. Robert Wyer's editions of Thomas Moulton's treatise are the most image-heavy, although only with generic woodcuts that Wyer and his successors used prolifically in many other works. At least one edition of the "Bisshop Arusiens" tract contained a generic astrological image on the first page, but most had no images at all. There might have been no obvious replacement for plague saints that English printers could offer. The most detailed image in an English plague text is the frontispiece of George Thomson's treatise, which purportedly shows Thomson's dissection of a plague victim (see figure 2.16). Of course, given the place of Thomson's tract in the polemic battles between traditional Galenists and chemical physicians, the dissection image carries much more meaning than a simple autopsy: it attacks Galenist reliance on humoral medicine and all the types of therapies that accompany it.

Plague tracts were not just texts: they were tangible objects that carried meaning. These meanings, and their target audiences, evolved as the physical features of the tracts changed. Although their contents were comparable, if not greatly similar, a richly illuminated and gilded vellum copy of John of Burgundy's treatise was not the same as one that was squeezed with cramped writing into the empty space at the bottom of a page of paper. The shift to small, cheap print opened the genre to a wider reading audience, while also enabling printers to advertise themselves as purveyors of the common good through their devices and their reuse of recognized woodcuts. The shift from manuscript to print also transformed the plague treatise from being an object created by one person to one in which many hands can be traced.

The different modes and places of production that demarcate English plague tracts from their French counterparts suggest that they were, at least for a time, different textual objects in the two kingdoms. The question that then arises is what impact these differences had on the ways in which the treatises discussed plague. This question is addressed in the chapters that follow.

CONCLUSION

Commenting on his own plague tract, the well-known French surgeon Ambroise Paré remarked "and furthermore, this little book is very useful because it is portable."[155] For Paré, the smallness, cheapness, and portability of his printed treatise contributed to its usefulness, "both to restore health to the sick, and to preserve those who are not yet at risk of the disease." Yet it was not only a book's format that mattered: its place of publication significantly influenced its fortunes. This meant not just the city in which a book was printed, but also the very shop. Early modern readers subconsciously transferred the perceived character of a printing house and its inhabitants, determined in part by the house's location, onto the books that the shop produced. A book published in folio around London's St Paul's Churchyard was perceived to have very different social connotations, value, and thus usefulness, than the same text printed in octavo or duodecimo in Moorfields, Smithfield, or Bartholomew Square. The ways in which printers represented themselves and their works were "therefore of central importance to the received credit of printed knowledge."[156] The value of a particular book was tied as much to its contents and its materiality as it was to the printer who produced it and where he or she lived.

For both manuscript and printed treatises, who produced them – and when, where, and how they did so – mattered, because it ultimately influenced local production of knowledge about plague. For hundreds of years, physicians and other writers produced plague treatises that were so similar in organization and medical content that the wide variety of small differences that distinguish them is easy to miss. Rather than addressing the formulaic structure the treatises share, I have focused instead on the factors that distinguish them, like the times and places of their production, the individuals involved in their publication, and their materiality.

Print technology not only facilitated the creation of more and less expensive treatises for a wider audience, but it also engaged an entirely new group of people in the production process. It is clear that printers and stationers drove changes to plague tracts in ways that were different from authors: in addition to textual changes, they controlled the physicality of the printed book and relied on typographical and formatting strategies to attract a wider readership.[157] Printers and stationers selected the treatises that made the transition from manuscript to print and the format in which they did so. These decision-making processes were not the same in England and France, however, due at least in part to the ways in which the two kingdoms' print industries evolved. The tight interconnectedness of the people involved in England's print industry arguably shaped which work(s) became popular and completely dominated circulation, while France's larger industry meant that authors and readers had more choice. The size of treatises differed between the two kingdoms, as did the use of images.

As we will see in the next chapters, these otherwise formulaic medical treatises respond to and reflect local contexts that were not exchangeable, especially after the turn of the sixteenth-century. France's decentralized print industry allowed a variety of voices and commentaries to appear in its tracts that was missing from the English ones. Religious turmoil existed in both kingdoms, but the visceral anti-Protestant rhetoric that appeared in some French treatises was largely absent in England (see chapter 4). French treatises were produced in many different cities, allowing authors in different places to emphasize the local and particular. A decentralized political system, a large regionalized population, and a multi-city printing industry worked in tandem, allowing nuanced local responses and reactions to plague to be apparent across both manuscript and print treatises.

While local linguistic nuances appeared in English manuscript treatises whose reproduction and dissemination was widespread, one really finds only reactions and opinions from London in the printed treatises. English writers and printers portrayed the city of London not just as the site of disease, but also as its source; because of London's demographic dominance and the concentration of printers there, authors (and printers) conflated the high mortality levels associated with epidemic outbreaks with the very nature of the city itself. As diverse as the tracts and their authors might have been, opinions and viewpoints from London drowned out voices from other towns. Vernacular diversity, which punctuated manuscripts and might have represented a resistance to the centralization of power in London, is lost in the printed treatises. In short, then, the patterns and trends of treatise production, and thus their contents, were specific to time and location.

Identifying and tracking small differences in production processes and practices, in local patterns and spaces of circulation and mobility, and in local encounters with plague contributes to a better understanding of the means by which the treatises' discussions of plague were socially and locally constructed by writers, translators, adapters, copyists, and printers. Together, these various agents and the numerous works that they produced helped to set both the language and the terms for understanding plague in England and in France, as that understanding evolved from the Black Death of the mid-fourteenth century through to the Plague of Provence in the early 1720s.

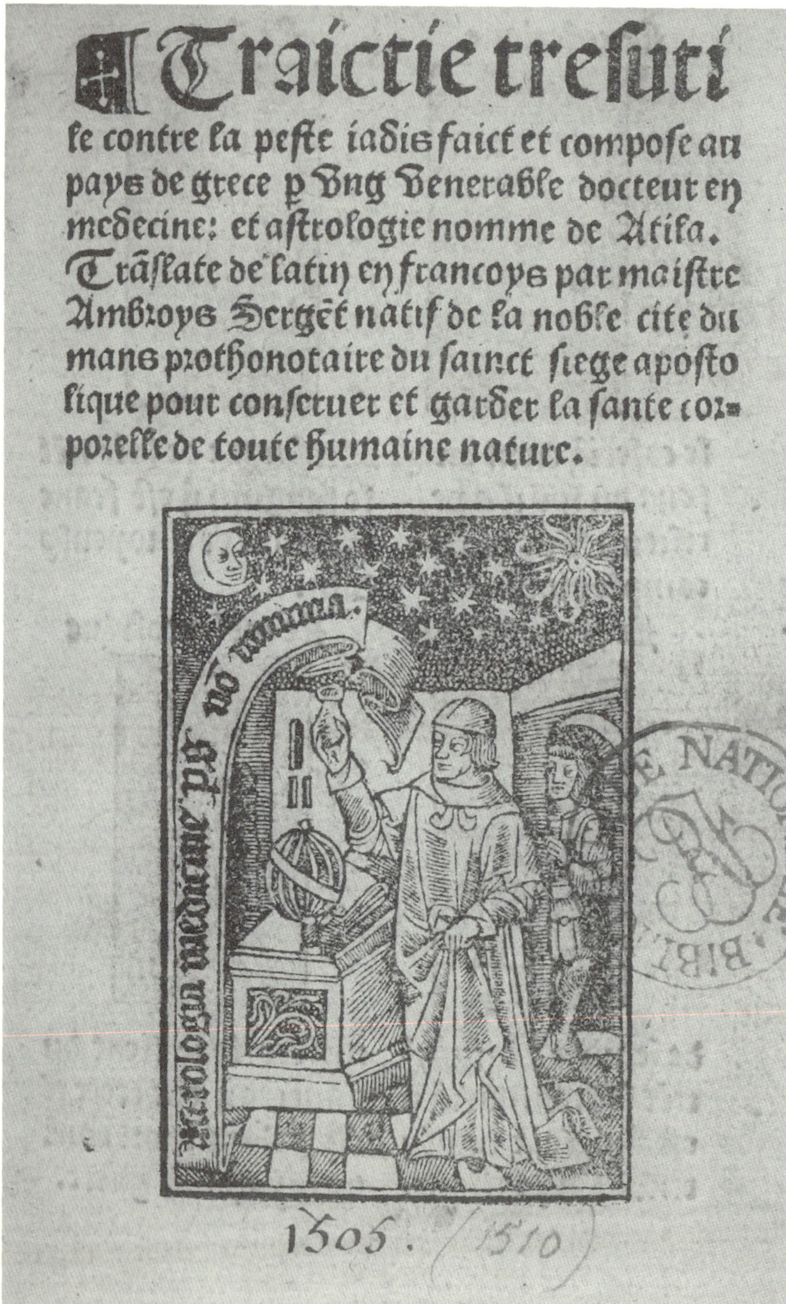

Traictie tresuti
le contre la peste iadis faict et compose au
pays de grece p ung venerable docteur en
medecine: et astrologie nomme de Atila.
Trāslate de latin en francoys par maistre
Ambroys Sergēt natif de la noble cite du
mans prothonotaire du sainct siege aposto
lique pour conseruer et garder la sante cor-
porelle de toute humaine nature.

1505. (1510)

2.1 Generic woodcut of a doctor examining a urine flask, in Atila, *Traictie tresutile contre la peste*, 1505.

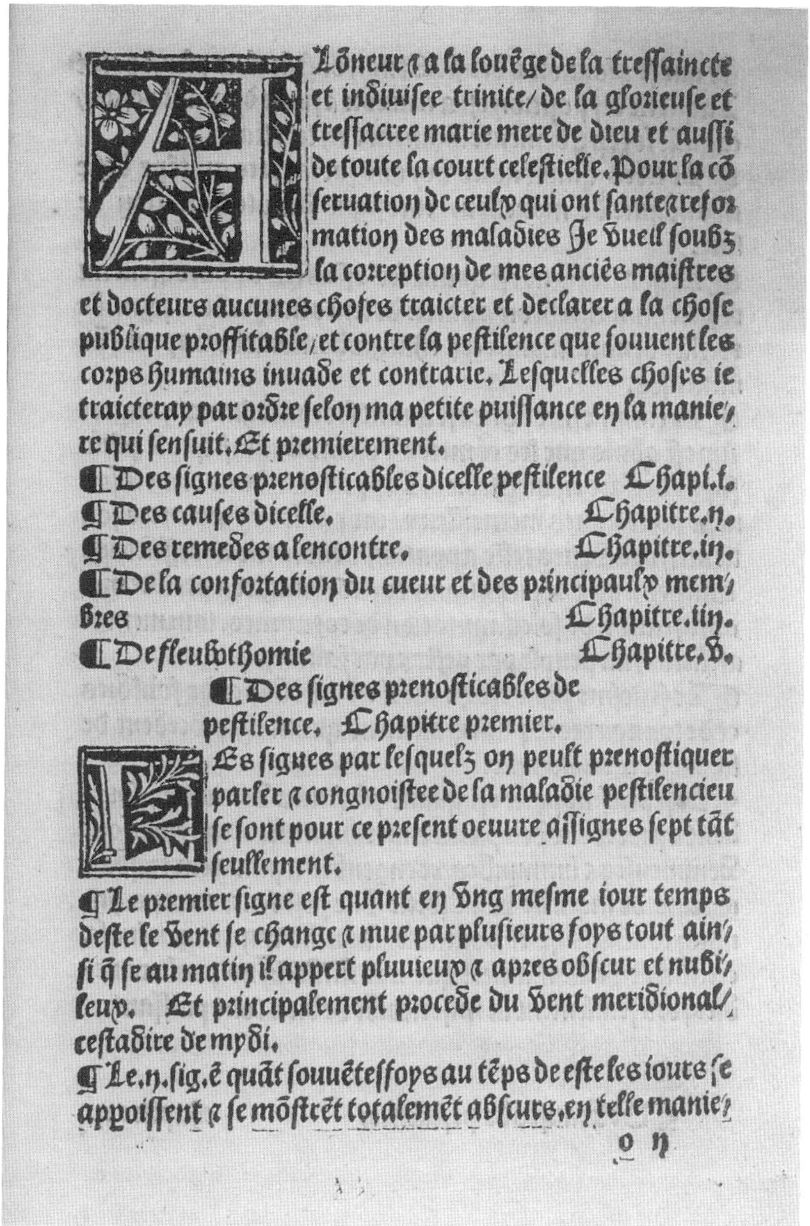

[H]Onneur & a la louēge de la tressaincte et indiuisee trinite/ de la glorieuse et tressacree marie mere de dieu et aussi de toute la court celestielle. Pour la cōseruation de ceulx qui ont sante & refor mation des maladies Je vueil soubz la correption de mes anciēs maistres et docteurs aucunes choses traicter et declarer a la chose publique proffitable/ et contre la pestilence que souuent les corps humains inuade et contrarie. Lesquelles choses ie traicteray par ordre selon ma petite puissance en la manie/re qui sensuit. Et premierement.

¶ Des signes prenosticables dicelle pestilence Chapi.i.
¶ Des causes dicelle. Chapitre.ij.
¶ Des remedes a lencontre. Chapitre.iij.
¶ De la confortation du cueur et des principaulx mem/bres Chapitre.iiij.
¶ De fleubothomie Chapitre.v.

¶ Des signes prenosticables de pestilence. Chapitre premier.

[L]Es signes par lesquelz on peult prenostiquer parler & congnoistre de la maladie pestilencieu se sont pour ce present oeuure assignes sept tāt seullement.

¶ Le premier signe est quant en vng mesme iour temps deste le vent se change & mue par plusieurs foys tout ain/si q̄ le au matin il appert pluuieux & apres obscur et nubi/leux. Et principalement procede du vent meridional/ cestadire de mydi.

¶ Le.ij.sig.ē quāt souuētesfoys au tēps de este les iours se appoissent & se mōstrēt totalemēt abscurs, en telle manie/

o ij

2.2 Anonymized French version of Johannes Jacobi tract, *Remède très utile contre fièvre pestilencieuse*, 1501.

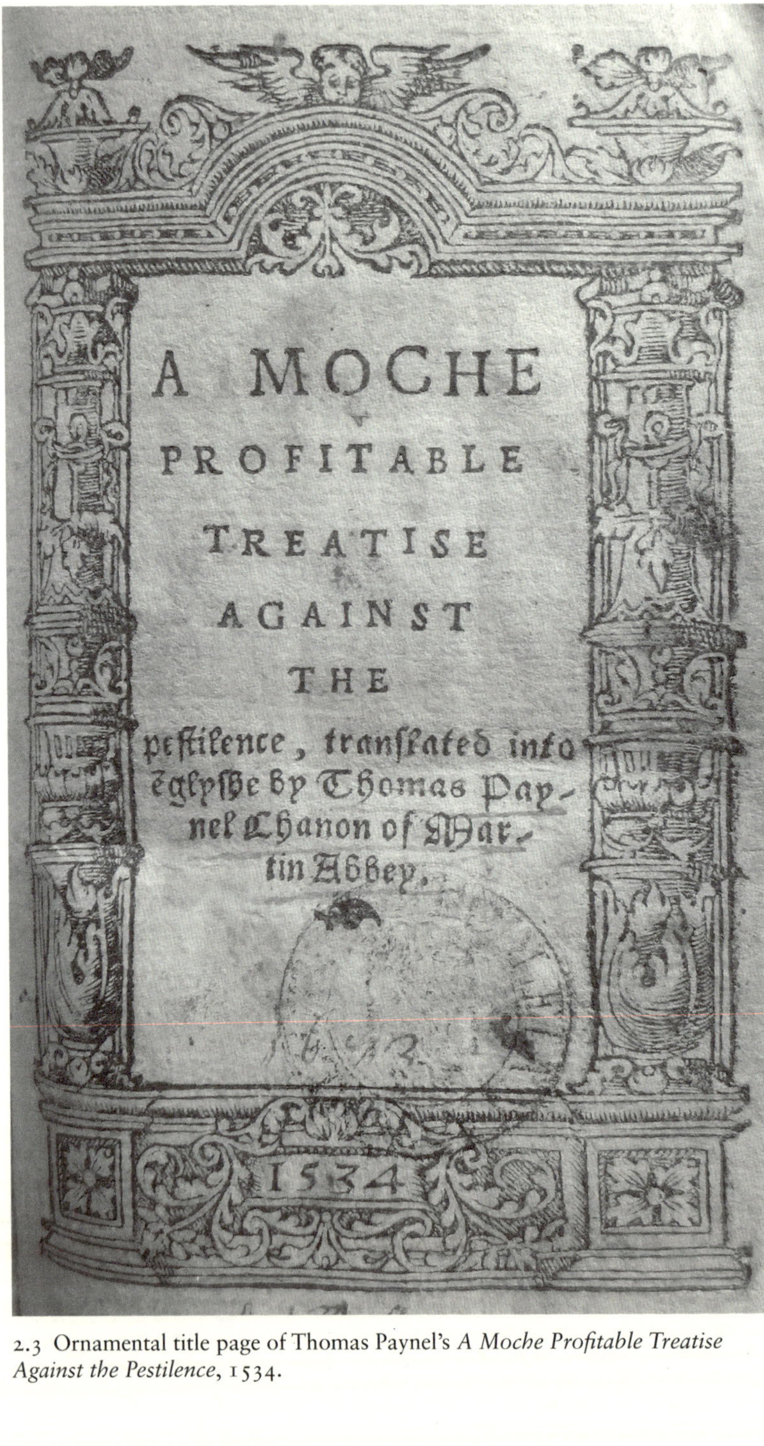

2.3 Ornamental title page of Thomas Paynel's *A Moche Profitable Treatise Against the Pestilence*, 1534.

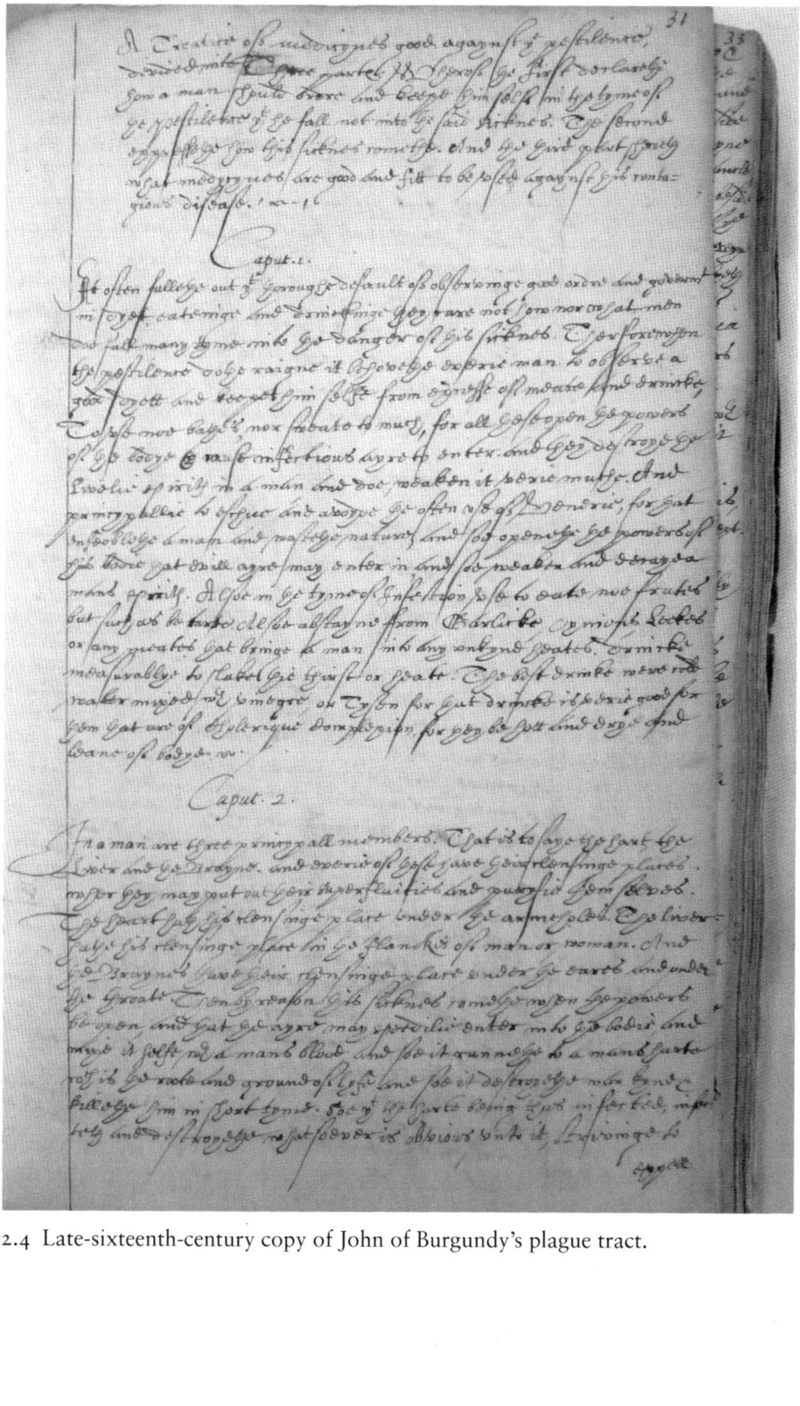
31

A Treatise of medicynes good agaynst the pestilence, devided into three partes. Whereof the first declareth how a man shoulde kepe and rule him selfe in the tyme of the pestilence that he fall not into the said sicknes. The second expresseth how this sicknes cometh. And the third plainly what medicynes are good and fitt to be used agaynst this contagious disease.

Caput. 1.

Caput. 2.

2.4 Late-sixteenth-century copy of John of Burgundy's plague tract.

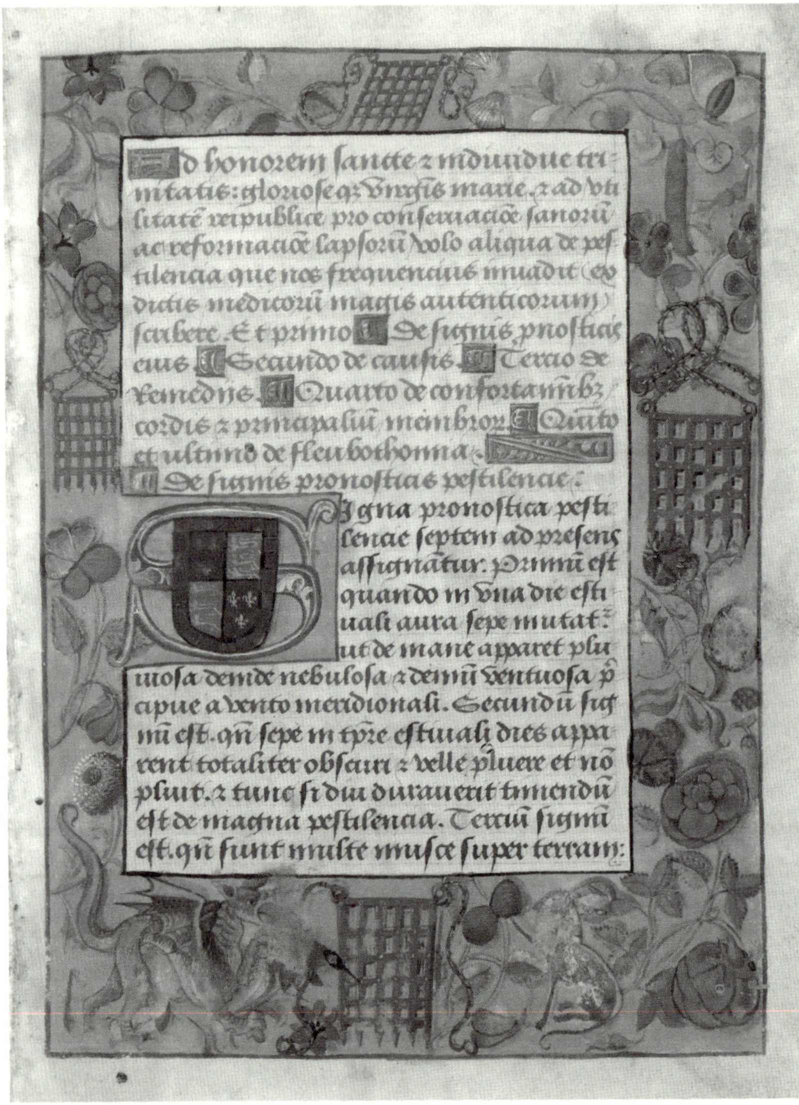

2.5 Illustrated folio from Lady Margaret Beaufort's Latin copy of "Bishop of Arusiens" (Johannes Jacobi) plague tract, 1485–1509.

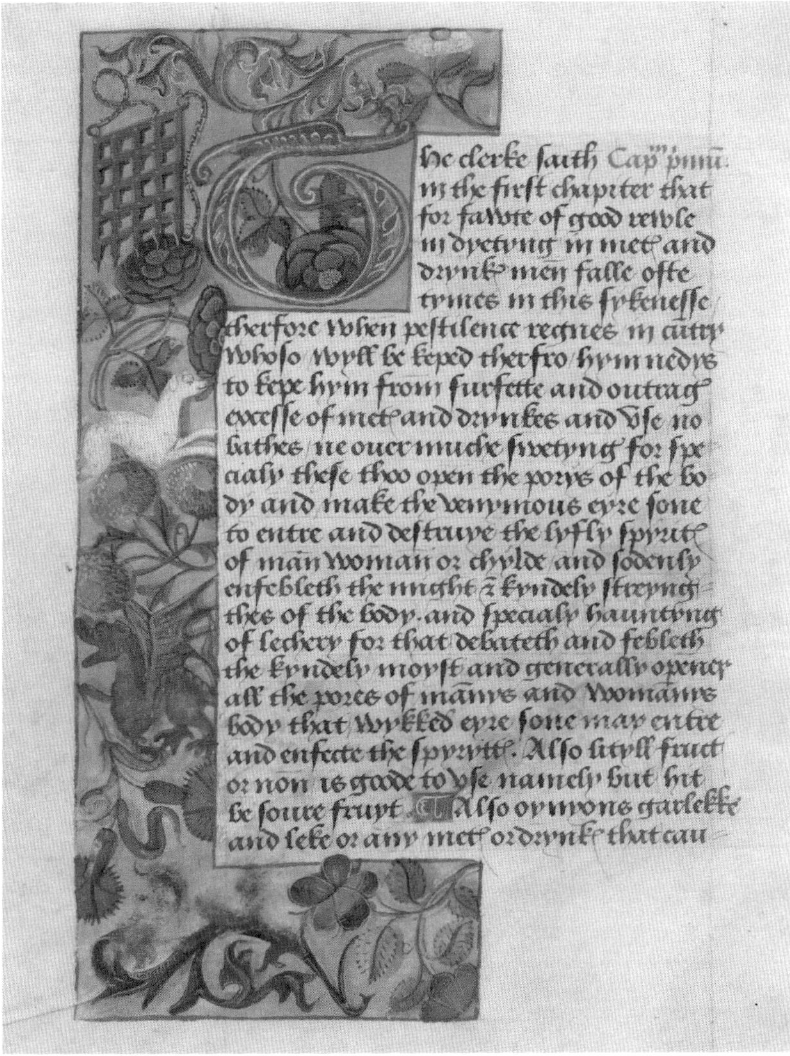
The clerke saith Cap^m primu
in the first chapiter that
for fawte of good rewle
in dyetyng in met and
drynk men falle ofte
tymes in this syknesse
therfore when pestilence regnes in cuntry
whoso wyll be keped therfro hym nedys
to kepe hym from surfette and outrag
excesse of met and drynkes and vse no
bathes ne ouer muche swetyng for spe
cialy these two open the porys of the bo
dy and make the venymous eyre sone
to entre and destruye the lyfly spyrit
of man woman or chylde and sodenly
enfebleth the myght & kyndely streyng
thes of the body. and specialy hauntyng
of lechery for that debateth and febleth
the kyndely moyst and generally openeþ
all the pores of manys and womanys
body that wykked eyre sone may entre
and enfecte the spyritt. Also lityll fruct
or non is goode to vse namely but hit
be soure fruyt. Also oynons garlekke
and leke or any met or drynk that cau

2.6 Illustrated folio from Lady Margaret Beaufort's copy of John of Burgundy's plague tract, 1485–1509.

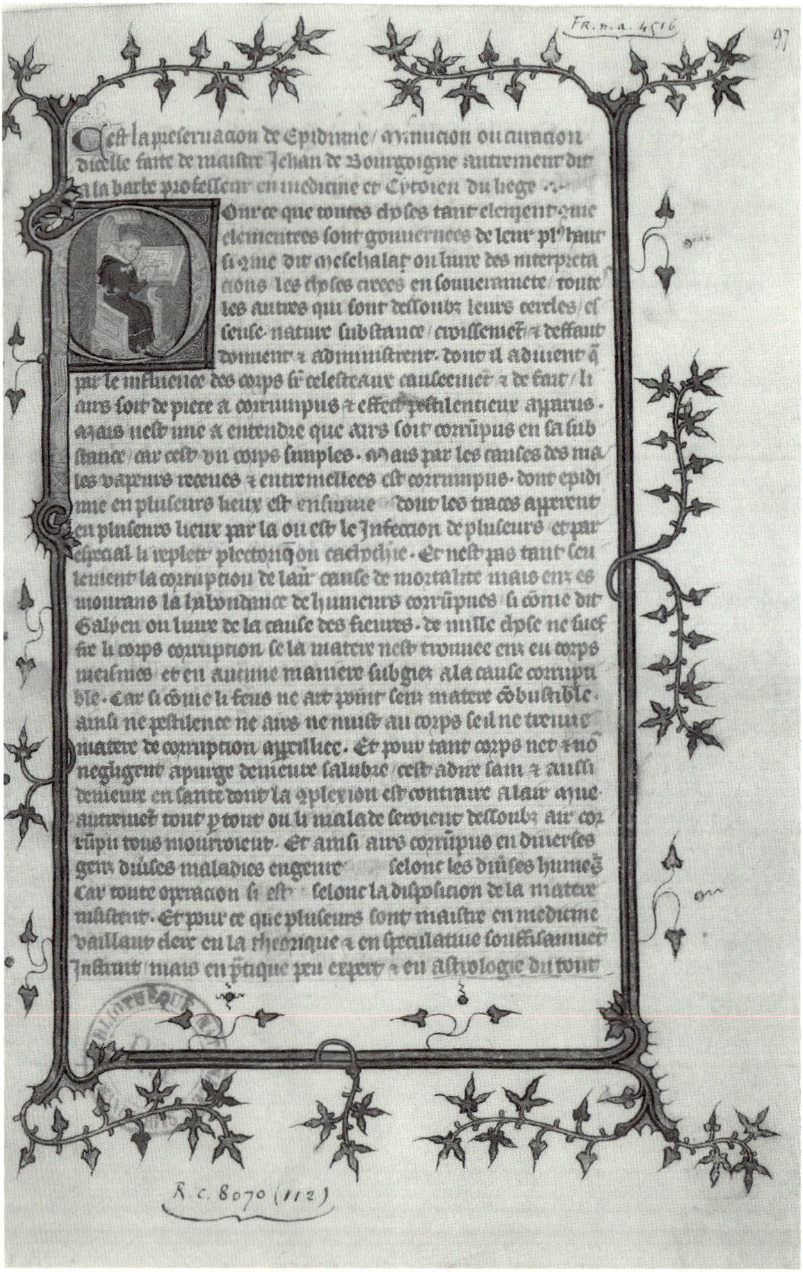

2.7 Illustrated folio from King Charles V's copy of John of Burgundy's plague tract, c. 1371, showing a miniature of a robed physician sitting at a writing desk.

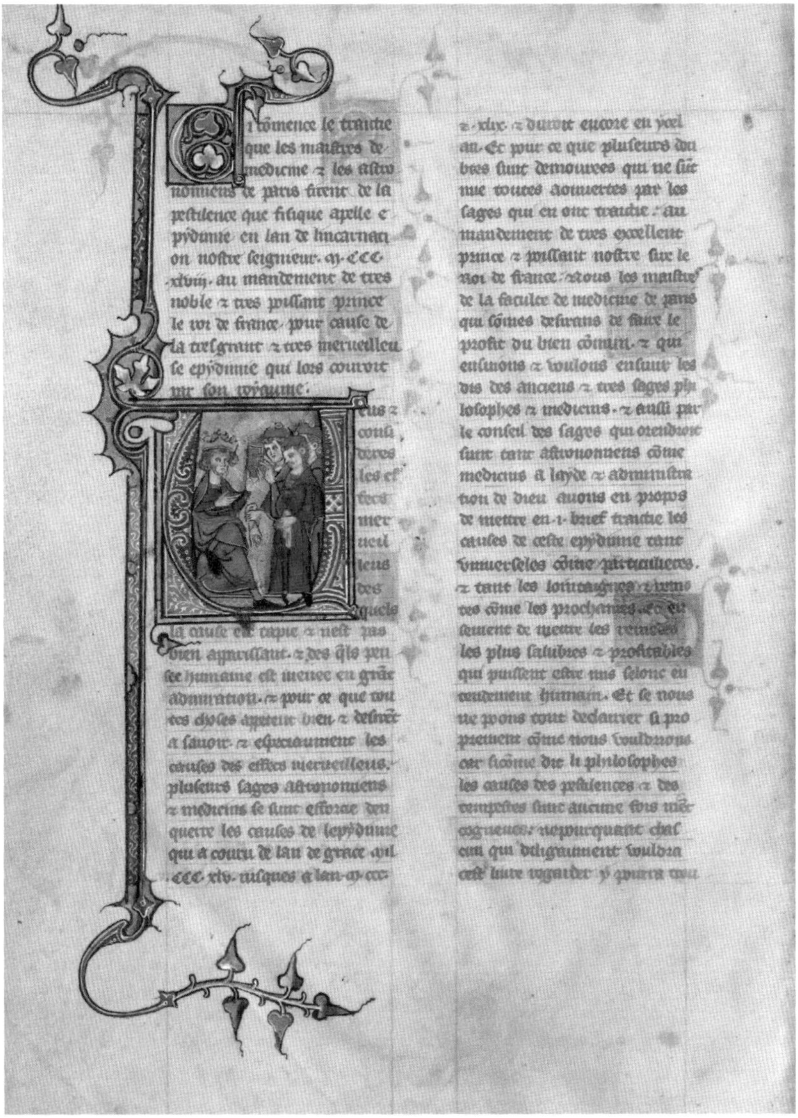

2.8 Illustrated folio from King Charles V's copy of the Paris Medical Faculty's plague tract, c. 1373, showing a miniature of a seated king being instructed by three robed physicians.

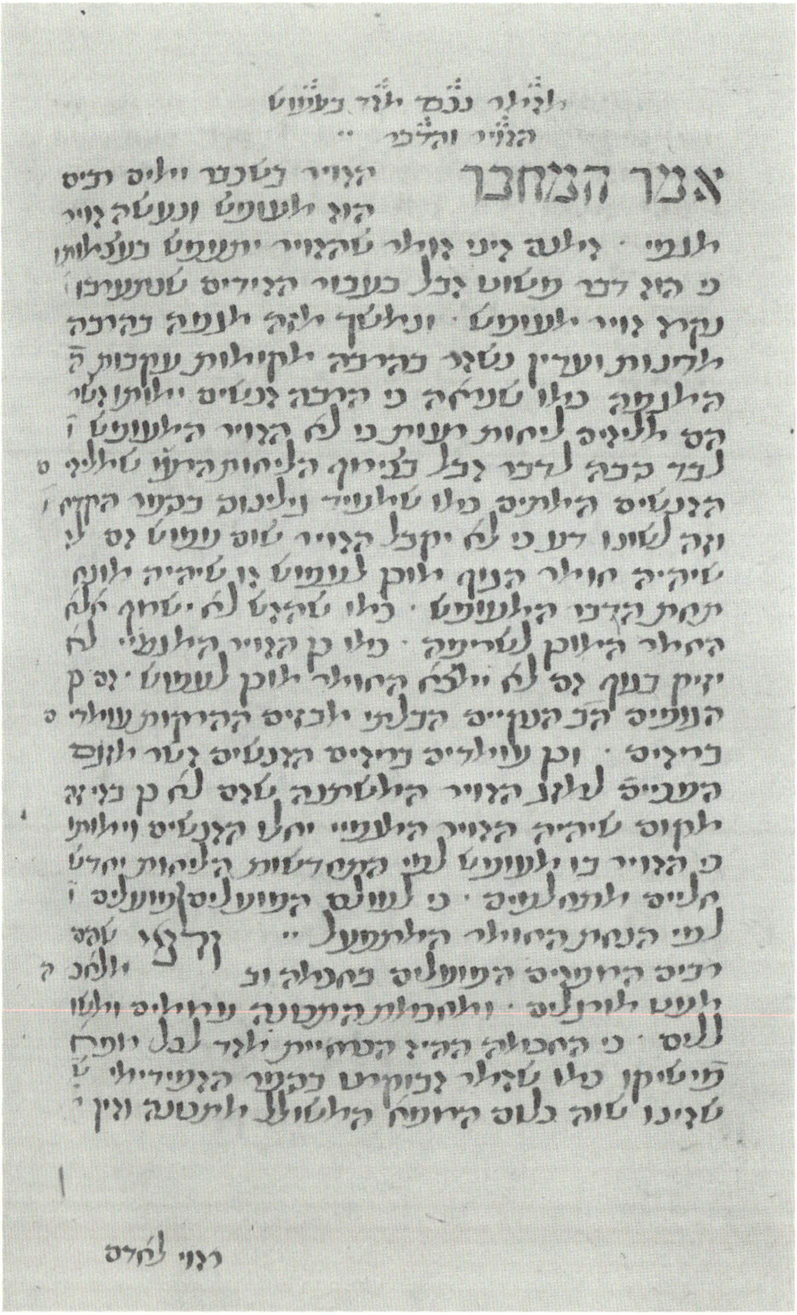

2.9 Fifteenth-century copy of Hebrew translation of John of Burgundy's plague tract, made c. 1399 by Benjamin bar Isaac of Carcassonne.

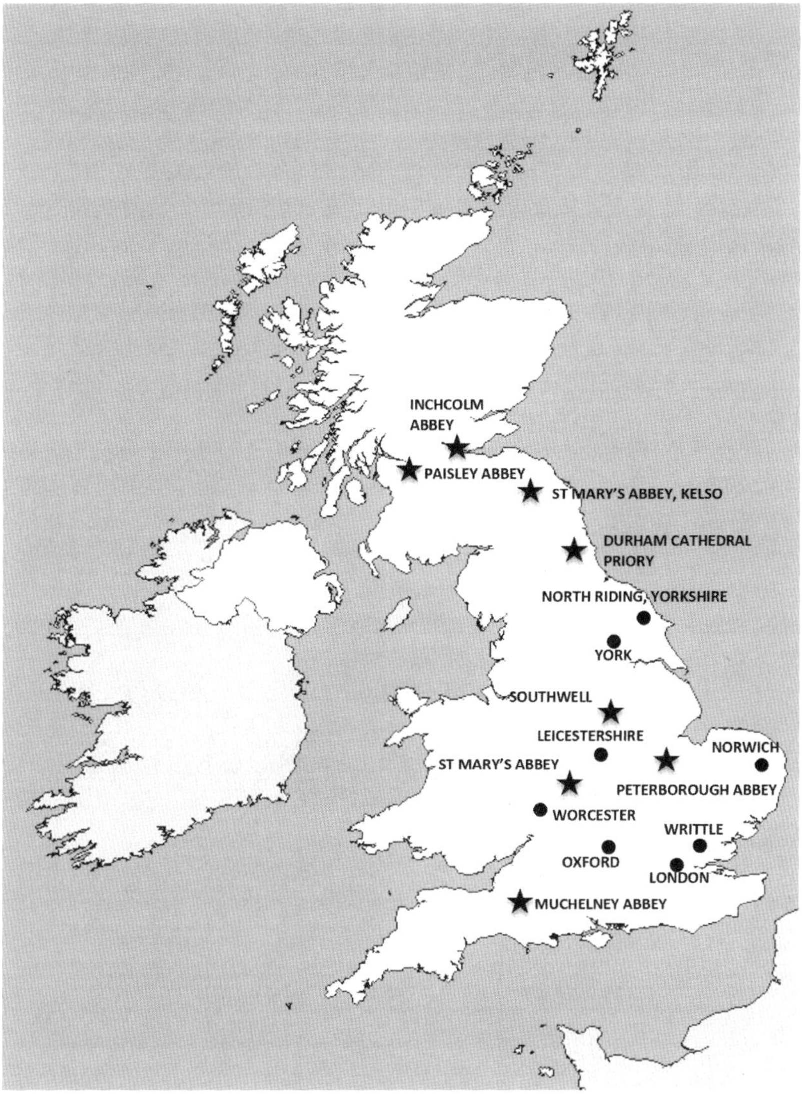

2.10 Sample of sites where manuscript copies of John of Burgundy's plague tract were produced in England.

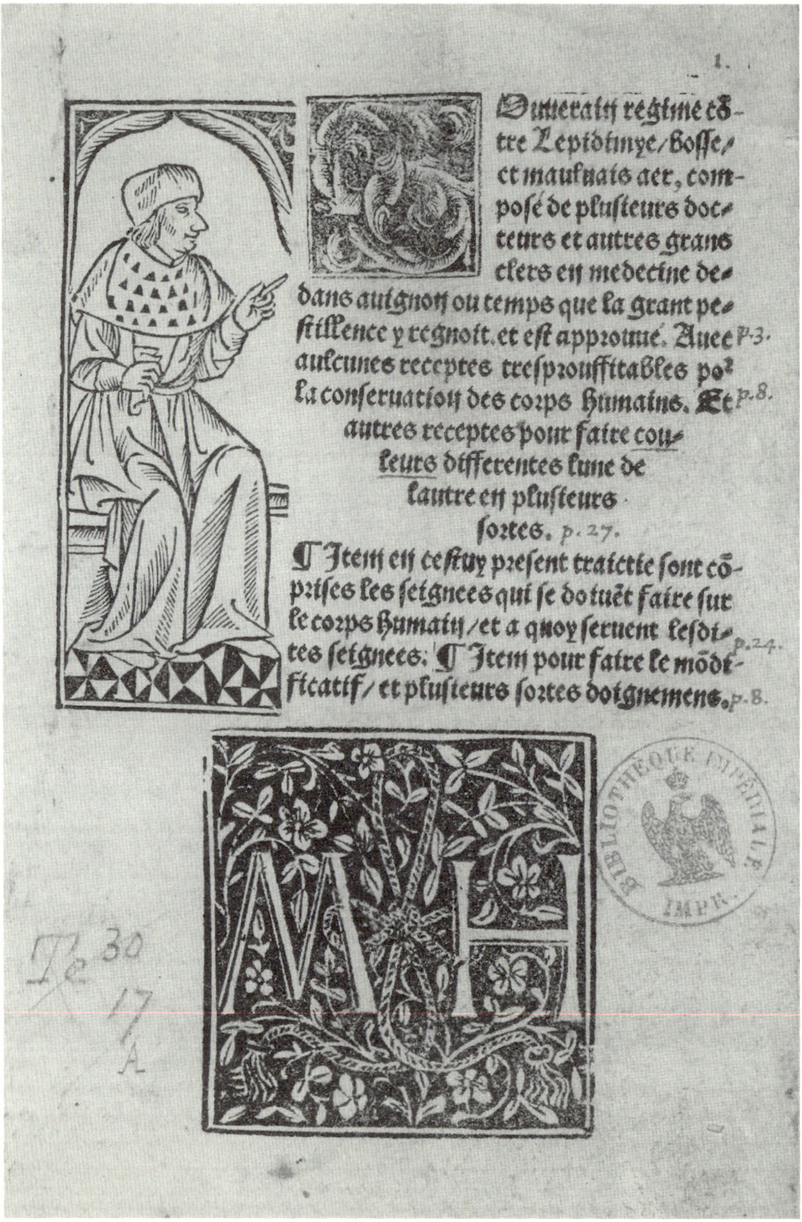

Souuerain regime co[n]-
tre Lepidimye/bosse/
et maulvais aer, com-
posé de plusieurs doc-
teurs et autres grans
clers en medecine de-
dans avignon ou temps que la grant pe-
stillence y regnoit. et est approuué. Auec
aulcunes receptes tresprouffitables po[ur]
la conseruation des corps humains. Et
autres receptes pour faire cou-
leurs differentes lune de
lautre en plusieurs
sortes.
¶ Item en cestuy present traictie sont co[m]-
prises les seignees qui se doiuent faire sur
le corps humain/et a quoy seruent lesdi-
tes seignees. ¶ Item pour faire le mondi-
ficatif/et plusieurs sortes doignemens.

2.11 First page from Anonymous, *Souverain remede co[n]tre Lepidimye bosse et maulvais aer*, c. 1501.

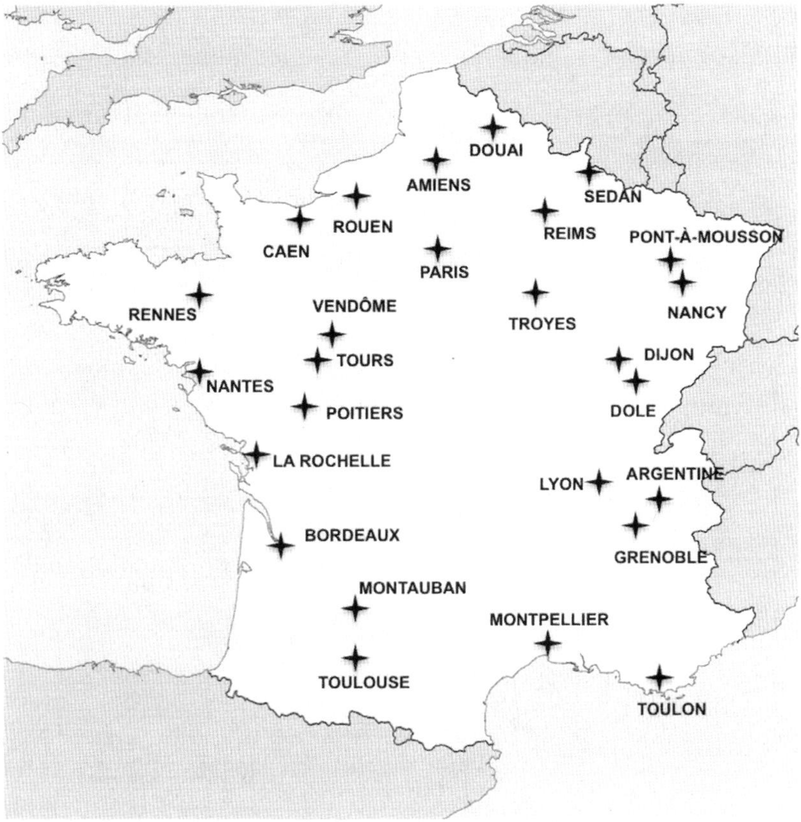

2.12 Location of printers of plague tracts in France.

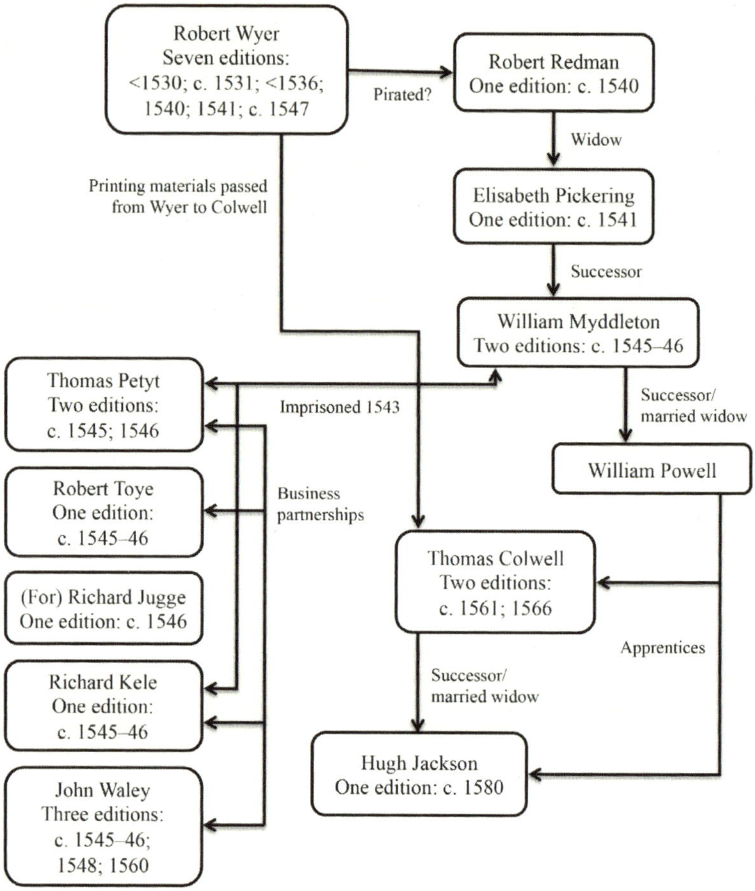

2.13 Commercial and personal relationships between London printers of *The Mirror or Glasse of Helthe*, c. 1520s–80, which contains Thomas Moulton's adaptation of John of Burgundy's plague tract.

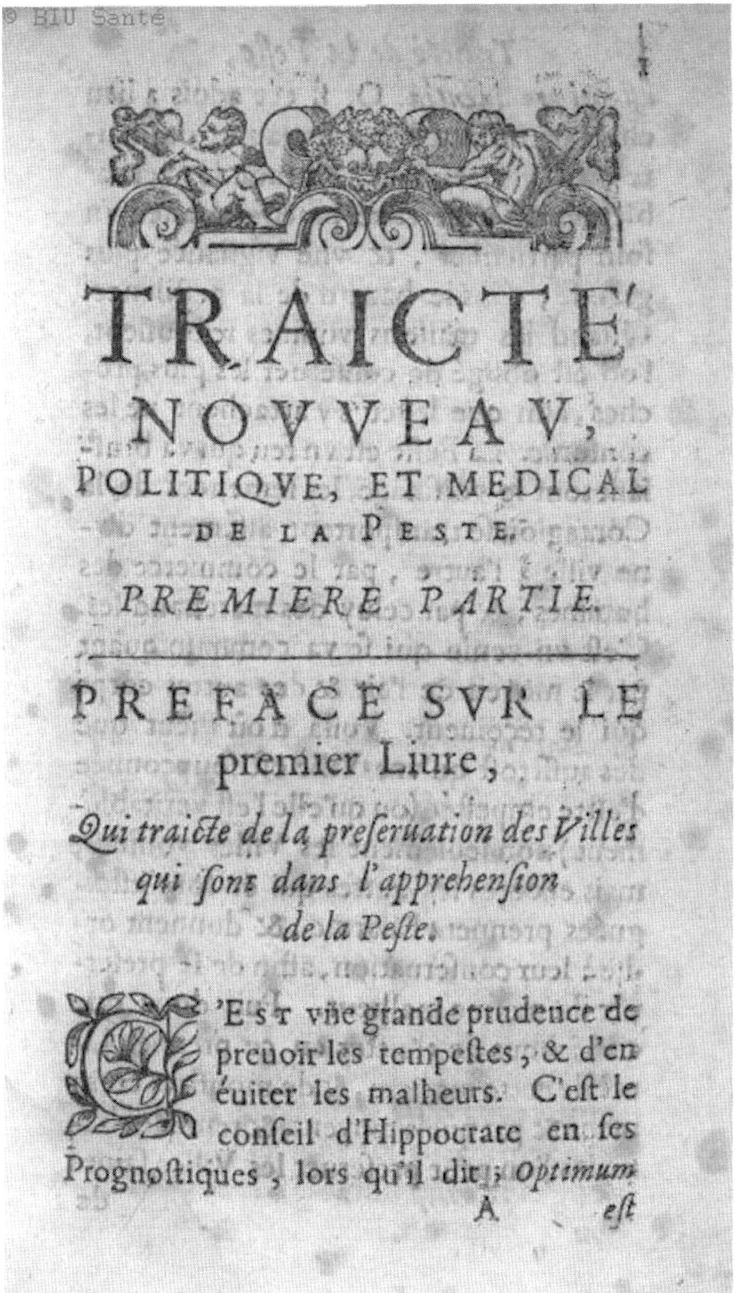

TRAICTE'

NOVVEAV,

POLITIQVE, ET MEDICAL

DE LA PESTE.

PREMIERE PARTIE.

PREFACE SVR LE premier Liure,

Qui traicte de la preseruation des Villes qui sont dans l'apprehension de la Peste.

C'EST vne grande prudence de preuoir les tempestes, & d'en euiter les malheurs. C'est le conseil d'Hippocrate en ses Prognostiques, lors qu'il dit; *Optimum*

A *est*

2.14 Page 1 from François Ranchin, *Opuscules, ou Traictés divers et curieux en medecine,* 1640.

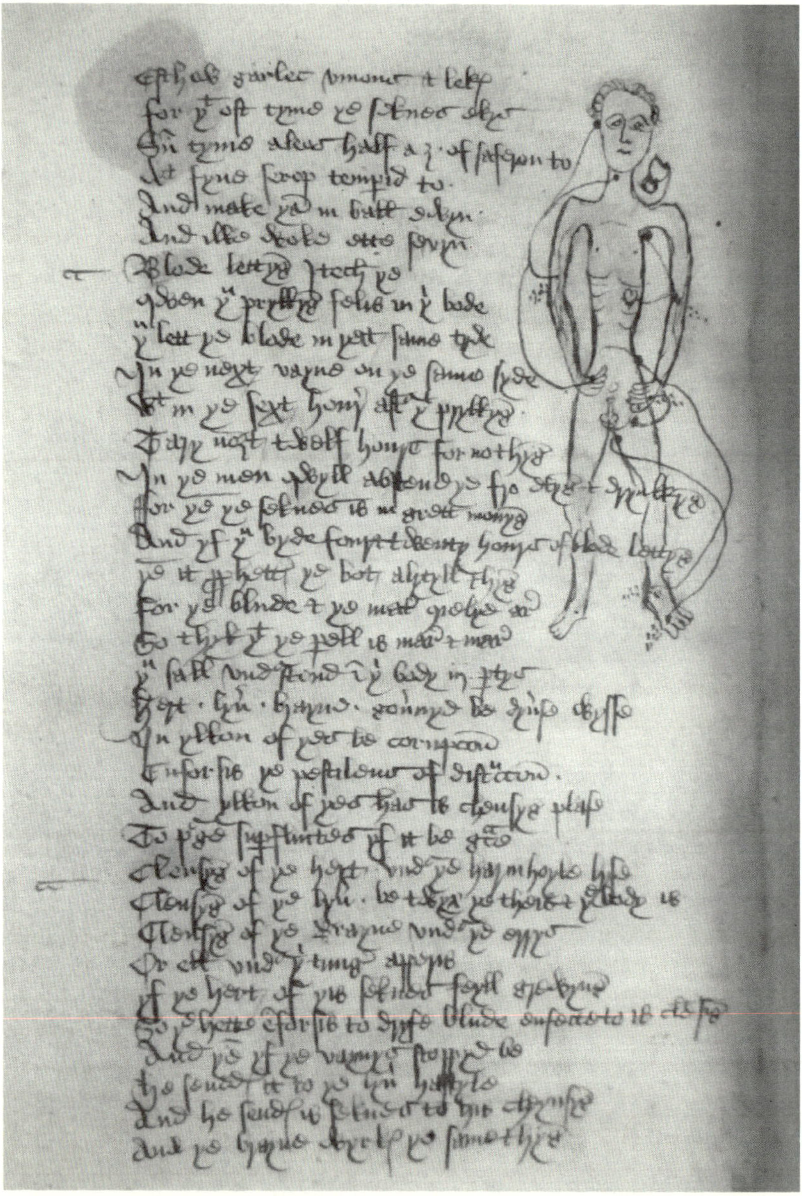

2.15 Phlebotomy Man with buboes in a versified version of John of Burgundy's plague tract, fifteenth century.

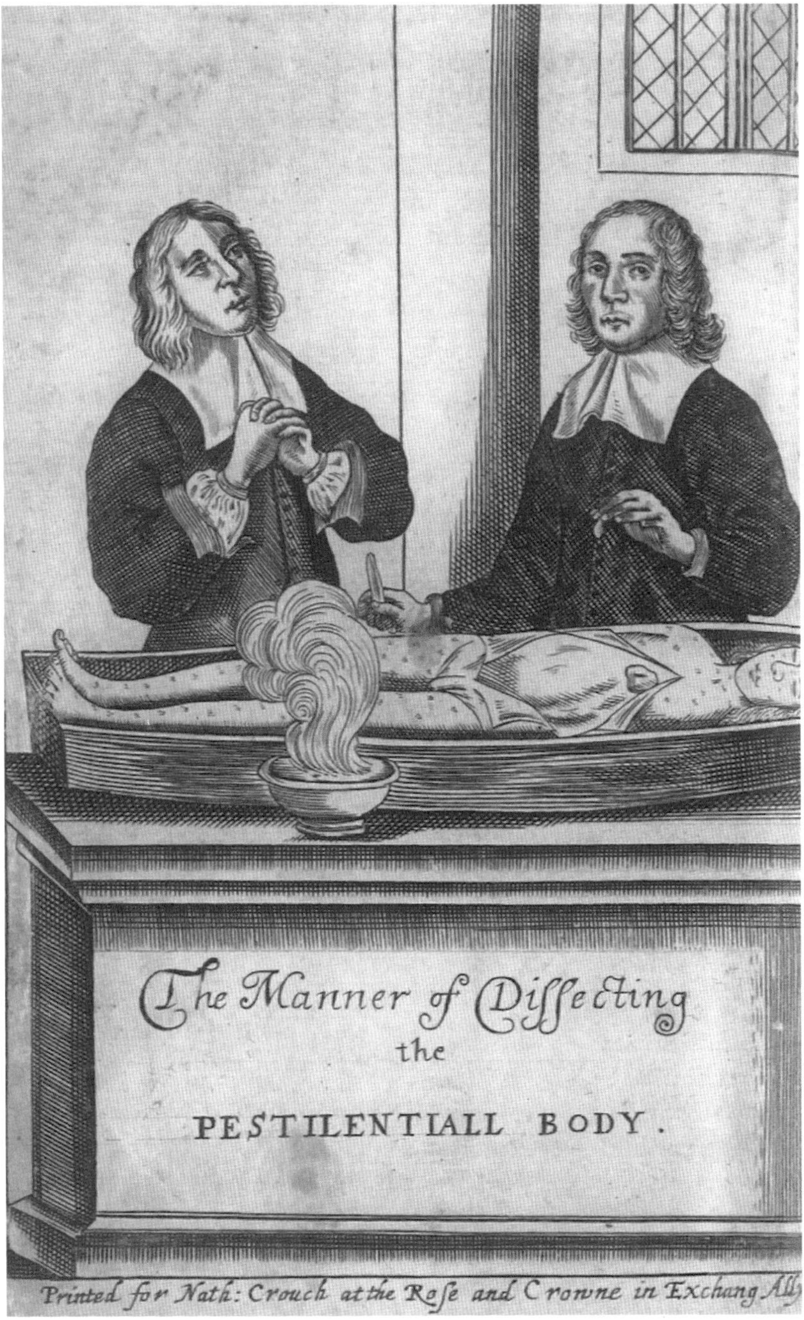

2.16 "The Manner of Dissecting the Pestilentiall Body," from the frontispiece of George Thomson, *Loimotomia, or the Pest Anatomized*, 1666.

3

Setting Plague in Time

From Never Before to Now, from the Past to the Present

If the Plague is, or lately hath been in any Neighbour Country, it doth not usually cease there, but travails from one Place and Nation to another, as Physitians and Historians do at large relate.

William Kemp, London, 1665[1]

WRITING PLAGUE'S PAST

As he witnessed London's devastating outbreak in 1665, English physician William Kemp turned to the plague tract format to publish his opinions about what had caused the disease, how one could recognize its signs, and how best to prevent and treat it. He recalled biblical and scriptural accounts of pestilences among the Israelites and Egyptians to argue that divine wrath and the hand of God was, and had always been, the ultimate source of the disease: "this not onely Jewes and Christians, but even Heathens, Priests, Poets, Philosophers, and Physicians, have acknowledged in their Writings."[2] Although Kemp insisted that no worldly medicine could protect mankind from divinely inflicted maladies, he nevertheless considered ancient authorities' explanations of and recommended treatments for them. He recounted in particular the remedies described by the tenth-century Persian polymath al-Rāzī and the twelfth-century "Arabian Physitians, *Avenzoar* and *Averroes*" to defend his preference for certain remedies.[3] He also turned to the canonical authors to ground his opinions about contemporary debates: whether or not plague was contagious and infectious, whether it might be spread through fear and imagination alone, and whether natural or supernatural factors were more likely to cause the disease.

Kemp's treatise was much like those written by both his contemporaries and his predecessors. Since the Black Death, writers had turned to the remedial advice of the medical canon – and especially in the sixteenth century, to the spiritual advice of the Church – to offer their readers as coherent and holistic an interpretation of plague as they could. Medieval and early modern societies were governed to a large extent by custom, traditional authority, and historical precedent. For religiously inclined writers, it made sense to place the Black Death and subsequent plague outbreaks into the context of other large mortality events of the past, including the Biblical plagues of Egypt, of King David, and of Ezechiel, or even the Great Flood. The Bible contained plenty of evidence of God's wrath, and its lessons provided sufficient proof that plague was a reminder of his power. For medical writers too, long-standing authority offered analogies: the plague of Athens and "the famous pestilence of the city of Crannon."[4] While acknowledging that their authorities may not have experienced anything quite like *this* pestilence, or that only modern advice was based on familiarity with the disease, medieval and early modern tract producers alike still relied on medical and religious traditions that had been handed down for generations. Ancient writing ruled – and often overruled – contemporary understanding and interpretation of health, illness, and disease until at least the sixteenth century.

Yet Kemp also explicitly drew from a type of material that treatise writers had begun to use with some regularity only a few decades earlier: narrative histories. In discussing the causes of disease, for example, he digressed to recount a seemingly well-known story from the previous century about how the death and burial of witches could generate plague. "[Though] it may seem fabulous," he contended, the tale about witches in Poland and Germany had come from most reliable sources: "the [learned] testimony of several famous men."[5] "[A] large Narrative" and other trustworthy and well-known "Histories" further supported the legend. Tract authors' adoption of a new kind of historical source signalled the emergence of different conceptions of where information about the disease could (and indeed should) be drawn, and of how stories about past epidemics could help negotiate present outbreaks. It was also part of a trend of changing ideas about the history of plague and its role in the human past.

This chapter explores how English and French tract writers used historical referents or precedents to explain plague, and how these evolved from the mid-fourteenth century to the mid-eighteenth. The tracts contain evidence of significant change over time in thinking about plague's long history. At the time of the Black Death, the first European writers to face this pandemic struggled to create a place in universal history for an ostensibly unknown disease absent from both medical and collective memory. Some authors resolved this problem by marking the disease as unheralded; others stayed silent, seeing in the epidemic shades of past catastrophes. The First Plague Pandemic, though, figured nowhere in these accounts, as surviving Latin narratives from earlier centuries had failed to remark on the widespread nature of the outbreaks. Those texts that did acknowledge the earlier plague's impact on what was called "the whole world" – and that underlay a more continuous tradition of plague writing in the Islamic Eastern Mediterranean – had been written in Greek and Syriac and were largely unknown in the late medieval West.

The next generations of fourteenth-century writers became increasingly familiar with both plague's devastation and its specific signs and symptoms. They were thus able to create a new historical space that plague could occupy, predicated on the Black Death as a marker of time. A turn to the local in the fifteenth and early sixteenth centuries followed, whereby writers – especially those in England – largely eliminated historical references and focused their tracts on the present. By the later sixteenth century, though, current outbreaks were integrated into the construction of local history, and recently rediscovered references to the First Pandemic facilitated the creation of a new, longer disease narrative that stretched to the Roman era and beyond. This history also played a role in creating an epidemiology for the disease, one that marked it as distinct from other illnesses.

Alongside these shifts, the chapter explores several critical questions: Which medical authorities continued to remain relevant, and which ones were relegated to the dustbin? How and why did non-medical, non-Biblical historical narratives become key to explaining plague's history? What role did these sources play in creating a historical-epidemiological setting for the disease? How did tract writers use them in their attempts to historicize plague as a disease that was, in fact, different from any other?

The new ways in which treatise producers incorporated concepts of time and history into their texts, starting in the later sixteenth century, mark changes in their understanding of disease and health. However, this shift reflects more than an increasing familiarity with the disease's regular and recurrent outbreaks. It also reveals broader socio-cultural change, including the rise of humanism and antiquarianism, the development of new medical assumptions and practices, access to historical Greek and Syriac documents about the First Pandemic long unknown in the West, and the emerging conception of history as a worthy (and hence authoritative) subject of study in its own right. Tracing the elaboration of plague's history through the pages of plague tracts, as well as its perceived place in human history, shows how understanding of and thinking about plague itself evolved. The construction, and constant reconstruction, of plague's history reflected an ongoing recalibration of experience and observation with accepted/acceptable knowledge, evolving writing practices, and available source materials. These practices and materials were not necessarily universal and, as such, the writing of plague's history occurred at a different pace in different places.

William Kemp's work elucidates several of these points. When Kemp wrote his work in 1665, plague was a familiar threat to London's population. The city's previous major epidemics of 1625 and 1636 were not so distant, and many of Kemp's readers had watched friends and family suffer and die or had heard details about the devastation from parents and older relatives. The single-page plague broadsheets circulating in 1665 clearly showed that lived experience followed from earlier outbreaks in 1603, 1592, and 1578. The popular *Remembrancers* also acted as a new form of easily accessible annal or chronicle, highlighting key events of years past. Plague thus connected Kemp's readers to the era of their great grandfathers and, as Kemp noted in his opening pages, this disease could be traced to Biblical times.

Despite this, Kemp claimed, most people were still unsure about what to do to protect themselves or, alternatively, could not afford to take the right precautions. Unable to see as many patients as he would like, and being frankly "almost tyred" of repeating the "plain and easy" directions for preventing plague with which he was "much satisfied [for their] good success," he offered his treatise "for the good of the people."[6] The treatise was not just the product of his own making, though, but was rather a collection of information that he acknowledged drawing out of older medical treatises, including both ancient texts and more recent works by Simon Kelway (1593), Giralomo Fracastoro (1546), Alexander Benedetti (1493), and Antonius Guainerius (d. 1440).

Kemp then turned to recent "Histories" to both supplement and validate his arguments, in effect harvesting personal-experience stories to rebuild plague narrative from anecdote. He referred to his and others' memories of past outbreaks in London in 1625 and in Bristol "about twenty years ago" to argue against the current practice of shutting up infected households. Everyone should know, he wrote, that during "last great Sicknesse [in] 1625 the people went promiscuously one among another, and the Houses were quickly fill'd with Inhabitants, and fresh comers out of the Country, and yet no new Infection followed."[7] Historical precedent therefore dictated against the much-maligned shutting-up policy. At the same time, he repeated warnings made by the sixteenth-century Italian writers Fracastoro and Benedictus about the danger of stealing the clothing and bed linens belonging to those who had died from plague.

Kemp likewise drew from "several credible Histories" to reflect on the causes of past outbreaks; alongside his account of witches in Central Europe, he pointed to stories circulating for some time about "Powders, Ointments, Mixtures, and Compositions dispersed by mischievous persons" and about corrupted vapours emanating from earthquakes.[8] Even older histories, such as those penned by the Roman writers Julius Capitolinus and Ammianus Marcellinus and the sixth-century Syrian scholar Evagrius Scholasticus, showed that plague arose from closed-up, infected air and "that many sound persons coming out of [such] infected places, did infect the Inhabitants, and brought the *Plague* among them."[9] These histories, Kemp argued, revealed not just plague's long existence but – more importantly for the present – that it was contagious and that people should flee from places where epidemics raged as quickly as possible, before they carried the infection with them. Kemp seemed somehow untroubled by the inconsistencies that marked his narratives: his conclusion that those exposed to plague could carry the infection with them directly contradicted his assertion that "promiscuous" dealings among households, even with new arrivals from the countryside, had not spread plague in 1625.

Kemp turned to the Plague of Athens (c. 430 BCE) both to suggest efficacious preventative measures – "Physitians, in the time of [past] great and grievous *Plagues,* have used several means, and tried divers wayes to clear and purifie the Air ... as *Hyppocrates* did in the *Plague* at *Athens* ... whereby he freed the City from *Infection*" – and, more pointedly, to draw moral lessons.[10] "Histories will tell you," he said, "that in the most grievous *Plague* at *Athens,* described by *Thucidydes, Socrates* the Phylosopher lived free and not infected" because he followed a temperate, and thus moral, lifestyle.[11] Unlike earlier writers' reliance on general Hippocratic remedies for epidemic disease, Kemp's references to the Plague of Athens were not about reiterating and validating traditional therapies. Instead, he used them to make observations of, and to write a narrative about, the parallels he perceived between the current outbreak and a similar event in the past. Rather than rely solely on ancient biblical and medical texts, Kemp turned to a *narrative* history of the Plague of Athens to describe, explain, and understand what he saw and experienced in the present.

In taking this approach, Kemp set his London outbreak of 1665 into an epidemiological narrative that linked past and present. For Kemp, as for other contemporary medical writers writing history, the past served not as "mere ornament or compliment" but rather as an integral part of his work's contextual and explanatory framework.[12] Kemp went further, invoking other events from the past to help explain the 1665 epidemic. He contended, for example, that the great wind that appeared "on the third of *September* [1658] when that detestable Tyrant and Traytor *Cromwell* died" corroborated a "large Narrative" and older "Histories" that there were obvious links between "Tragedies and Troubles" and great outbreaks of plague.[13] He likewise turned to the mythical destruction of Troy by "a Wooden Horse, whose Belly was full of armed *Greeks*" to provide a direct analogy of the many otherwise harmless items through which one could unwittingly become infected by the disease: "a pair of Gloves, a Periwigge or a Muffe, or any Apparel; your destruction may be brought upon you by your Meat from the Shambles, by your Wine from the Tavern, by your Bread from the Bakers, by your Drink from the Brewers; it may come in a Nose-gay from the Garden, in Herbs from the Fields, in Fruit from the Market; it may be handed to you by the Water you wash in, it may be drawn in by the Air you breath in; and as at other times you are so frail, that your breath (so in times of *Infection* your Death) may be in your Nostrils."[14]

Kemp's turn to historical narratives for his medical text did not occur in a vacuum but was an early modern phenomenon. The construction of a long timeline for plague that incorporated a wide range of historical narratives and analogies first appeared in European tracts during the last quarter of the sixteenth century. Although Kemp did not purposefully engage in writing history, it was important to him that the observations and lessons learned from "History [about how plague moves from one infected place to another] be remembered to be done [i.e., considered and applied] in later years."[15] History, and especially *written* history, provided both precedents and lessons for the present.

Making recourse to historical precedents to comprehend current events was not, of course, a new concept in the sixteenth and seventeenth centuries. Nor was setting current events into a series of historically comparable incidents. Societies of all eras used, manipulated, called upon, or submerged collectivized or even manufactured memories of the past to create desired images of their present.[16] Contemporary social memories of plague itself were also created to serve political or economic ends.[17] The development of histories of disease in the nineteenth century built upon these same traditions, sometimes taking them at face value, all the while building in new biases about what was important. Among the first such, and one of the most influential, was German medical historian Justus Friedrich Karl Hecker's 1832 *Der schwarze Tod im vierzehnten Jahrhundert* [*The Black Death in the Fourteenth Century*]. Before then, wrote Benjamin Guy Babington (Hecker's English translator), "Dreadful as was the pestilence here described ... our modern historians only slightly allude[d] to its visitation."[18] For him, the value of translating Hecker came as much from learning about "one of the greatest natural calamities that ever afflicted the human race" as from understanding a variety of theories about what caused "general pestilences ... [and] universal disease." The real inducement for Babington in making Hecker's work more widely available was the recent emergence, threat, and terror of the cholera pandemics. This was perceived as a "new pestilence [that] has attained almost an equal extent, and though less formidable, [it] has partly produced, partly indicated, similar phenomena" to plagues of the long ago past.[19] Faced with the prospect of another universal disease, the experiences and lessons of the Black Death held particular appeal for nineteenth-century European authors.

Although he recognized the importance of the Black Death in human history, Hecker saw little historical value in plague treatises. While promoting Hecker's work, Babington too perceived only "quaint and amusing" opinions in the tracts. However, both Hecker and Babington failed to look beyond the seemingly formulaic contents of these sources. Doing so now shows identifiable trends in the conception, discussion, and portrayal of plague's history. Reading across the tracts also exposes the shifts that took place between the mid-fourteenth and mid-eighteenth centuries in the types of authorities on whom treatise writers relied to validate and explain their observations.

CREATING A FIRST HISTORY FOR PLAGUE

A Disease without a History

> Seeing things which cannot be explained, even by the most gifted intellects, initially stirs the human mind to amazement; but after marvelling, the prudent soul next yields to its desire for understanding … To attain this end we have listened to the opinions of many modern experts on astrology and medicine about the causes of the epidemic which has prevailed since 1345.
>
> Paris Medical Faculty, Paris, 1348[20]

The sudden and catastrophic arrival in mid-fourteenth-century Western Europe of an epidemic disease that had distinctive yet unrecognizable physical symptoms – a disease that reports suggested was affecting people from one end of the earth to the other – taxed the reasoning powers and historical memories of religious and medical writers alike. Simply noting the arrival of the pandemic was insufficient; the Paris Medical Faculty, like its peers, sought to make sense of the phenomenon through close scrutiny of traditional and modern expertise. As it discovered, attempts to understand this unfamiliar epidemic posed a challenge to all that its members knew about the world and its history, in a way that no other disease had done in living memory. For those, like members of the Paris Faculty, who had not even seen the disease yet, the task was that much more challenging.

For many lay and religious authors, attributing the disease to an act of divine retribution was natural. Just as God was the ultimate cause of everything on earth, so too was the Bible the written record of all human history. Medieval writers in Christian lands typically framed their stories of epidemics within biblical or prophetic frameworks. The early plague tract authors, however, tended to offer more astrological or natural explanations than religious ones; most acknowledged that plague reflected divine will, but did not postulate moral or divine causation. Instead, some struggled to identify historical precedents for the epidemic. The emergence of the plague tract genre can be read, in part, as their attempt to make sense of what they were witnessing in the absence of solid historical or medical parallels.

This was not just a problem in France. Although he initially thought that the plague epidemic might be similar to others that he had experienced or read about, Italian physician Gentile da Foligno quickly changed his mind, stating in 1348 that "the famous pestilence of the city of Crannon, or that which Thucydides or Galen or Avenzoar wrote about, do not seem comparable in their evil to [this] pestilence."[21] The Granadian physicians and scholars Ibn Khātimah and Ibn al-Khatīb agreed, claiming that historians offered no solution, since "never before has a catastrophe of such extent and duration occurred. No satisfactory reports have been given about it, *because the disease is new.*"[22] Foligno, Ibn Khātimah, and Ibn al-Khatīb's suggestions that the Black Death was incomparable to anything previously known is reflected in Francesco Petrarch's emotional lament: "When at any time has such a thing been seen or spoken of? Has what happened in these years ever been read about … Consult historians, they are silent; ask physicians, they are stupefied; seek the answer from philosophers, they shrug their shoulders, furrow their brows, and with fingers pressed against their lips, bid you be silent."[23]

Even historians, it seemed, offered nothing helpful. Perhaps recognizing but not wanting to admit this gap in their knowledge, only a small number of writers made specific references to the disease's nature or directly compared the Black Death to other outbreaks. Although some pointed to the epidemic's wide reach as evidence that it was much greater than anything recorded, attempts to place the epidemic into a broad historical context were largely absent.

Perhaps writers simply perceived the pandemic as a particularly devastating example of known phenomena.[24] Whatever they thought, they offered scant discussion of clinical symptoms and fitted their observations into existing theories and disease classifications. Montpellier physicians attempted to assimilate what they observed to traditional theory by explaining the emergence of buboes in terms of humoral pathology; one anonymous author in that city called the bubo "the sign of this disease."[25] Few others writing in the midst of the Black Death openly pointed to the bubo as a signature of this new pestilence; French physician Pierre de Damouzy went so far as to avoid talking about them: "of the other signs that have not yet appeared among us [but that are indicated by other writers], I will say nothing."[26] Overall, tract writers' focused on what they knew and accepted through their academic training and practice; direct experience took a decidedly second place. Their general silence about plague's uniqueness reflected an unwillingness to state categorically that they were observing something that ancient authorities had not already explained. There was little inclination to point to plague's lack of historical antecedent because there might be, somewhere, a precedent of which they were not aware; acknowledging a gap in their knowledge could be harmful to their own status.

Given their reliance on medical precedence to manage the epidemic, most writers provided a list of authorities on whose advice treatment and precautionary measures could be based. Damouzy, for example, offered therapies from al-Rāzī, noting somewhat hopefully that no one suffering from plague had yet died from such remedies. The Paris Medical Faculty called on the wisdom of Albertus Magnus, Aristotle, Hippocrates, Haly Abbas, and Avicenna, among others. Physician and astrologer Geoffrey de Meaux began his treatise "with the basics, as set forth by the wise authors, philosophers and astrologers who have had things to say on such matters," including Ptolemy and Roger Bacon.[27] Other early French writers followed suit.

Despite their efforts to stretch existing knowledge to account for the disease's unusual nature, some of these same French authors emphasized the need to consult with and draw on the opinions of modern experts as well. The Paris Medical Faculty noted that although the "ancients, notably Hippocrates ... [and] numerous wise men who are still remembered with respect" were aware of the various signs that foretold the emergence of local epidemics – having "experienced them themselves" – lack of textual evidence demonstrated that they had neither direct experience with nor personal knowledge of an especially widespread disease. As such, the medical canon could only go so far to explain the cause of plague or to provide treatments for it. As the Faculty noted, even the opinions of modern experts left "room for considerable uncertainty," since they too were dealing with what seemed to be an unknown phenomenon. It thus felt compelled to rely on the combined "opinions of the most brilliant ancient philosophers *and* modern experts, astronomers as well as doctors of medicine."[28] For Alfonso de Córdoba, "experience teaches us" that traditional explanations were inadequate and incorrect "in *this* pestilence." This was why, he explained, "the wise counsel of doctors does not profit or help those in the grip of this most cruel and pernicious disease."[29]

Considering the Black Death with the benefit of hindsight, later fourteenth-century chroniclers and the next generations of tract writers placed much greater emphasis on the disease's unparalleled nature. Once enough time had passed, they were able to share and compare their experiences in a way that made it clear that *this* disease was distinctive from all others known to mankind.[30] Writing about a decade after the Black Death, French Carmelite friar Jean de Venette asserted, "nothing like it has been heard or seen or read about." The chronicle of the Grey Friars at Lynn (Norfolk) retrospectively noted for the year 1348 that sailors had arrived from Gascony "infected with an unheard of epidemic called pestilence." Scottish chronicler John of Fordun likewise claimed in 1385 that "so great a pestilence and plague among men … from the beginning of the world even unto modern times, had never been heard of by man, nor is [it] found in books."[31] Biblical precedents still prevailed in many chronicles, but even they did not seem to match how writers had come to view the Black Death.

Although these lay authors emphasized the Black Death's uniqueness, they used language similar to Thucydidean accounts of the Plague of Athens – almost verbatim in some instances – to describe the disease's effects. Indeed, tropes about streets lying deserted except for rotting corpses, communities being emptied of life, insufficient people being left living to bury the dead, the abrogation of civic-minded behaviour, and widespread fear and chaos are commonplace in narratives of all large-scale epidemics.[32] Such tropes may have helped survivors of the Black Death deal with the horror of the unknown. They filled the gap between people's direct experiences and their inability to adequately describe them: the Black Death had no equivalent "in living memory … [or] in historical testimony" and thus became labeled as an event without a history.[33]

Plague tract authors writing in the decades after the Black Death faced the same challenge: trying to account for the sudden appearance of the Black Death. Unlike their immediate predecessors, many were willing to claim that the pandemic was unparalleled. Alongside "wider intellectual perspective and calmness,"[34] statements about the absence of historical precedent reflect the lack of contemporary experience of large-scale epidemics with such high and widespread levels of mortality. At least nine disease epidemics are noted in contemporary English documents between 1257 and 1340 (with similar records elsewhere), but between the late eleventh and early fourteenth centuries, before the Great Famine (c. 1315–22), Western European populations were by and large the healthiest that they had ever been.[35] Large-scale outbreaks of animal disease (sheep-scab and rinderpest) received scant attention in contemporary records.[36]

Crucially, fourteenth-century writers were almost completely unaware of the First Plague Pandemic of the mid-sixth to mid-eighth centuries as a widespread historical event. Numerous accounts did survive, including the narratives of sixth-century Byzantine and Syriac authors Procopius, Agathias, Evagrios Scholastikos, and John, Bishop of Ephesus, and the Latin writers Gregory of Tours, Paul the Deacon, and Bede.[37] But knowledge of Greek had declined considerably in the West following the eleventh-century schism that separated the Western Roman and Eastern Orthodox churches; it was really only revived to a substantial degree with the flight of Byzantine Greek scholars and other *émigrés* from Constantinople around the time of that city's sacking by the Ottomans in 1453. Procopius's extensive Greek account of "a pestilence, by which the whole human race came near to being annihilated" was largely unknown in the West before the fifteenth century.[38] John VI Kantakouzenos' (Byzantine Emperor in Constantinople) Black Death report was, in many respects, an adaptation of Procopius's account, and his literary production would not have been unknown in contemporary regions of Italy with enduring Greek heritage, nor was it unfamiliar to his Catalan trade partners. But beyond those circles, awareness of his work was scant.[39] While the Western chronicle tradition had knowledge of some Greek accounts, medieval readers primarily knew only those Hellenistic texts that had passed through the hands of Islamicate scholars and translators, such as the partial medical works of Hippocrates and Galen.[40] And, crucially, knowledge of Islamicate writings on plague, which had continued throughout the inter-pandemic period, was also lacking in the Christian West.[41]

Latin texts about plague were better known than their Greek and Syriac counterparts, but only the latter had pointed to the First Pandemic's apparently unprecedented nature and its "dreadful newness."[42] Latin authors were concerned chiefly with local events and concerns, and writing solely about their local outbreaks, they offered little sense of having witnessed anything like the epidemic that fourteenth-century authors faced.[43] Pope Gregory I's sixth-century intercession against plague was, of course, well known to fourteenth-century readers, being a key story in Jacobus Voragine's popular thirteenth-century *Aurea Legenda* (*Golden Legend*). The liturgical practice that Gregory instituted during the Roman outbreak of 591 – the *Litania maior* – included a great procession on 25 April that, it was claimed, had ended the epidemic; it subsequently became an integral part of the Western Christian liturgy. Its alleged success in ending outbreaks in other cities likely influenced the idea that past epidemics had been manageable, unlike the Great Mortality of the mid-fourteenth century.[44] No medical writers who had produced accounts that described the First Pandemic's symptoms in any detail or provided any sense of its devastation or scope were well known in the later Middle Ages. This pandemic, then, appeared in neither the inherited plague trope nor the traditional medical canon.

Whatever did or did not happen in assigning historical uniqueness to the Black Death at the time that it occurred, by the time the second epidemic wave passed through in the 1360s, tract writers emphasized the exceptionality of their experiences. Guy de Chauliac claimed that the Black Death had been great and "unprecedented": none of the historical outbreaks known to have occurred in Thrace or in Palestine or discussed by Hippocrates or Galen or experienced by Pope Gregory, he said, were "as great as this one."[45] Raymond Chalin de Vinario, a physician at the Avignon court in the early 1380s, asserted that ancient medical authorities had only "transmitted incomplete and superficial explanations" of large-scale epidemics "because they knew neither what caused the disease nor what action to take"; therefore, he argued, it was necessary to "look to the writings of various modern doctors" instead.[46] John of Burgundy, a Liège-based physician, was even more explicit about the lack of historical precedent for the Black Death and, consequently, the need to rely on modern expertise to explain and treat it. "I make bold to say," he wrote around 1365, "not in criticism of past authorities, but out of long experience in the matter, that modern masters are more experienced in treating pestilential epidemic diseases than all the doctors from Hippocrates downward. For none of them saw an epidemic raging in their time, apart from Hippocrates in the city of *Craton* and that was short-lived ... Galen, Dioscorides, Rhazes, Damascenus, Geber, Mesue, Copho, Constantine, Serapion, Avicenna, Algazel and all their successors never saw a general or long-lasting epidemic, or tested their cures by long experience."[47] Ancient masters had relied on their own observations to describe and treat the diseases prevalent in their times; John argued that since modern practitioners (i.e., in the 1360s) had already lived through more than one plague outbreak, they were the experts in treating this disease.

Despite plague's apparently exceptional nature, some authors did attempt to link it to specific incidents, in a sense using history as a defense against the unknown. The Paris Medical Faculty's tract was the first, in October 1348, to provide a historical explanation for plague: the conjunction of Saturn, Mars, and Jupiter at one hour after noon (presumably Paris time) on 20 March 1345. Astrologers had predicted this particular conjunction long before it happened, and studied it intensely thereafter for anticipated malignant effects.[48] The Paris Faculty was the leading institution of astronomical science in Western Europe, and its influence led many other treatise writers – but not those in Montpellier, who were their rivals – to adopt its astrological arguments for centuries thereafter (admittedly not without debate).[49] John of Burgundy repeated common predictions about "great wars, mutations of kingdoms and of sects ... the pauperization of many of the rich ... [and] the destruction of the Saracens," adding that "this [great] pestilence" had resulted directly from the Saturn–Jupiter conjunction of 1345.[50] Vinario and John of Burgundy also tied subsequent outbreaks in the 1360s and 1370s to the conjunction's after-effects. While the Black Death itself was without a history, then, at least its cause could be linked to a recorded astrological event.

Plague Gains a History

This current epidemic is one that has newly returned here.

John of Burgundy, Liège, c. 1365[51]

Anyone who had survived the Black Death and then witnessed a succeeding outbreak of plague believed that they were seeing the same disease, and described it as such. The return of the disease within a single generation – not just once, but several times – also meant that the first epidemic, if unprecedented in historical terms, was no longer unique. Rather, return of the disease seemed possible and even probable. In the course of no more than a decade, between the early 1350s and the second wave of epidemics in the late 1350s and early 1360s, treatise writers became convinced that the emergence of plague signalled a new, unparalleled challenge to traditional notions of time, history, and the natural order of the world. They described the Black Death as unprecedented, while establishing a historical trajectory that descended directly from it. In their minds, the great mortality might have been unique, but subsequent outbreaks proved that it was the precedent for all that followed.

For writers such as John of Burgundy, plague's recurrence made it necessary to explain more than just the disease's initial appearance or even its first return: he also felt compelled to discuss plague's propensity to come back repeatedly. Large-scale plague epidemics reappeared in France and England every decade for the rest of the fourteenth century, quickly establishing the Black Death as the starting point of a long line of outbreaks.[52]

Plague chronologies are most evident in later fourteenth-century chronicles. For 1361, the Leicester-based Augustinian canon Henry Knighton recorded "a widespread mortality, known as the Second Plague, [that] overwhelmed the people."[53] His contemporaries concurred, utilizing a sequential numbering system that recorded a "third pestilence" in 1369, a "fourth pestilence" in 1374–75, and so on.[54] Others made direct comparisons between the Black Death and subsequent outbreaks: the Grey Friars at Lynn claimed that the second outbreak was "much less serious" than the one in 1348, while Thomas Walsingham, a monk at St Alban's Abbey, described an outbreak in 1379 as being "on a scale never seen before"; in 1391, he said, the outbreak of plague in Norfolk was "thought [to be] as bad as the great pestilence."[55] The *Petit Thalamus* of Montpellier likewise referred to 1348 as "the year of the great mortality" and then linked succeeding decadal outbreaks to it.[56] Since most of these chronicles were written around the turn of the fourteenth century, their compilers had the benefit of having survived more than one of the outbreaks that they described. Living memory and immediate experience of plague's recurrent visits combined to create a disease chronology.

The second, third, and subsequent generations of tract authors similarly understood the large outbreaks of the century's later decades as continuations or repetitions of the mid-century epidemic. In his opening paragraphs, John of Burgundy explained that astrological conjunctions had "recently corrupted" the air and "made [it] pestilential," the result being a widespread epidemic (i.e., the Black Death) whose traces had reignited the disease to generate subsequent outbreaks. Later in the text, to account for his second-wave treatise, John specified that the same disease had newly returned. By his reckoning, the initial pandemic had not spent its force; rather, it had left traces of itself behind and was rekindled some years later. Guy de Chauliac likewise began his discussion of plague with a recounting of the Black Death "which appeared to us in Avignon in the year of our Lord 1348."[57] He then noted that "After [1360] the mortality revisited us." Chauliac discussed the ways in which the second wave of plague differed from the first, notably that its victimology had shifted from the common people to the wealthy and the young. Even so, he emphasized the symptomatic similarities between the two outbreaks, insisting that they were the same disease.

Raymond Chalin de Vinario stated that the malevolent Saturn–Mars–Jupiter conjunction of 1345 was responsible for an outbreak of the disease in 1373 (although he attributed the cause of the 1382 outbreak to a comet).[58] By tracing outbreaks of plague from the mid-century pandemic to a large national epidemic in 1382, he provided the longest and most explicit chronological discussion of the disease in the later fourteenth-century French tracts. Even where direct references to the Black Death or to plague's recent history did not appear, the idea of disease recurrence was at the forefront of almost all French treatises before the fifteenth century. Johannes Jacobi claimed that he felt the need to write something about the pestilence because it "invades us more frequently than the ancients."[59] Montpellier medical faculty chancellor and court physician Jean de Tournemire pointed out that the disease had occurred previously. Each new outbreak added to plague's chronology and offered additional insight into its nature and its uniqueness.

As it became a historical precedent, the Black Death also gained a potential future. As early as 1348, the Paris Medical Faculty had speculated that the southern winds "may perhaps continue [to carry the epidemic] in future."[60] John of Burgundy wrote his tract, he claimed, because "this current epidemic ... will continue to return in the future because it has not yet reached its end."[61] For him – as for Guy de Chauliac, who stated that the Black Death had been "so remarkable" that he felt compelled to describe it "as a guide in case it comes again" – plague outbreaks were part of a pattern that stretched from the past into the future.[62] Jean de Tournemire referred to plague as the pestilential disease that "had been, is, and will be" problematic.[63] Already by the 1360s, then, the Black Death's novelty was complemented by the more immediate problem of its experienced – and notably its anticipated – recurrence.[64]

Later fourteenth-century writers also linked post-Black Death epidemics by discussing their personal experience with multiple outbreaks of the same disease. This allowed them to make observations about epidemic patterns. John of Burgundy, for example, claimed to have written a treatise "at the beginning of this epidemic" in which he differentiated plague from other diseases. He also claimed to have gained "more than twenty years of experience in many places where the epidemic has reigned."[65] Guy de Chauliac noted that the disease became less deadly toward the end of the epidemic. Indeed, he attributed his very survival to the fact that he was infected late in the epidemic's course. In this sense, the epidemic itself was acquiring a history, a narrative that changed over time, from onset, to peak, to end, to aftermath. Johannes Jacobi and Jean de Tournemire likewise offered testimony of their own experiences avoiding or treating plague.[66] Claims of having "long-time" experience were commonplace in medical treatises to add credibility to their therapeutic recommendations. In plague treatises, such claims also served to create a short chronology for the recurrent epidemics by connecting current outbreaks to ones the authors had already survived.

The clearest link between these various epidemics was plague's defining physical signs, notably the bubo. Later fourteenth-century writers blended their observations of plague's signs and symptoms with existing medical theory to create what were, in essence, new categories of fevers and poisons. Regardless of the category into which they situated plague, the disease's signs distinguished it from all other illnesses, and the recurrence of those signs meant that subsequent outbreaks could be linked. By the second epidemic of the early 1360s, the majority of writers who penned new tracts pointed specifically to buboes as an indication that someone was infected with plague.[67] Chauliac provided a recognizable description – "apostemes and carbuncles and tumours" that were primarily located in the armpits and groin – before noting that the second appearance of the disease in the early 1360s was characterized by similar "swellings, carbuncles, and tumours."[68] The title of Jean de Tournemire's text, *Prevention and cure of apostemic anthrax according to the Master Jean de Tournemire*, also emphasized the importance of the bubo as an identifying characteristic. After the turn of the fifteenth century, writers continued to emphasize the bubo as one of the disease's symptoms; indeed, "even long after the *living* memory of the Black Death had ceased, physicians [and hence tract authors] saw buboes as evidence of plague."[69] Direct association of the bubo with plague, and hence with the Black Death, allowed treatise writers to create an implicit historical chronology in their works.

CREATING A SECOND HISTORY FOR PLAGUE

Plague Made Current

þe first [chapiter] tellis how a mane sall kepe hym in tyme of pestilens þt he fall noght in tyll þt yvell.

John of Burgundy, English adaptation, late fourteenth century[70]

Recurrent epidemics marked the fifteenth and sixteenth centuries throughout Eurasia. Yet explicit reference to the Black Death, either as a unique event or as a historical precedent, quickly faded from European plague tracts. Some fifteenth-century Italian authors specifically mentioned earlier outbreaks (Antonio Guaineri, for example, made reference to the outbreaks of 1402 at Pavia and 1416 at Chieri), but did not relate them to what transpired in 1348. Flemish physician Jacques Despars, who was a rector at the Paris Medical Faculty early in the fifteenth century, likewise mentioned the Parisian outbreak of 1400 in his larger commentary on fevers, suggesting that preventive measures should include quarantines and barriers like those instituted by the Duke of Milan in 1399.[71] A century later, the opening pages of a c. 1505 French tract adapted from Johannes Jacobi's fourteenth-century treatise claimed that a harsh disease marked by "l'apostume" had come often in the previous century.[72] For the most part, though, such historical discussions were rare.

It is not clear why a chronology of past outbreaks no longer found a place in the most successful plague treatises produced in England and France in the fifteenth century. The dominance of the adapted version of John of Burgundy's tract in England, which omitted all historical referents, and the predominance of Montpellier-origin tracts in France, which focused more heavily on the terrestrial causes of disease than on any historical astrological event, may have led to the deletion of old references. Perhaps familiarity with the disease's symptoms and memory of its numerous outbreaks created an understanding that it had been around for a long time. Overt discussion of the bubo also made it unnecessary to mention historical cues.

Whatever the reason, what was important for readers by this time was not reading about the history of plague but knowing what dietary and lifestyle choices they should make to avoid becoming ill. Tract producers continued to provide explanations of the disease's causes, and to vigorously debate them, but they largely stopped making direct references to either the Black Death or to previous epidemics. Some scribes even deliberately removed such references from older texts as they continued to copy them. In other words, after the turn of the fifteenth century, plague treatises largely addressed their audiences in terms of current and problematic "tyme[s] of pestilens."

This purposeful relegation of plague's history to the background accords with the argument that "the distance, and tension, between the space of experience" and the present dictates the sense of importance attached to past events.[73] In the immediate decades after the Black Death, that epidemic remained a touchstone. After the turn of the fifteenth century, plague still occupied a critical place in national and local memories in both France and England but its regular, somewhat less deadly appearances no longer called to mind the catastrophic event that it once had been. It was, in fact, now a familiar affliction – even a banal reality occupying "a central place in the social imaginary" – that stretched beyond living memory.[74]

By the end of the fourteenth century, chroniclers had already begun to replace their longer, more descriptive entries of the Black Death and its immediately successive outbreaks with increasingly cursory comments.[75] Most mentioned nothing more than the fact that an outbreak had occurred, if they mentioned it at all. Henry Knighton, who left behind one of the most detailed descriptions of the social and economic impacts of the Black Death in England, passed over the post–1361 outbreaks even though his chronicle extended to 1396.[76] The later additions to the *Grandes Chroniques de France* focused almost entirely on matters of state, monarchy, and national identity, and especially on expressions of kingship, dynastic continuity, and the creation of "royal myth."[77] Post-Black Death outbreaks were not noteworthy unless someone of high status died from the disease.

Fifteenth-century chronicles often continued to highlight the Black Death, numbering the ensuing two to four major outbreaks, but thereafter made fewer and fewer references to any but the largest or most disruptive epidemics. The chronicle of the Grey Friars of London noted only three "grete pestelens" outbreaks for the entirety of the fifteenth century (1434, 1478, and 1500). Even these it mentioned only in relation to other events such as a great frost, the deferral of term, or a dearth. In the group of fifteenth-century secular works known collectively as the London Chronicles, plague outbreaks are noted in passing, and are far less detailed than regal activities, battles, and legal and religious events in and around the City of London.[78] A Parisian chronicle covering the years 1405 to 1449 mentioned only three of that city's major outbreaks: 1418, which it called an epidemic crueller than anyone had seen or heard of before, 1421, and 1432–33.[79] After a half century and more of regular epidemics, chroniclers perhaps felt that they had nothing to add to discussions of a disease that was "[e]tched deeply into contemporary consciousness."[80] Plague had become a part of life that required little mention, especially in a form of historical writing that was already fading in both attraction and output.

Fifteenth-century English administrative records typically indicated when government business was adjourned or the court and parliament moved due to an outbreak. The laconic phrase "on account of the pestilence" belied the challenge posed by recurrent outbreaks but, like the chronicles, suggests that people no longer perceived plague as a catastrophic threat to either life in general or political functioning. Instead, those working in public life came to view the disease as a temporary hazard and inconvenience. Sessions of parliament were regularly adjourned as a precautionary measure during outbreaks in London and Westminster, but only once, in 1439, did the commons request that the time-honoured practice of kissing the king during homage rituals be suspended "now that a sickness called pestilence, [generally] common through this your realm more commonly reigneth [now] than hath been usual before this time."[81] Although persistent warfare was perhaps a greater concern than plague outbreaks in northern French cities in the first half of the fifteenth century, in both kingdoms the regularity of plague outbreaks mattered more than its history; indeed, its history could be taken for granted.

In this context of ever-increasing familiarity, writers adjusted their rhetoric about the disease. Rather than talking about plague as a disease that had emerged at a particular moment in time, one that was historical, they began to distinguish what they called "tyme[s] of pestilens" from all other times. Some treatise writers as early as the 1370s and 1380s, such as Jean de Tournemire and an anonymous Parisian writer, had already situated their prophylactic advice for use "in times of epidemic."[82] These earlier authors used such phraseology, however, in the context of discussing outbreaks that they presented as being linked to the Black Death and part of a historical chain. The turn of the fifteenth century, by contrast, marked a shift away from this historical accounting. Specific references to earlier epidemics disappeared almost entirely from plague tracts, with only few French writers still recalling the Great Mortality.[83] Adaptations made to John of Burgundy's plague treatise in the late fourteenth century as it moved from Liège (or perhaps from France) to England provide a particularly clear example of this shift. In the tract's earlier version, John commented directly and at length on plague's astrological and temporal origins, the Black Death's traces, its subsequent and projected recurrences, and the long line of medical authorities whose knowledge and experience had little to offer concerning this new disease. This version was largely supplanted in England by a shorter edition that removed all these historical references. Instead, the new English version concentrated almost entirely on prophylaxis and treatment, advising its readers to be moderate in all things in order to avoid becoming ill "in tyme of pestilens" and "whene pestilens regnes."[84] This adaptation targeted people living through recurrent epidemic outbreaks, and as such it focused on the present, not on the past.

Thomas Multon's late fifteenth-century comprehensive rewrite of John of Burgundy's treatise opened with the assertion "Here bigynnes a trety that is nedefull and necessarie ayenst the pestilens that *nowe is regnand* [i.e., reigning]."[85] Multon still blamed plague outbreaks on a Saturn–Jupiter conjunction, but since he did not explicitly date the conjunction – and notably omitted mention of Mars – it could have easily referred to any such recent occurrence. The later printed edition of "Moulton's" treatise likewise offered advice to mitigate the effects of "the vengeaunce and corrupcion of the pestylence *that nowe is reygnynge*."[86] Some temporal specificity can be ascertained through one minor yet telling adjustment that later printers made to the text: replacing the phrase the "Kynges liege people" with "Quenes liege people" after the coronation of Queen Elizabeth, and then again with "common liege-people" during the Commonwealth.[87] For the most part, though, the tract remained largely ahistorical, its nod to a plague outbreak that ostensibly affected readers "nowe" remaining intact as the treatise was reprinted repeatedly over a half century.

The same emphasis on current (or very recent) outbreaks is found in numerous other tracts of the fifteenth and sixteenth centuries. Some authors used specific dates to frame their discussions of plague: the authors of yet another version of John of Burgundy's treatise claimed to have written it in Oxford during a plague outbreak in 1407.[88] In the late 1540s, Jehan Guinter d'Andernach, a former royal physician and professor of medicine, wrote a tract because

"I see that the present time is heading towards the same problem" with plague that he had written about previously.[89] Most tracts, though, offered temporal contexts that were less specific. The English version of Johannes Jacobi's treatise attributed to the "Bisshop of Arusiens" and published in 1485, opened with the vague statement "Here after ensuith a little treatise very necessary & behouefull as well to preserve the people from the pestilence," which, it says, "oftentimes infects us."[90] English physician Thomas Phayer lamented suffering that was "dayly sene where the sayde dysease raygneth."[91] Jean Thibault, a physician and astrologer to Holy Roman Emperor Charles V and French King François I, explored how and why plague outbreaks returned repeatedly.[92] Many English and French tract titles in the sixteenth and early seventeenth century responded to readers' needs in times of pestilence since, as the English translator Thomas Paynel noted, plague "dothe very often invade, trouble, and vex mens bodys."[93] Largely generic titles – "Remedies against the plague" or *Traicté tres utile contre la peste* – appeared on many printed tracts between the late fifteenth and early seventeenth centuries.

If one looks at treatises from the perspective of readers who sought medical advice during recurrent outbreaks, this lack of temporal specificity helped make such advice appear timeless. Remedies continued to present a blend of long-standing and apparently well proved therapies alongside more recent proprietary medicines. In a society in which "written information came to be of increasing value … for practical purposes,"[94] there was a significant increase in the production of practically oriented texts. The more theoretical treatises that had appeared during the fourteenth century no longer met readers' expectations, especially as that readership itself expanded in response to rising literacy rates. Instead, the plague tracts of the fifteenth and early sixteenth centuries were to a large extent "practical manuals of traditional wisdom." [95]

Plague Rehistoricized

This place of Sedan is being rudely assailed by the plague for the second time.

François de Courcelles, Sedan, 1595[96]

In a few instances, tract writers between the late fifteenth and mid-sixteenth centuries included some type of recent historical discussion. In his discussion of the meaning and nature of epidemics, for example, the late fifteenth-century Norman physician Thomas le Forestier recalled both a deadly "pestilential catahhr" in Montpellier in 1387 and England's sweating sickness outbreak in 1485.[97] Jacques Guerin, a physician and surgeon in the Walloon city of Enghien, drew on his experience during a terrible outbreak in the region around Utrecht in 1558 to provide advice during an outbreak in his own city almost ten years later.[98] Yet, it was really only in the later sixteenth century that history re-emerged as a serious consideration in English and French tracts. The treatises' practical component remained intact, as did their ongoing debates about the causes of the disease. However, longer prefaces provided local context and authors began to incorporate relatively detailed personal reflections on recent outbreaks to demonstrate not only that they had expertise to offer but also that current "tymes of pestelens" were part of a longer historical narrative.

Reacting to the second outbreak to hit the Huguenot Principality of Sedan in a short period of time, for example, physician François de Courcelles painted a dismal picture of a town surrounded and besieged by both pestilence and religious enemies. For Courcelles, Sedan's great distance from the sea and its lack of harmful "exposure to the south" – as well as its Christian provision of refuge for beleaguered French Protestants – should have protected it from repeated outbreaks of plague.[99] Nevertheless, the city was once again at the mercy of the disease, and Courcelles sought to explain its nature and its causes while providing recommendations for the most efficacious preservatives and therapies. In its explanations and recommendations, Courcelles's tract echoed both the contents and the tone of other treatises of its time: since plague had natural and supernatural causes, remedies must include an appropriate mix of spiritual and physical treatments. In its commentary on a specific previous outbreak in the same place, however, Courcelles's work reflected a re-emerging trend: situating current outbreaks into a historical chronology, just as late fourteenth-century authors had linked the outbreaks that they faced with the Black Death.

More than simply creating a new chronology, however, French and English writers also began once again to interweave personal testimonials into discussions of the origins, trajectories, and progression of local plague outbreaks.[100] Individualization through place naming and the incorporation of longer first-person narratives are important markers that distinguish the early modern treatises from those of the late medieval era. This kind of historical comparison between a current outbreak and earlier ones had been largely absent from the tract genre for more than a century and a half, at which point the Black Death itself had been the primary point of reference. Some of the fourteenth-century treatise writers had also incorporated personal vignettes or discussed their outbreaks in the context of those that had preceded them; what was unmistakably different about the early modern treatises was the "emergence [and incorporation] of written histories of local plagues" that served to add an individualized narrative – a kind of "imposed, literate memory" – to the genre.[101] Historical re-engagement in the treatises coincided with the integration of history into medical writing more broadly, and with a turn to historical analysis as a mechanism for understanding the present.

By the early sixteenth century, there was growing awareness that socio-economic, political, and religious changes were "extending beyond the normal range of mutability in human affairs."[102] These changes were not only significant in and of themselves, but were also believed to be negatively affecting the "just ordering" of affairs and to be causing a "fraying of customary expectations." Recognition of economic and social change led influential English writers such as Sir Thomas More (*Utopia,* 1515–6), Sir Thomas Smith (*Discourse of the Common Weal of the Realm of England,* 1549), and William Harrison (*Description of England,* 1577) to consider the impact of longer-term historical change. Well before the 1600s, there was a common sense that the present "is so very different from what it was 150 years ago."[103]

In France, too, although there were a number of reforms in the first half of the sixteenth century, the second half was engulfed in religious wars that precluded the opportunity to discuss modernity or a disconnect with the past. Of course, literary and artistic debates within the early seventeenth-century Académie française between Ancients and Moderns (*la querelle des Anciens et des Modernes*) offers a partial comparison, but those battles had less to do with changes experienced over the recent past than with determining the respective superiority of ancient or modern writers.[104]

This tendency to notice and write about historical change reflected two major intellectual shifts. The first relates to the significant transformation in historiographical practice that took place in the late sixteenth century, when nearly a century of European travel and exploration and the beginning of the European colonial enterprise gave rise to a nascent sense of the "whole world," its peoples, and its history. This, in turn, changed conventions in history writing, fostering an inclination to frame it within a broad discussion of all places in the known world. This new sense of history contrasted with the universal history of the European Middle Ages, which was much more limited in its geographical, and thus historical, scope.[105]

The second intellectual shift, which becomes evident in plague tracts earlier, was the spread of humanism in the fourteenth through sixteenth centuries. Humanism provoked a transformation in medical knowledge as well as greater scholarly and professional enthusiasm for history and antiquarianism. Along with other learned disciplines, medical writing changed. By the early sixteenth century, Italian physicians began to use the word *historia* – suggesting a historical narrative that blended empirical observation with authoritative texts – in the titles of their anatomical books. The beginning of medical case histories can also be traced to this era.

Jean Bodin's 1566 *Methodus ad facilem historiarum cognitionem*, on the *ars historica*, demonstrated the value of historical information for interpreting and understanding contemporary societies and events; he also asserted that reading history could "cure all illness of the body and the mind."[106] Numerous physicians tried their hand at writing a wide range of historical works, including biographies of historical medical figures, medical treatises, formal essays, and even civil chronicles and grander historical narratives. As history gained greater academic value across Western Europe in the sixteenth century, medical writers began to incorporate a wider range of historical sources, such as first person and chronological narratives, records, case studies, and other types of "memories from the human past," into their medical treatises, including those on plague.[107]

Over the course of the sixteenth century, *historia* became a key aspect of medical writing and fostered the creation of *historia anatomica* and *historia medica* genres. Italian medical knowledge provided an influential model for other authors across Europe, who then began to place greater emphasis on description and narrative in medical texts of all kinds, alongside empirical investigation and greater consideration of material evidence. For some writers, this meant integrating descriptive and historical narratives into discussions of current local epidemics. It also meant deliberately creating "powerful official histor[ies] about the nature of the plague" in the places where treatise authors wrote.[108]

These changes are first and most noticeable in the French tracts, and appear as temporal localizations. While the English titles typically remained generic, providing practical remedies for recurrent times of pestilence, by the second half of the sixteenth century some French treatises either indicated directly which epidemic had inspired their composition, or at least pointed to a specific time in the present. Some tracts still used general phrases such as "the plague of this present year" or "of this time" to indicate that they were writing about specific outbreaks, but others included actual dates in their titles and/or contents. The title of Claude de Rubys's treatise, which responded to an epidemic in 1577, indicated that it was about "the plague that was in Lyon this present year."[109] Municipal physician Guillaume Briet's tract title was precise: it was about the "plague in Bordeaux, this year 1599."[110] As his title suggests, for Jesuit writer Jean Grillot plague was the most memorable event in the city of Lyon between August 1628 and October 1629.[111] No such specificity appeared in English tracts at this time.

Some French writers also compared or linked current outbreaks to ones recently past that were either part of their personal memories or the lived experiences of older contemporaries.[112] Claude de Rubys, the Lyonnais *échevin* (local magistrate), recalled a time from his Padua university days in 1555 when a foreign man was throttled after being accused of purposely spreading plague. For Rubys, this was but a precursor to the violence that he witnessed (and indeed encouraged) in his own city in 1564 and again in 1577.[113] Laurent Joubert, chancellor of the University of Montpellier, also referenced the Lyonnais outbreak of 1564 to demonstrate how plague could erupt in a single house before spreading through an entire town.[114] While discussing the pending arrival of plague in Tours in 1581 and tracking its advance from Paris, physician Nicolas de Nancel anticipated that the devastation caused by the "evil beast" would be like that which other people had experienced some fifteen or sixteen years previously in the city of Trent.[115] In a less common English example, clergyman and medical writer Thomas Brasbridge opened the second edition of his treatise by recounting his childhood experiences with plague and his later encounters with the disease when he was studying in Oxford and London. He then contrasted those memories to observations of the outbreak in 1578, which had inspired him to write his treatise.[116]

Some authors, again more typically French than English before the mid-seventeenth century, provided chronological timelines for local outbreaks, tracing plague's progress as it moved toward and then through their towns and thus revealing epidemic patterns. I discuss this in more detail in chapter 4. Others used historical references to make particular statements. While providing an overview of four separate outbreaks in Paris, Guillaume Potel made a pointed complaint that barber-surgeons such as himself had been treating the city's plague patients "since 1596 until now without pay."[117] Surgeons elsewhere in France had all been duly and regularly compensated for their work, and so, Potel protested, Parisian officials must pay local surgeons who had risked their lives during all four recent epidemics. Furthermore, Potel claimed that the remedies he proposed could be verified by their successful use in previous outbreaks and their promotion by other treatise writers over the past fifty years. Guillaume Chevalier argued that having "possessed perfect health" for about forty years, the Lyonnais had forgotten the terrors of the outbreak that they had suffered in the 1580s before plague returned in the late 1620s and several more times in the 1630s.[118] This lack of historical memory, he lamented, had left them totally unprepared to deal with the disease and as a result, many more died than should have.

Some sixteenth- and seventeenth-century writers went so far as to incorporate references to other historical events to establish context. In France, the situation was especially dire in the sixteenth century: the entire reign of Henri III (r. 1574–89) was marked by serious religious, political, and economic problems. The king's authority faced constant challenge from political and religious parties supported by foreign powers. Dynastic contest, conspiracies, and political discontent arose from within his own family, and his relationships with the old noble families, the wider court, and the *parlement* were strained, confrontational, and adversarial.[119] Despite the apparent initial willingness of the crown (or rather, the regency until 1563) to accommodate Protestantism, to "the *parlementaires*, [Protestant] heresy … threatened the political and social order; in their view, protestantism and revolution went hand in hand."[120] Tract authors Jacques Aubert, Nicolas Houël, and Guillaume Briet each claimed that underlying plague epidemics in Lausanne, Paris, and Bordeaux respectively, was the tumult generated by France's civil and religious wars.[121]

Writing in 1582, Esaïe le Lievre, a surgeon from Vermandois in Picardy, opened the address to his readers by explaining that only two things could bring down the monarchy: war and plague. Civil wars were as dangerous as foreign wars, he said, and when combined with plague, they could bring utter destruction. After providing several historical examples, le Lievre noted that it was not necessary to look to the past to understand such miserable events, since France was currently in the midst of one of its own. "For the past five or six years," he said, "Paris, the very heart of France, can render faithful testimony of the inconvenience and loss that the cruel contagion brings ... and those who live there are plunged more and more into it" while the wars continue.[122] To fight the disease, he pointed out, it had been necessary to employ a number of "excellent and tranquil" persons to erase from the hearts of men their tendency toward discord and war and to emphasize the utility and benefits of peace.[123]

In 1665, the English physician William Kemp metaphorically likened plague to "an Enemy which the Undaunted Valour of the Invincible English Nation, is neither able nor willing to encounter."[124] Here, Kemp suggested that despite English victories in the Anglo-Spanish Wars and the first Anglo-Dutch War, and despite having survived its recent civil war, the kingdom was still incapable of forestalling plague. The disease was its greatest enemy. In an era in which there appeared to be a growing and uncomfortable sense of changing times, it is not surprising that treatise writers linked together events of an unsettled present and past.

If early modern English tracts were less likely than their French counterparts to reflect specific epidemics, they did circulate alongside or even in conjunction with popular *Remembrancers,* weekly plague mortality broadsheets, and other civic records that made specific reference to previous outbreaks. The *Remembrancers* were a form of annal in narrative or poetic form; some provided chronological lists of major events, such as coronations, political and religious conspiracies, and serious plague epidemics. Samuel Clarke's seventeenth-century *Remembrancer*, for example, included the following heading for the year 1603: "A Great Plague began at *London.* Prince *Charles* created Duke of *Albany,* Marq. *Ormond, &c.*"[125]

George Wither's religiously poetic *The History of the Pestilence* – published in 1628 in *Britain's Remembrancer* alongside "a declaration of the mischiefs present; and a prediction of judgments to come" – also focused on London's plague outbreak of 1625.[126] The long poem opens as a battle between Mercy and Justice over England's fate in the face of God's wrath, and provides a detailed description of plague and its progress through London. It also sets the outbreak into a longer historical context: England had been free of the religious wars that wracked Continental Europe, had created a worldwide trading and colonial empire, had been led by a virtuous queen (Elizabeth I) and king (James I) who ruled through holy discipline, and had survived previous corrective plague outbreaks. Yet in the midst of their advantages, Wither wrote, England's people had forgotten their righteous ways and a more grievous plague epidemic was required to turn them around. In addition to castigating his fellow citizens for their sinful ways, Wither had a distinctly historical purpose in mind: he dedicated his work "(for the glory of God) to Posteritie and to *These Times*."[127]

By the sixteenth and seventeenth centuries, it was customary in London and other English towns such as King's Lynn, Norwich, and Yarmouth to post broadsides in public places that recorded the number of local deaths during plague outbreaks.[128] These single page prints, commonly known in London as *Red-Crosses* or *Lord Have Mercy Upon Us* after their banners, offered basic advice for both spiritual and physical health. They also typically contained a variety of death-related images and religious verse or prose narratives about the causes and impacts of plague (see figure 3.1). These were not one-off productions: successive copies of each broadsheet offered updated mortality figures. Printers did not expect people to continuously buy new broadsheets, though: most included blank spaces into which purchasers could write their own updates and thereby create personalized chronicles of the outbreak.

Surviving copies indicate that people did just that, both adding information and annotating what was already there.[129] In effect, the broadsheets "helped construct a model of plagues as ontologically distinct and thus quantifiable, constituting them as visitations of a disease which could be tracked through time, measured and compared."[130] Many also provided annual death counts from previous epidemic years, alongside diagrams that captured the mood and actions taken by Londoners during plague outbreaks. *Londons Lord Have Mercy Upon Us* printed by Thomas Lambert in 1636, for example, included weekly mortality statistics for the years 1592–93, 1603, 1625, and 1636. Much like the City of London's official bills of mortality that had enumerated weekly deaths by all causes since the early sixteenth century, these privately published broadsheets used plague mortality statistics to generate local knowledge about the disease's history. Readers of the bills and of the broadsheets could use the cumulative enumeration of plague deaths, both past and present, to identify patterns in plague deaths and to compare those patterns from one outbreak to another, stretching back almost half a century. One of the consequences of the concurrent official and unofficial collection and distribution of such data in the sixteenth and seventeenth centuries was an increased interest in, and ability to create, a quantitative history of plague in particular localities at particular points in time.[131]

By the mid-seventeenth century, men such as John Graunt were doing exactly that. Graunt published several works that compared, contrasted, and analyzed the "four greatest plagues in London … within this generation, or one hundred years."[132] To set the then-current outbreak of 1665 into a longer historical context, he used bills of mortality statistics and other contemporary sources to assess its relative devastation against those of 1592, 1603, 1625, and 1636 (see figure 3.2). Graunt determined that although the total number of deaths was greater in 1625 (which he said in another book "was ever since called *The Great Plague*"), the epidemic of 1603 was actually worse because a larger proportion of people died from plague than from other causes.[133] Other contemporary commentaries on the weekly bills of mortality provided similarly detailed examinations of the number of plague deaths from the 1590s to 1665, sometimes with annotations that resembled plague tracts by providing information about the disease and how to avoid it.[134]

English plague tract writers did not refer often to the mortality statistics that the broadsheets and bills provided. Yet by drawing on a blend of personal, community, and social memories they too started to note and compare local and regional outbreaks in the seventeenth century. Writers more often alluded to the dates of previous or current outbreaks than stated them explicitly. Medical writer and practitioner Thomas Thayre remarked in 1603 "it is not yet ten yeares since this Citie of *London* was visited and afflicted with this sicknesse."[135] An anonymous treatise printed in 1625 provided remedies and recommendations "whiche have (heretofore) beene well Tryed and Experienced, *in the last heavy and greivous time of the Pestilence.*"[136] William Boghurst was more specific, noting in his preface to the reader that he was writing specifically about his eighteen months experience with plague "viz., from the 7th of November 1664, to the latter end of this May last past, 1666."[137]

Burial registers were common in many other European cities, but these were for official government use; public records of death (and cause of death) like those produced in England were much less common. Such

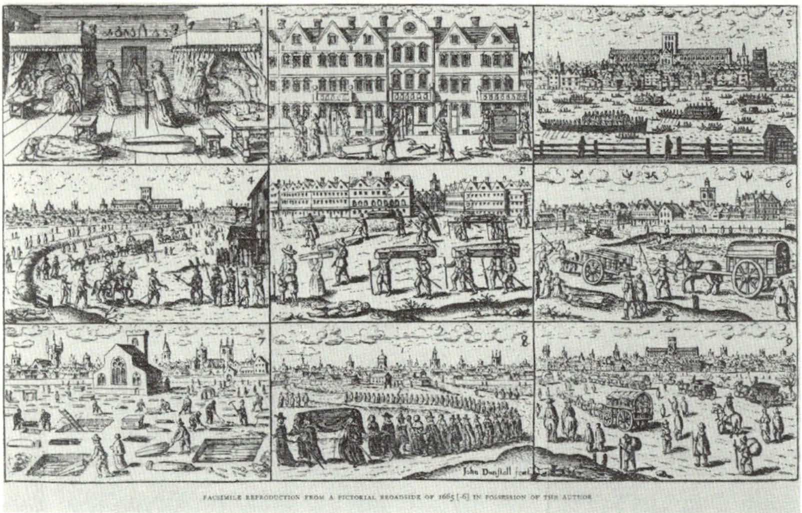

3.1 Detail of plague broadsheet comprising nine scenes relating to the 1665 outbreak in London, John Dunstall, 1666.

public reports were rare in France and were not widely disseminated, nor were they systematically produced before the eighteenth century. In only a few French cities, during specific outbreaks, were registers that included statistical information about the places and people affected by plague made public. Detailed reports on plague deaths by neighbourhood and by house appeared in Dunkerque and Gravelines in 1666, for example. During an outbreak in Rouen and its suburbs in 1668–69, magistrates published weekly bulletins that listed plague deaths by parish for public use and information; in this case, the bulletins also noted the occupations of those killed by plague to demonstrate that it was mostly the labouring classes who were affected, not the city's elite.[138] The primary purpose of these bulletins was not to inform residents about the progress of an epidemic, however, but rather to mitigate rumours about the presence of plague and its purported victims and to demonstrate that the government was responding. In addition to their rarity, a key difference between these French bills and those produced in England was the fact that when they appeared, they were issued by the central authority and were meant to serve specific political and commercial objectives.[139]

In fact, officials in many French municipalities actively delayed publishing news of impending or active plague outbreaks or making direct reference to past outbreaks to explain current ones.[140] They did

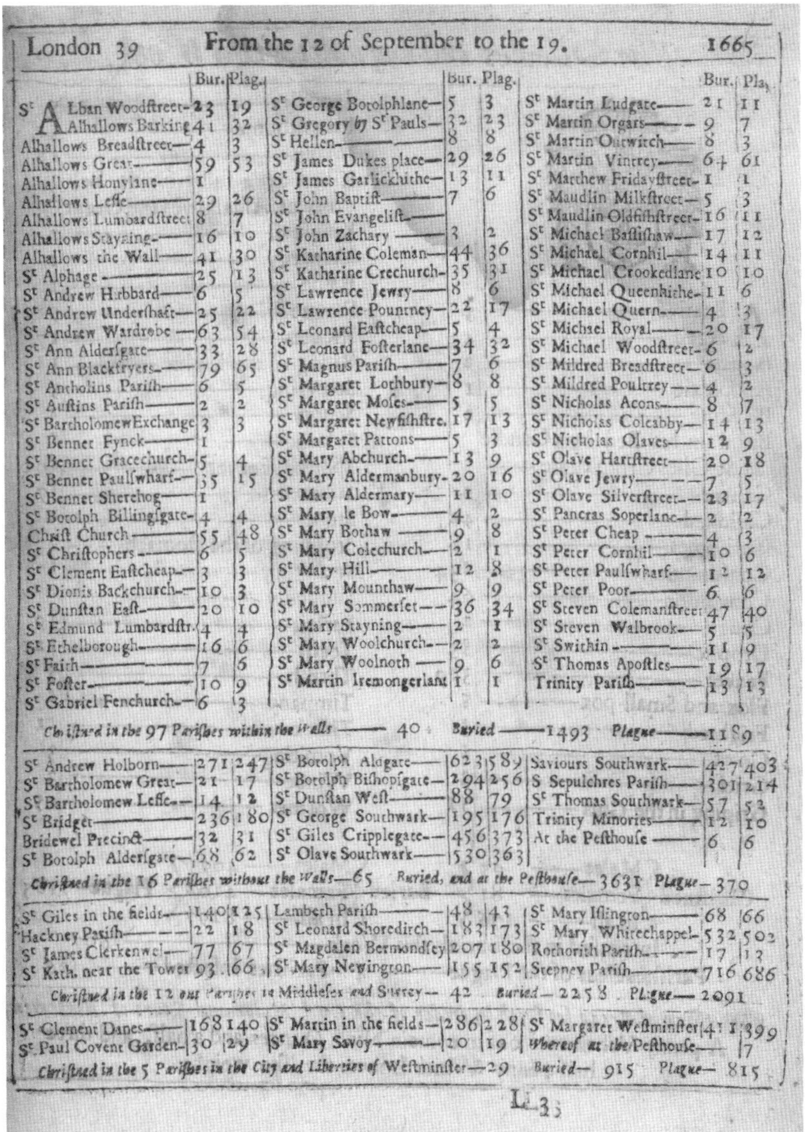

London 39 | From the 12 of September to the 19. | 1665

	Bur.	Plag.		Bur.	Plag.		Bur.	Pla.
St Alban Woodſtreet	23	19	St George Botolphlane	5	3	St Martin Ludgate	21	11
Alhallows Barking	41	32	St Gregory by St Pauls	32	23	St Martin Orgars	9	7
Alhallows Breadſtreet	4	3	St Hellen	8	8	St Martin Outwitch	8	3
Alhallows Great	59	53	St James Dukes place	29	26	St Martin Vintrey	64	61
Alhallows Honylane	1		St James Garlickhithe	13	11	St Matthew Fridayſtreet	1	1
Alhallows Leſſe	29	26	St John Baptiſt	7	6	St Maudlin Milkſtreet	5	3
Alhallows Lumbardſtreet	8	7	St John Evangeliſt			St Maudlin Oldfiſhſtreet	16	11
Alhallows Stayning	16	10	St John Zachary	3	2	St Michael Baſſiſhaw	17	12
Alhallows the Wall	41	30	St Katharine Coleman	44	36	St Michael Cornhil	14	11
St Alphage	25	13	St Katharine Crechurch	35	31	St Michael Crookedlane	10	10
St Andrew Hubbard	6	5	St Lawrence Jewry	8	6	St Michael Queenhithe	11	6
St Andrew Underſhaft	25	22	St Lawrence Pountney	22	17	St Michael Quern	4	3
St Andrew Wardrobe	63	54	St Leonard Eaſtcheap	5	4	St Michael Royal	20	17
St Ann Alderſgate	33	28	St Leonard Foſterlane	34	32	St Michael Woodſtreet	6	2
St Ann Blackfryers	79	65	St Magnus Pariſh	7	6	St Mildred Breadſtreet	6	3
St Antholins Pariſh	6	5	St Margaret Lothbury	8	8	St Mildred Poultrey	4	2
St Auſtins Pariſh	2	2	St Margaret Moſes	5	5	St Nicholas Acons	8	7
St Bartholomew Exchange	3	3	St Margaret Newfiſhſtre.	17	13	St Nicholas Colecabby	14	13
St Bennet Fynck	1		St Margaret Pattons	5	3	St Nicholas Olaves	12	9
St Bennet Gracechurch	5	4	St Mary Abchurch	13	9	St Olave Hartſtreet	20	18
St Bennet Paulſwharf	35	15	St Mary Aldermanbury	20	16	St Olave Jewry	7	5
St Bennet Sherehog	1		St Mary Aldermary	11	10	St Olave Silverſtreet	23	17
St Botolph Billingſgate	4	4	St Mary le Bow	4	2	St Pancras Soperlane	2	2
Chriſt Church	55	48	St Mary Bothaw	9	8	St Peter Cheap	4	3
St Chriſtophers	6	5	St Mary Colechurch	2	1	St Peter Cornhil	10	6
St Clement Eaſtcheap	3	3	St Mary Hill	12	8	St Peter Paulſwharf	12	12
St Dionis Backchurch	10	3	St Mary Mounthaw	9	9	St Peter Poor	6	6
St Dunſtan Eaſt	20	10	St Mary Sommerſet	36	34	St Steven Colemanſtreet	47	40
St Edmund Lumbardſtr.	4	4	St Mary Stayning	2	1	St Steven Walbrook	5	5
St Ethelborough	16	6	St Mary Woolchurch	2	2	St Swithin	11	9
St Faith	7	6	St Mary Woolnoth	9	6	St Thomas Apoſtles	19	17
St Foſter	10	9	St Martin Iremongerlane	1	1	Trinity Pariſh	13	13
St Gabriel Fenchurch	6	3						

Chriſtned in the 97 Pariſhes within the Walls — 40 *Buried* — 1493 *Plague* — 1189

St Andrew Holborn	271	247	St Botolph Aldgate	623	589	Saviours Southwark	427	403
St Bartholomew Great	21	17	St Botolph Biſhopſgate	294	256	S Sepulchres Pariſh	301	214
St Bartholomew Leſſe	14	12	St Dunſtan Weſt	88	79	St Thomas Southwark	57	52
St Bridget	236	180	St George Southwark	195	176	Trinity Minories	12	10
Bridewel Precinct	32	31	St Giles Cripplegate	456	373	At the Peſthouſe	6	6
St Botolph Alderſgate	68	62	St Olave Southwark	530	363			

Chriſtned in the 16 Pariſhes without the Walls — 65 *Buried, and at the Peſthouſe* — 3631 *Plague* — 370

St Giles in the fields	140	125	Lambeth Pariſh	48	43	St Mary Iſlington	68	66
Hackney Pariſh	22	18	St Leonard Shoreditch	183	173	St Mary Whitechappel	532	502
St James Clerkenwel	77	67	St Magdalen Bermondſey	207	180	Rothorith Pariſh	17	12
St Kath. near the Tower	93	66	St Mary Newington	155	152	Stepney Pariſh	716	686

Chriſtned in the 12 out Pariſhes in Middleſex and Surrey — 42 *Buried* — 2258 *Plague* — 2091

St Clement Danes	168	140	St Martin in the fields	286	228	St Margaret Weſtminſter	411	399
St Paul Covent Garden	30	29	St Mary Savoy	20	19	*Whereof at the* Peſthouſe		7

Chriſtned in the 5 Pariſhes in the City and Liberties of Weſtminſter — 29 *Buried* — 915 *Plague* — 815

L 3

3.2 London plague statistics for 12–19 September 1665, from John Graunt, *London's Dreadful Visitation: Or, a Collection of all the Bills of Mortality for this Present Year*, 1665.

so in an effort to avoid the economic and social disorder that would ensue once they were forced to acknowledge the local presence of the disease and the need to implement what were, in many instances, rather expensive and unpopular prevention measures: mandatory reporting, quarantine and isolation, conversion of buildings into pesthouses and the requisition of goods to support inmates, destruction of infected property, killing of domestic animals, travel bans, hiring of medical personnel, and so on. Ongoing debates in the plague tracts and among municipal medical and administrative authorities in France about the actual cause of the disease, its mode of transmission, and its clinical signs and symptoms also led to confusion, indecisiveness, and even paralysis. Similarly, the far-reaching consequences for individuals, families, and entire communities once the disease was diagnosed sometimes stayed the hand of those responsible for investigating and announcing the presence of plague.

The risk to families and communities (and to magistrates) of mistaken diagnosis was actually played out in French plague tracts and had significant implications for municipal officials: during an outbreak in Rouen in 1620–22, the local plague doctor, David Jouyse, was accused by another physician, Jean de Lamperiere, of having misdiagnosed a recently deceased plague victim. That mistake led to the entire house being contaminated. Jouyse, in his defence, argued in his treatise that other physicians had seen the victim while he was still alive, and they had not given a diagnosis of plague. By contrast, Jouyse said, he and an accompanying surgeon had in fact reported a likely case of plague to the magistrate, who in turn had marked and shut up the house. Lamperiere responded with a new version of events: that it was only the surgeon who diagnosed plague and not Jouyse himself, as he had remained undecided. It was this indecision that had condemned the entire family – which until that point had not been infected – because plague was subsequently brought into the shut-up house by a servant tasked with providing food. The original deceased man, then, had not had plague and Jouyse, simply following along with the surgeon's misdiagnosis rather than being competent to diagnose correctly himself, had led the magistrate to act incorrectly.[141]

The local implications of acknowledging, announcing, and officially tracking an outbreak were formidable. In the face of medical controversy, and confronting reluctance among citizens to report their symptoms (for fear of being isolated) and pushback from both ecclesiastical authorities (who resented having public masses banned) and economic leaders, municipal authorities tasked with managing outbreaks in French towns were slow to announce the presence of plague publically. When they did so, they did not turn to bills of mortality to keep track of an epidemic's progress. And thus, neither did French plague tract writers. Instead, as we will see next, they turned to other kinds of sources to track plagues through time.

HISTORICIZING PLAGUE AS PLAGUE

Rediscovering Old Sources

> This is what the Ethiopians are believed to have done, in the terrible Plague of Athens, that Thucydides recites.
>
> Oger Ferrier, Lyon, 1548[142]

To explain the cause of the plague epidemic that was devastating Lyon in 1548, Auger (Oger) Ferrier – physician to Catherine de Medici and judicial astrologer – turned to a variety of sources. Of those who had studied such things, he said, some said that plague was a rod of God (*verge de Dieu*) while others said that it came from infected air. Still others said that it was a contagious and popular malady, one to whose diverse causes they paid little regard. Ferrier came to the conclusion that all these possible causes (and several others) were correct: sometimes one, sometimes the other played the primary role in generating an outbreak of this deadly disease.

To show how this was possible, that plague had multiple causes and that each outbreak was its own unique manifestation, Ferrier relied on a mix of traditional religious and medical figures together with Ancient Greek philosophers, biographers, and historians. Thus, alongside the Bible, Hippocrates, and Galen, we find among his sources Demetrius, Plutarch, Proclus, Thucydides, and Herodotus. From philosophers, Ferrier adopted the idea that demons or spirits engendered mutations in the air. From the stories of past epidemics told by historians, he drew parallels with the outbreaks of his own day: evil and cruel men could, whether through vengeance or in the hope of profit, collect and spread infected filth, just as Thucydides said the Ethiopians had done to the Athenians. Or, as Herodotus recounted in his *Erato*, God could send plague not as a punishment, but rather as a portent or omen of a forthcoming misfortune like that faced by the people of Chios.[143]

The historical commentary incorporated into early modern tracts did not focus just on the near past. By the sixteenth century, interest in historical knowledge in general, and in historical medical knowledge specifically, had broadened substantially. Fourteenth-century authors had, of course, relied on Hippocrates and Galen, but the full Hippocratic corpus became readily available only after its publication in Latin in the early 1500s, and the complete works of Galen (in Greek) appeared only in 1525.[144] Ferrier was, in fact, the first French tract writer to re-employ the Hippocratic categories of external versus internal causes of disease, and the subsequent mid-sixteenth century turn to a Hippocratic (rather than solely Galenic) framework allowed tract writers to better see the parade of great epidemics over time.[145] This, in turn, enabled them to put their current outbreak into a timeline that weighed its relative importance across history. At the same time, humanist developments in historical thought and learning, and their incorporation with other disciplines, irrevocably altered medical thinking, practice, and writing. Ever-increasing amounts of historical narrative made its way into medical texts of all kinds, including plague treatises. Like Hippocrates and Galen, Thucydides and the Plague of Athens had had their role to play in the earliest tracts, but no author was able to offer much detail or engage in sustained analysis of these sources until the sixteenth century.

The humanist movement and the turn to ancient sources emerged in tandem with the flight of Byzantine scholars and their manuscripts from the eastern Mediterranean in the early fifteenth century. After the Ottoman conquest of Constantinople in 1453, this westward flight of *émigrés* increased significantly. New knowledge of the Gothic Wars, described so vividly by Procopius, also provided Italian and northern humanists with information about the early histories of Italy and the Germanic states. With access to such materials, Western acquaintance with and interest in the knowledge and events of the near and distant past expanded exponentially, as did exploration of the social and cultural aspects of that past. Growing interest in the practice of history followed, along with distinct changes in the way that political, military, and ecclesiastical histories were both written and used to understand the present.[146]

The rediscovery of and new access to centuries-old texts opened treatise writers to the realization that the disease they regularly faced was not simply a product of their own times. References to greater numbers of and more detailed Biblical analogies also appeared in the treatises, as Protestant writers tied their perceptions of a currently sinful world to the errors recounted in and lessons learned through the Bible. Thomas Brasbridge, for example, argued that it was important to take notice of the pestilences that befell the Israelites, since such things "are written for our learning ... as an example to us ... lest their plagues fall upon us."[147] More importantly for the discussion here, treatise authors started to draw heavily from sources such as Homer, Aristotle, Plato, Thucydides, Livy, as well as late medieval writers like Giovanni Boccaccio and Matteo Villani. In doing so, they began the process of creating a longer chronology for plague, one that established a direct connection between current outbreaks, the Black Death, and even the First Pandemic. Curiously, though, they rarely turned to medieval medical writers or plague treatises for guidance; while medieval literature was an acceptable source of historical information, humanism was predicated in large part on the dismissal of medieval scholastic (and hence, medical) knowledge.[148]

Like the full works of Hippocrates and Galen, ancient texts that discussed past epidemics, such as Procopius's descriptions of the First Pandemic, only became generally available in Western Europe in Latin in the fifteenth century and in vernacular translation in the sixteenth. Other texts that had been known indirectly in the West for much longer, such as Thucydides's description of the Plague of Athens, saw a surge of interest, translation, republication, and integration into new texts, including plague treatises. Thucydides's *History of the Pelopponesian Wars* had been available in Latin only since the mid-fifteenth century, and the first vernacular edition appeared in French in 1527. For most contemporary scholars, the primary value of Thucydides's works lay in the lessons they provided for modern monarchs and politicians, but his description of the Plague of Athens also drew significant attention. The story of Athens's epidemic was best known in seventeenth-century England from Thomas Hobbes's translation. Thomas Sprat, the future Bishop of Rochester, also published a popular poetic account of the epidemic in English.[149] Although Sprat stated that the specific disease about which Thucydides wrote was unknown to him, much of what Thucydides described about the ramifications of the illness (which Sprat contextualized in a more contemporary fashion) was familiar to seventeenth-century readers: both the symptomatic fever and the attendant social disruption and loss of hope were well understood. Indeed, portrayals of plague as "a [still] new and inexplicable disease [that] continues remorselessly not only to conquer but to consume" were commonplace.[150] Many sixteenth- and seventeenth-century treatise authors included Thucydides in their long list of historical sources, since his narrative format provided much more information about, and lessons learned from, the disastrous outbreak of disease in Athens than did Hippocrates's medical works alone.

In his 1557 commentary on the Hippocratic treatise *De flatibus*, the Parisian physician and author Adrien l'Alemant compared Thucydides's account of the Plague of Athens, contemporary narratives of the Black Death, and records of a local outbreak in 1514 to determine if the effects were similar enough to consider them to have been the same disease. A few years later, the Italian polymath Girolamo Cardano provided another history of plague epidemics, including in his list both the major outbreaks of the First Pandemic, especially in Constantinople, and the Black Death.[151] Access to new historical sources, combined with the fresh emphasis on the value of historical narrative, likewise provided writers with both greater historical awareness and a plethora of examples of older epidemics (plague or otherwise) that they then used to trace plague across time.[152] The English sweating sickness (*Sudor anglicus*) of 1485, and its subsequent outbreaks in the sixteenth century, appeared in almost all plague treatises that engaged in historical discussion. In short, the epidemics of the present were now not just traceable to the recent past: they could also be understood as part of a much longer human experience with disease.

In 1577, the Lyonnais *échevin* and self-described historian Claude de Rubys turned to the Black Death-era writings of historian Matteo Villani and writer Giovanni Boccaccio to discuss "the great pestilence that happened in ... Italy" in 1346–49.[153] Rubys was among the first French post-Black Death tract authors to refer to these texts and to re-establish a longer, and more historically evidenced, lineage for the plague outbreaks of his day (Laurent Joubert, one of Henri of Navarre's physicians, had contended in a Latin treatise ten years earlier that some plagues were universal, "like the one described by Guy de Chauliac ... that circled almost the whole world"[154]). Rubys also referred to a great outbreak in Rome during the First Pandemic, which he placed in the time of Pope Pelagius II (r. 579–90), although it was more commonly associated with his predecessor, Gregory I. That same year (1577), Italian philologist and physician Girolomo Mercuriale wrote a tract full of historical references, beginning with an excerpt from Thucydides's description of the Plague of Athens. Thereafter, he cited examples of numerous epidemics taken from the accounts of "all the historians," including Thucydides, Procopius, and Evagrius, to argue that history clearly demonstrated that an outbreak of one disease could eventually evolve into "true plague."[155] This apparently vindicated his complete misreading of an outbreak the previous year, since he now claimed that at the time of his consultation, the epidemic in Venice had not yet turned into "true plague." For Mercuriale, the narrative descriptions of centuries of past epidemics were "*historiae*, which ought to be the highest form of reasoning for us on this topic."[156] The medical canon and direct experience were no longer sufficient to explain plague; they needed to be supplemented with historical narrative. Subsequent tract writers hailed Mercuriale as an authoritative source.

Shortly after Mercuriale and Rubys wrote their tractates, Laurent Joubert translated Guy de Chauliac's 1363 *Grande Chirurgie*, which contained a long commentary on plague, into French; this helped to make knowledge about the 1348 and 1360 epidemics more widely known. Other treatise writers did not immediately pick up these references, though, and even Rubys did not make much of the historical outbreaks. Within a few decades, however, references to the Black Death were commonplace.

In its 1606 treatise, the College of Surgeons of Paris mentioned two great outbreaks in Rome, one that was reported in the Ecclesiastical histories and the other by St Gregory. A printed marginal notation in the College's treatise specifically marked the latter outbreak as "notable history" worthy of attention.[157] J.S. de Saincte-Hillier, a royal physician, drew from a variety of historical sources to define plague and its variants; in addition to Thucydides, he referred to Lucretius, Eusebius, Procopius, Sabellicus, and others. He also spoke about a great epidemic that began in 1385 and continued for five years, "taking half of the world."[158] Jean Vigier, a physician and surgeon in Castres, offered an etymological analysis of plague, listing the variety of names by which peoples throughout time had known the disease: to the Latins it was "*Pestis à Despacendo*," to the Greeks "Loimos," to Homer "le Dard d'Apollon," to the Fathers of the Church "l'Ire, le flambeau & la vengeance de Dieu," to the Hebrews "Dauar."[159]

Although it began somewhat later, a similar pattern can be seen in English writings. Henry Chettle's *True Bill* not only accounted for plague deaths in London, Westminster, and Norwich in 1603, but also recounted plagues from the years 81, 188, 254, 530, 540, 1348, and 1359, along with more recent outbreaks in England.[160] John Gadbury's mid-seventeenth-century astrological account began in 1348, a year in which "the chronicles tell us" that a great plague occurred throughout the world.[161] An anonymous English tract that disputed the validity of shutting up the homes of infected victims noted that "In the years 1346. 1348. 1350. there was a great plague all over the world ... such as was never remembered to be in any place before."[162] Although not actually a plague tract, John Graunt's reflections on the *Bills of Mortality* are also important here because they influenced how other English writers perceived the temporality of plague. The Black Death, he said, began in 1346 and was "the greatest [mortality] that ever we read of since the Universal deluge." He then provided a narrative description of post-Black Death outbreaks, including one in 1362 "which was called *The Second Pestilence,*" two each in the fifteenth and sixteenth centuries, and all those in the seventeenth century until 1665.[163] An anonymous commentary on London's *Bills of Mortality* in 1665 included a discussion of pestilential outbreaks from the third and sixth centuries, noting that "In the year 540, there began a universal plague all over the world that continued 50 years with great violence."[164] This appears to be one of the earliest accounts in English of the First Pandemic. It was not until the eighteenth century, however, that English tract writers took up longer-term historical writing.

Enlightenment Discourse

> We may observe that the Contagion now spreading it self in Foreign Parts, has nearly the same Symptoms that were observ'd in the late Plague at London.
>
> Richard Bradley, London, 1721[165]

The practice of creating local plague histories gained momentum in the eighteenth century, when placing current outbreaks into first a short and then a longer historical timeline, and tracing the progress of local epidemics, became an integral part of efforts to explain both the disease and how it should be managed. After the 1665 outbreak in London, English tract writers no longer had large local epidemics to historicize. They thus began writing about epidemics that were happening abroad. No outbreak spurred them to turn again to the tract genre in large numbers until the one in Provence in 1720. More than half a century without large-scale epidemics meant that the disease was becoming, for these eighteenth-century writers, a historical relic, albeit one that still had the power to instil great fear.

Many of the new English tracts produced between 1720 and 1722 were marketed as historical accounts of the French epidemic. These writers typically described the similarities between the Marseille outbreak and the London epidemic of 1665; some also compared it to other large outbreaks that had afflicted the city since the late sixteenth century. The naturalist and botanist Richard Bradley, for example, inserted into his tract "some Observations taken from an Original Manuscript of a Graduate Physician, who resided in London during the whole Time of the late Plague, *Anno* 1665" as the centrepiece of a short history of epidemics in London.[166] For Bradley, the year 1665 was "the Last Time that we can say the Plague raged in *London*."[167]

Spurred by "the last Foreign Advices" that had "given us something particular relating to the Pestilence" – these being letters he had received from fellow physicians in southern France full of descriptions of ghastly plague symptoms and of societies crumbling under the weight of the disease – Bradley felt confident that Marseille's plague was the same disease that had cast its shadow over London more than fifty years earlier.[168] It stood to reason, then, that successful seventeenth-century medicines and anti-plague measures utilized in London should work once again, both to deal with the epidemic in Marseille and to prevent the disease from spreading to England. 1665 was not, of course, the only year in which plague had assailed London; Bradley incorporated pages from the seventeenth-century Bills of Mortality to demonstrate that plague mortality had waxed and waned in London, both on its own and in comparison to other diseases, during the outbreaks of 1592, 1603, 1625, 1630, and 1636. These Bills, he said, served both "as a Memorandum to the Curious" and as a practical tool.[169]

That the same disease caused these epidemics was not in doubt. The fact that the Bills recorded plague as a distinct cause of death was not questioned; recurrent experience with the disease showed that the same signs and symptoms caused high mortalities in the same months of the year. It was a straightforward exercise for tract writers to detect the same patterns in historical outbreaks.

For other eighteenth-century English writers, to comprehend a no-longer experienced disease and to understand its history in relation to that of other diseases, it was critical to look at both the tracts and other historical texts of prior generations. English physician Richard Brookes produced a plague tract whose purpose, alongside dispensing advice for appropriate treatments and prophylactics, was to provide readers with a succinct history of all the major epidemics that had happened in Europe over the previous three hundred years. Believing that to understand present diseases one must turn to what had been written previously, Brookes compiled his history by bringing together information from a "Variety of Books … which before were scattered here and there."[170] Although he admitted to making "considerable Contractions" of the material that he consulted, Brookes assured his readers that "I have omitted no material Circumstance that would either explain the Nature of the Disease, or the Manner of its Cure; and if my Authors had been more particular, I might have been so too." Most importantly, Brookes wanted his readers to understand that he had not set out to write "an *entire* History of Pestilential Distempers."[171] Instead, his purpose was to demonstrate how historical authors had distinguished between plague and other kinds of disease, and how and why this distinction mattered. Differentiating plague as its own sort of disease was critical if "endeavours to weaken its Force or stop its Progress" were to have any hope of success.[172]

Brookes began his historical account with the sweating sickness, a supposedly "new Distemper … call'd by Authors Sudor Anglicus" that was first observed in 1486.[173] After discussing its signs and symptoms, Brookes commented on the disease's recurrences in subsequent years while also claiming that it had continued in England almost constantly for forty years. Following a detailed discussion of treatment regimens for the sweating sickness, he then moved further back in time to "that terrible Pestilence which raged in the Year 1348," which, he said had "made dreadful havock all over the World, scarcely leaving the tenth part of Mankind alive."[174] Repeating Black Death-era contentions, he wrote "it's probable no Age ever saw the like [epidemic]."[175] The remainder of his tract addressed various "Epidemical disease" outbreaks in the sixteenth and seventeenth centuries. Most of these occurred in Germany – likely a reflection of Brookes's apparent reliance on German sources such as one Shenckius of Graffenberg – and included pneumonic diseases, smallpox, measles, spotted fever, dysenteries, other malignant fevers, and an unknown malady that he called the "Hungaric Disease." None of these were to be confused with plague.

Other English tract authors wrote with the same ideas in mind. John Quincy declared in 1720 that the "Histories of Physick abound" with stories of pestilential outbreaks, including those by Thucydides, Livy, and the second-century Greek historian Appian of Alexandria.[176] To discuss and explain outbreaks of all pestilential infections in England over the previous one hundred years, Joseph Browne drew on the "Rules and Methods" of what he called "the Product of the most learned Physicians of the Age they lived in, whose Names are far from being unknown to you, as [Théodore de] Mayerne, [William] Butler, [George] Bate, [Andrewes] Burrel, [Hieronymus] Fabritius, [Nathaniel] Johnson, [Thomas] Rudgeley, [Henricum van] Rhede, Tulpius [Nicolaes Tulp], [Thomas] Gibson, [William] Harvey, [Jonathan] Goddard and [Charles] Scarburgh."[177] These were mostly sixteenth- or seventeenth-century physicians, whose medical writings and practices – and likely experience with plague in the previous century – Browne invoked to refute Richard Mead's assertion that the disease was transmitted via trade and merchandise. In doing so, he also highlighted the features that distinguished plague from other types of diseases, including "the Black and Yellow Jaundice, Itch, Leprosy, Measles, SmallPox, [and] Venereal Lues."[178] Neither the signs and symptoms nor the mode of transmission of these diseases could be observed with plague. To make this argument, and having no direct experience of his own with plague, Browne repackaged the observations and conclusions of writers and physicians mostly from the time of Kings James I and Charles I – "the most Learned Physicians, in the Two great Plagues before that of 1665."[179]

Richard Mead, for his part, had advocated for the implementation of preventative measures that were "very different from the Methods taken in former Times among Us," arguing that newer approaches were more "agreable to Reason."[180] The implication was that measures historically enacted during outbreaks of plague were insufficient. Prior misunderstanding of the disease needed to be replaced by greater clarity and knowledge; such insight could only be attained by assembling, reviewing, and analyzing documents from the past. In the ninth edition of his plague treatise, issued in 1744, Mead contended that "There is in all ancient History no Account" of any plague outbreak worse than that in Constantinople in 543. This, he said, he had learned from "The History of it [that] is very well told" by Procopius, Evagrius, and others.[181]

Even some three decades after the outbreak in Marseille, the English surgeon Dale Ingram found it useful to write a treatise on "the most remarkable plagues that have appeared ... which I have taken from the Histories."[182] For Ingram, though, the purpose of his treatise was "not so much to shew its [plague's] antiquity" as to disprove the contagionist theories of his predecessors and contemporaries.[183] Ingram claimed to have "strictly searched the journals of the Plague at Marseille" for real evidence of contagion there; in doing so, he contended that the historical records showed all assertions of plague's contagious nature to have been false.[184] As such, he argued, although history was important for informing later writers about the long historical presence of plague, it nevertheless had to be read and interpreted carefully.

Experience with plague was perhaps a little fresher in mind for some French writers in the 1720s. The physician Jean-Baptiste-Nicolas Boyer de Paradis assumed that plague was "a disease that the whole world should know well enough" because of its long presence and widespread familiarity.[185] Ordered by Regent Philippe d'Orléans to assist with the epidemic in Marseille, Boyer soon had the opportunity to put his knowledge to the test. Some writers, like Abbé Martin Gaudereau, claimed to be relying upon personal experience with multiple plague outbreaks, while others drew from what earlier authors had written.

Pierre Baux, a physician from Nîmes and doctor of medicine at the University of Montpellier, dismissed the geographic indicators that physicians usually relied on to distinguish between various types of "*Peste.*" Instead, he pointed to the importance of particular symptoms such as the bubo. This, he said, marked plague as "a genre, and not a species of disease."[186] To prove his point, Baux differentiated between the plague epidemic of 1348, described by Guy de Chauliac, an outbreak in France in 1557 "that was called *Coqueluche* [pertussis]," and the English sweating sickness in 1486–87. Each of these forms of disease were called "*Peste*," he argued, but each had its own history. Relying on the accounts of Procopius and Evagrius, he set the origins of the bubonic plague in the sixth century. Swiss physician and medical writer Jean-Jacques Manget claimed that sixteenth- and seventeenth-century writers' experience with plague "in their times" provided sufficient proof that the outbreak in Marseille was the same disease he found described historically.[187] In dedicating his tract to "all the young physicians and surgeons destined to help plague victims," Jérome Jean Pestalozzi compared the arrival of the disease in Marseille to the experience of Toulouse in 1607 and Lyon in 1628.[188] Other writers had a different take: they believed that ancient histories that discussed the cause of disease had misled modern writers into accepting "outrageous" ideas such as contagion.[189]

Jean-Baptiste Bertrand's account of the 1720s outbreak in Marseille claimed to provide a historical account of everything that happened, including how the disease had been introduced into the city. Much like Nathaniel Hodges in London the previous century, Bertrand charted the progress of the Marseille outbreak from one city quarter to another, delineated distinct phases of the epidemic, and then provided a detailed commentary on previous outbreaks as points of comparison. He also traced a long history of outbreaks in that city, beginning in the first century CE and moving through the sixth-century First Pandemic (as Gregory of Tours had reported it, he said) and on to the Black Death. Bertrand concluded that the recent Marseille epidemic – the twentieth outbreak in the city's history – was the most destructive of all time: "One dares to affirm," he wrote, "that of all the cases that historians report, that medical writers describe, and that our merchants and seamen have seen in different countries of the Levant, none has ever progressed so rapidly or been so violent as this one."[190] Bertrand's exceptionally long treatise also suggests that the troubles and disorders of plague, and the extreme desolation that it caused, "were a subject well worthy of a historian."[191]

If humanism introduced tract writers to the value of historical narrative and provided them with access to a wide range of sources, it still took a surprisingly long time to achieve consensus about the impact of the Black Death. Once an acceptable story of plague across two time periods was forged, other factors influenced how tract writers used this history. New intellectual trends – such as growing interest in geography, local climates, and foreign customs brought about by overseas exploration – as well as closer to home military and imperialistic threats, coloured treatise writers' interpretations of past epidemics. In addition to recasting plague's history, these authors began to reconsider the disease's geographical locus. In doing so, they bound together plague's longer-term temporality and spatiality in a way that both reflected and responded to contemporary political and religious concerns. At the same time, the Ottoman threat generated interest in the West about the history of the Byzantine Empire that the so-called Turks were now supplanting. I discuss the creation of a historical geography for plague in chapter 5. First, though, it is important to establish how plague's contemporary geography evolved, which is the subject of chapter 4.

CONCLUSION

"This part of medical history, which has such a manifold and powerful influence over the history of the world," claimed Benjamin Guy Babington in the opening preface to his translation of Justus Friedrich Karl Hecker's 1832 historical narrative of the Black Death, "is yet in its infancy."[192] For Babington, a physician, epidemiologist, and translator of medical works, the plague narrative was "an important page of the history of the world" that highlighted the universality of human frailty. "History … offers," he said, "even for pestilences, an inexhaustible, though scarcely explored, mine of facts."[193] The facts that Hecker had mined in producing his history book came from what he called "authentic" sources, including the testimonies of Byzantine writers, Guy de Chauliac's account of plague in Avignon and Boccaccio's of it in Florence, numerous chronicles, seventeenth- and eighteenth-century general histories (themselves largely summaries of earlier chronicles), and a variety of antiquarian collections.

Of contemporary medical sources about the Black Death, Hecker claimed, it was possible to find only two adequate discussions, the ones by Chauliac and Vinario. He did, however, quote extensively from the Paris Medical Faculty's plague tract, if only to ridicule its "strange precepts."[194] In the later part of his narrative, Hecker explored subsequent outbreaks of plague in a rather cursory fashion, focusing for the most part on the public health measures that were taken (or not) across Europe to forestall the disease. Plague treatises, he believed, offered nothing of value that would enable him to grasp how contemporaries had understood the disease or how they perceived its history.

By not reading the treatises for clinical descriptions and by looking past their "strange precepts," I offer here a deeper reading of plague histories. The tracts contain evidence of significant change over time in thinking about plague's long and local histories. Experience with recurrent outbreaks and access to new information and knowledge were crucial to this evolution, not only because they shaped ideas about the historical origins of the disease, but also because the ways in which experiences and knowledge were interpreted ultimately shaped how people understood plague itself. As people's perceptions of the world around them changed, so too did their perceptions of history.

Each successive outbreak built a new history for plague, but the incremental nature of this history-building, and its general absence as an narrative feature in the fifteenth and early sixteenth centuries, has made it easy for scholars to overlook or even dismiss it. Rather than reading the treatises for remedies and therapeutic advice, I have concentrated instead on the cycles and evolution of ideas that are woven through them about plague's place in history: initially in the history of the known world, then in the history of specific places, and finally again in the history of an expanded world. By exploring in this chapter the different ways in which references to plague's history (or purported lack thereof) entered into English and French tracts, I have evidenced a unique record of changing attitudes about plague's history.

The focus here on English and French tracts complements existing work on Italian treatises that recognize the second half of the sixteenth century as a transition point in plague tract writing. Furthermore, I have extended that observation back in time and shown how treatise writers utilized concepts of time and history over a multi-century period to better explain the historicity of plague in their societies.

As inheritors of a long period of relative human healthiness – or at least freedom from epidemic disease – the earliest writers assumed that the Black Death was a unique historical event. Subsequent epidemics became part of a recognized series of outbreaks. In the sixteenth century, English and French treatise writers began to implement a two-pronged – short-term/local and long-term/global – recreation of plague's history. It was only under the intellectual and material influences of sixteenth-century humanism, including the new availability of ancient texts and the authoritative lustre given to history writing, that writers began to explore the much longer history of plague. Authors interpreted and manipulated those sources according to their worldviews. The treatises themselves thus must be read with their specific historical context in mind and we, as later readers, must "recognize that much of the material that we use to understand past plagues is drawn from memory" – memories retold to serve their authors' wider purposes.[195] One perhaps curious side-note to this contemporary memory building is that, while the devastating plagues of the 540s and 590s, the 1340s through 1390s, and the later sixteenth and seventeenth centuries all make regular appearances in the humanist tracts, aside from reference to *Sudor anglicus* and French pox, the fifteenth-century experience all but disappeared. It is no wonder, then, that it is also largely invisible in modern plague studies.[196]

Plague contributed to empirical thinking and historical writing in the early modern era more than most other diseases because of its long existence in human communities. Only *sudor anglicus* (English sweating sickness) and *morbus gallicus* (French pox or syphilis), both of which seemingly appeared out of nowhere in the late fifteenth century, generated similar, albeit much shorter, reflections. Placing the study of plague treatises within this broader context of the rise of historical writing, especially such writing that was undertaken by physicians and other medically oriented writers, is crucial for understanding the nuances that exist in discussions of plague's temporality. Here, too, we might note that aside from Jean-Baptiste Bertrand, none of the tract writers were able to provide a historical account of disease in his own city that stretched back beyond a century or so. Plague did gain a very long history in these texts, but it was largely a universal one, not a local one.

Carefully tracing and comparing how treatise writers portrayed plague's history over time pinpoints a number of distinct transitions in those discussions. Some of the transitions are incremental, while others are transformative; together they belie any suggestion that plague treatises are static and interchangeable. Looking at how tract writers discussed plague's history is important for better understanding how they constructed the role of the disease in their societies. It also shows us how they set the terms by which plague itself was understood across almost four centuries of recurrent outbreaks and how we still understand it, as a historical force, today.

4

Seeing Plague in Space

From Elsewhere to Everywhere, from Here to There

We almost never remark on either the progress or the duration of the plague in a territory. No word is said about the many places that are afflicted [at the same time or sequentially]. This makes it appear that we are speaking of several plagues, when it could be the same one that has passed from one city or kingdom to another, or that has been renewed because it was not sufficiently extinguished.

Pierre Baux, Nîmes, 1722[1]

WRITING THE SPACES OF DISEASE

At the height of the Provençal outbreak in July 1721, Nîmois physician Pierre Baux complained that other writers had ignored the geographical origin of plague and the route by which it travelled. Of course, as he acknowledged in his subsequent plague tract, at first he had not thought it necessary to know these things either: such information did not help physicians treat the sick.[2] However, ignoring the various places affected by plague meant that not only were medical practitioners oblivious to the fact that they could all be facing and treating the same disease, but they also failed to recognize its contagious nature and did not put preventative measures in place to forestall its movement. Many doctors had fled Nîmes in fear, but Baux remained in the city to treat the afflicted despite his conviction that plague was contagious.[3]

Baux argued that by not acknowledging that plague moved – for example, by disregarding outbreaks apparently reported in Syria – Marseille officials shamefully were caught by surprise when it appeared in their city in 1720. This directly led to the dire situation that physicians faced throughout southern France. It was clear, he contended, that a ship had carried plague to Marseille. That vessel had not just moved commercial goods and men from one place to another; it had also transported a contagious disease.[4]

Geography underpinned Baux's discussion of plague. One key to understanding the disease was its apparent association with specific places. Drawing from ancient Hippocratic and Galenic traditions, medieval and early modern medical culture accepted that a direct relationship existed between particular geographies and topographies, corrupted air or miasma, and the generation of specific diseases.[5] In the centuries prior to the Black Death, numerous medical texts – including authoritative works by Ali ibn Abbas al-Majusi (Haly Abbas), al-Rāzī (Rhazes), and Ibn Sīnā (Avicenna) – and popular regimens alike addressed the link between place and disease, noting, for example, locations that generated unpleasant smells and were thus unhealthy.[6] Therefore, it was thought that particular features of rural and urban landscapes such as marshes, sluggish waterways, damp and dark valleys, slaughterhouses, tanneries, and garbage heaps were local sources of disease because of their propensity to emit corrupted air. Some regions of the world were believed to be unhealthier than others because they embodied more of these sources of disease. It was evident to centuries of tract authors, like Baux, that plague resided or erupted in particular spaces and spread from them to infest other (previously healthy) places.

Despite Baux's contention that other writers ignored plague's movement, some of the earliest had, in fact, paid close attention to this issue. As the Black Death arrived in the Mediterranean region in 1348, these authors considered the disease's origins and observed its propensity to spread from one place to another. The extensive nature of an epidemic whose steps one could trace was, in fact, one of the pandemic's early defining features. As outbreaks localized over time, writers turned to investigating their more immediate surroundings. Regardless of whether they took a wide or narrow geographic focus, these authors questioned both the places in which plague originated and how it had come to be in the spaces where they lived and wrote.

I argue here that the treatises' underlying explanations of plague were inherently spatial, and that writers fitted their epidemiological observations to their geographical preconceptions, rather than the other way around. They used astrological and religious considerations to interpret and explain plague's apparent universality, environmental and terrestrial features pointed both to particularly unhealthy places and to the disease's geographic movement, and human susceptibility and individual temperaments clarified why people in one place could become infected while their neighbours did not. There was more to their geographic thinking, though, as these explanations blended and reworked ideas about the respective contagiousness of places. The placement of plague's locus was slowly and subtly shifted first inward and then outward. Each explanation for plague's appearance and spread evolved in response to changing perceptions of the complex relationships between place and disease. Unpacking these shifts points to changing medical norms and the influence of broader socio-cultural and socio-political imperatives on geographical thought, including increasing (and increasingly concentrated) urban poverty, religious conflict, and global trading relationships.

This chapter explores how treatise authors used geographic considerations to discuss plague from the mid-fourteenth century until the mid-eighteenth. It first examines the Black Death-era construction of references to a so-called "universal" plague, as writers attempted to conceptualize the pandemic in geographical terms. French authors all commented in one way or another on plague's widespread nature. Many noted that it appeared in numerous places, either at the same time or following an identifiable pattern; some traced the disease's progress as it moved ever closer to their homes. The pandemic nature of plague also required physicians to distinguish between this universal pestilence (*pestilencia universal*) and the more familiar (and more localized) particular pestilence (*pestilencia particular*) that they were used to treating. In the face of subsequent outbreaks, however, most tract writers stopped talking about universality, instead shifting their attention to local recurrences. In England, this meant using generic, non-specifying terminology: speaking of unnamed places throughout the kingdom allowed the same tract to appeal to a diverse readership scattered across the realm. In France, by contrast, more specific geographic localization appears in plague tracts by the 1360s: Avignon, Liège, Montpellier, and Paris all make an appearance. Over the course of the sixteenth and seventeenth centuries, an increasing number of French cities and towns are named as places infected by plague. Most, but not all, accord with the presence of local print industries. In England, however, London takes centre stage. As the heart of the kingdom's print production, the city also acquired the reputation of being its locus of plague. In fact, London and plague became inseparable in the pages of many English treatises by the sixteenth century.

Aside from ubiquitous local spaces of disease, such as swamps and the foul-smelling industrial sections of town, English and French writers also notably diverged by the early sixteenth century when it came to assigning blame to the peopled spaces that they considered to be disease-generating: in England, plague came to be associated with the poor, while in France religious tensions spilled over into discourses of the places of plague. In the seventeenth century, the local was displaced in its turn, at least partially, by allusions to hemispheric disease. The new medium of newspapers facilitated readers' ability to trace an epidemic's movements, first across domestic regions and then across other kingdoms and countries; this fostered the idea that plague was not, in fact, a local disease, but rather one that was imported from outside. While Black Death-era writers had pointed to an eastern source for their plague, three centuries later this easterly glance took on a different meaning: it did not take much intellectual effort for humoral-based susceptibility to a locally-generated disease to become recharacterized as the flaw of a social, religious, and geographic Other.[7] This chapter demonstrates that ideas about plague's geography did not remain static over time, but evolved alongside experience, observation, available knowledge about the world, and medical thinking. As with its history, then, the recreation of plague's geography reflected people's changing worldviews and intellectual influences.

Geography certainly plays out in Baux's treatise. It was clear to him that plague was not a disease that originated within Marseille: "if Marseille had been the centre of infection," he argued, "mortality should have been greater there, or it should not have been [so] considerable in the places that were far away from it."[8] Given the outbreak's catastrophic effects throughout Provence, it was foolish to suggest that only those places closest to Marseille had suffered. Instead, the disease affected all towns in southern France, some at quite a distance. This was not, as some wanted to argue, because each city contained its own, individual, source of infection; rather, this was a disease that actively moved. Plague's power seemed to grow in strength as it spread: Baux pointed to the town of Arles, which was located some twenty leagues (111 kilometres or 69 miles) away from Marseille but was affected worse than Marseille itself. Furthermore, the disease's movement was not uniform: places as far northwest as La Canourgue were infected, while towns that lay between it and Provence appeared unscathed. The pattern of spread suggested to Baux that plague was both contagious and portable, able to be picked up, carried, and then dropped somewhere else.

For proof, he contended, one needed only to look at plague's progress through the places where it "made its harvest": the disease's advance could easily be traced from one household to another, from one neighbourhood to the next.[9] On a larger scale, its arrival in and movement through France in 1720 could be tracked: "We see the plague enter France; we see it moving from town to town, from province to province."[10] So too could its earlier progress towards the French coast be mapped, he argued: the ship that carried plague had arrived in Marseille only after stopping at Sidon, Beirut, and other ports where the disease was reportedly reigning with full force.[11] The last major plague epidemic in southern France, in 1649, had shown a similar, methodical advance, entering first through Marseille, then successively attacking cities and villages in Provence, before spreading into Languedoc and finally slipping into Nîmes.

Baux also argued that medical writers' traditional method for distinguishing pestilences – as general when they affected a large part of the world, as particular when they afflicted a single kingdom, province, or city, or as local when they did not extend beyond their point of origin – was not useful for understanding plague. Instead, he said, plague outbreaks had the potential to evolve from one type to the other. It was thus critically important to recognize that outwardly unrelated local outbreaks might not be isolated but could be part of a widespread epidemic. Recognizing geographical patterns was thus necessary to forestall the spread of disease. Baux pointed to individual outbreaks of the previous century, before 1649, convinced that they would have clearly shown a geographical pattern if only someone had taken the time to consider them as parts of a single epidemic: 1606–07 in Poitiers; 1620–23 in Paris; 1626–28 in Lyon, Toulouse, and across Languedoc; 1629 in Montpellier; 1629–30 in Aramont and finally in Nîmes.[12] To Baux, these outbreaks were evidence that plague moved in traceable patterns. The geography of disease mattered.

Some 100,000 people died of plague in Marseille and across Provence between 1720 and 1722. Half of those deaths occurred outside the city, and in some small towns the death rate exceeded 50 per cent. The epidemic reached as far as Aix-en-Provence, Arles, Apt, and Toulon, and spread into the Comtat-Venaissin, the foothills of the Alps, and the Massif Central. Some cities experienced more than one outbreak over the two-year period, while others were spared entirely.[13] Quarantines and *cordons sanitaires* failed to keep the disease in check, and may have actually increased local mortality; they did, however, help to contain its spread further north.[14] All of these facts, if not known immediately by Baux, were suggestive enough to inform his perception that plague was a disease whose spatial implications – its foreignness, its portability, and its contagiousness – had to be recognized, even if such knowledge meant nothing in the end to those who suffered and died from it.

The roles and meanings given to and derived from spaces and places have underscored a significant amount of scholarship since the mid-1970s. Such studies have explored, among other things, political, legal, socio-cultural, and religious spatial practices, the fluid definition and use of public and private spaces, and the juxtaposition of healthy and diseased spaces.[15] In terms of the latter, urban and empire planning processes from the medieval to the modern eras have implicitly, and sometimes explicitly, integrated notions of the opposing states of well-being – not simply in the medical sense of health and disease, but also in terms of creating harmonious social interactions. Deciding what constitutes healthy or diseased spaces in any given place or time has been as much a reflection of socio-political and cultural constructions as of geographic realities.[16]

The conceptual links between space and plague are perhaps most evident in the classic prophylactic advice *cito, longe, tarde* ("flee early, go far, and return late"). They also exist in religious processions to forestall an epidemic, pest houses, quarantines, *cordons sanitaires*, and the hotly debated practice of shutting up the houses of the infected to contain an epidemic. In each case, authorities created or designated specific spaces to protect, remove, isolate, hold at bay, or otherwise separate the diseased from the healthy. All required a significant level of religious, civic, and/or military administration, and all were met with varying degrees of opposition.

Each of these socially-defined diseased or disease-free spaces also embodied a geographic reality: replications of Pope Gregory I's sixth-century procession through Rome, which many believed had ended a serious plague outbreak in that city, followed predefined paths through the streets for spiritual cleansing.[17] Pest houses, like other hospitals, were typically (although not always, especially in their early days) placed in liminal spaces outside a city's walls or, where none existed, beyond the towns' densely inhabited areas.[18] Quarantined ships and goods were likewise relocated and stored in spaces away from the sites where economic transactions took place. *Cordons sanitaires* included the stationing of soldiers and other military *materiel* along boundary lines between infected and uninfected regions; their regular adjustment revealed plague's geographic progression.[19] Seventeenth-century critics of shutting-up policies argued that enforcing household isolation as soon as one member fell ill, with doors nailed shut and guards posted outside, both created a diseased space that doomed an entire family to death and "actually spreads [the disease] as people [break out and] flee."[20] Recurrent outbreaks of plague and other diseases also spurred attempts to clean and improve natural and built environments and encouraged ongoing examinations by physicians and topographers of the relative healthiness of particular places.

Contemporary ideas also held that plague itself was generated in, occupied, and moved from specific places. A close reading of a broad sample of English and French plague tracts shows that thinking about where those places were located evolved over time, and was not always conceived in the same way in the two kingdoms.

GEOGRAPHIES OF PLAGUE

A Universal Disease

> I, Alfonso of Cordoba, master of the liberal and medical arts, have examined with much study the cause and nature of the pestilences which have arisen and begun in the present year of our Lord 1348 … [and which are] spread throughout all the regions of Christendom.
>
> Alfonso de Cordoba, Montpellier, 1348–49[21]

In contrast to the invention of a historical narrative for plague, wrestling with concepts of place and space was fundamental to the original treatises. In one of the earliest tracts, Alfonso de Cordoba, a student at or medical practitioner affiliated with the University of Montpellier, echoed his contemporaries by pointing to the epidemic's broad extent. Even though he wrote before plague had spread throughout Europe, it seemed clear that it would affect the entire Christian world, east and west, north and south. When the Paris Faculty of Medicine had issued its tract a few months earlier, the epidemic had not yet reached Paris. It was, however, anxiously anticipated. Stories circulated widely about the devastation that this great mortality was causing as it moved steadily westward and northward, from Provence to Avignon and throughout le Midi, after arriving on France's southern coast some months earlier. The Faculty's treatise was thus predicated on its "fear [of] a future pestilence here [in Paris]."[22] By now, it noted, plague had to be recognized as a universal epidemic.

Black Death-era French treatises noted that plague appeared in many different places, either at the same time or following an identifiable geographical pattern. Some writers like the Paris Medical Faculty and Pierre de Damouzy could write only about what they heard from nearby regions and towns because plague had not yet reached them.[23] Others – perhaps having better access to information brought by merchants, pilgrims, or travellers from further afield – took a wider geographical view. French physician and astrologer Geoffrey de Meaux, writing in 1349, sought to understand why "this general pestilence ... affected so many countries."[24] Simon of Covino's allegorical poem spoke to a pestilence that was depopulating the whole earth. An anonymous treatise likewise sought to explain the pestilential epidemic "which now prevails in the world," wondering why towns situated so far apart could be affected by the same epidemic at the same time.[25]

In England, plague tracts were not yet circulating; even so, before the epidemic reached the kingdom's shores, religious leaders such as Robert Hathbrand, prior of Christchurch Canterbury, pointed to "the pestilences and wretched mortalities of men which have flared up in other regions" and called for processions and prayer to "save and protect the king's realm of England from these plagues."[26] In a letter to his officials in July 1348, William Zouche, Archbishop of York, wrote of the "great mortality, pestilence, and infection of the air [that] are now threatening various parts of the world."[27] Statements about the outbreak's apparent universality are also found in many other contemporary texts. Petrarch lamented the death of "peoples throughout all the world ... [which has caused] nearly the whole world – not just this or that part of the earth – [to be] bereft of inhabitants."[28] Gilles li Muisis, Abbot of St Giles at Tournai, wrote that "the mortality grew strong in Rome, the Romagna, Sicily, Tuscany, Italy, Gascony, Spain and various other countries, at last entering France in 1348." Two years later, in 1350, he expanded his description of the pandemic, writing "there were persistent reports of a mortality which had begun in the East, and spread throughout India and all Christian and pagan countries from East, North and South, as was attested by the travellers and merchants who regularly visited those distant countries."[29]

Centuries earlier, chroniclers and historians of the First Plague Pandemic had made similar observations about plague's universality. The sixth-century Byzantine historian Procopius wrote "it did not come in a part of the world nor upon certain men ... but it embraced the entire world ... [it spread] in either direction right out to the ends of the world."[30] He further exclaimed: "the plague came, seizing in its grip the whole civilized world and especially the Roman Empire."[31] Other sixth-century Greek and Syriac writers wrote of witnessing an analogous event that passed "from one land to another."[32] A few contemporary Latin writers used comparable terminology to describe the outbreaks that they faced – the Illyrian chronicler Marcellinus Comes, for example, wrote of "a great pestilence [that] ravaged the land of Italy, and also the Orient and Illyricum which had been already similarly affected" – but most focused on their own regions.[33] Gregory of Tours offered the most detailed Latin narrative of epidemics between the 540s and 590s, but although he noted outbreaks in different regions and places, his information and thus his discussion was largely "geographically constrained" to a region centred on Clermont (south-central Gaul).[34] Corippus, Bede, and Paul the Deacon also each wrote of plague outbreaks as if they were localized rather than widespread events. Stories attributed to Pope Gregory the Great likewise were geographically specific, centred on Rome.[35] Other First Pandemic-era texts that addressed plague's clinical characteristics, such as Isidore of Seville's *On Medicine* and *De natura rerum*, did not place the first pandemic into a geographical or spatial context at all.[36] Without access to the Greek and Syriac accounts, Black Death-era treatise writers were largely unaware of the First Pandemic's reach; although some recalled reading about great epidemics from the days of Hippocrates, Galen, and Pope Gregory I, they categorically dismissed these earlier outbreaks as less universal than the one that they faced.[37] Thus, they struggled to understand plague as it moved ever closer to them, seeing its apparent global extent as unprecedented.

Such descriptions of a widespread disease outbreak as "universal" might be explained as a literary trope or cliché, much like calling it "unprecedented" or "unheralded." Even when using terms such as "universal," "everywhere," or "the whole world," of course, writers in both the sixth and fourteenth centuries meant, for the most part, only their own immediate regions and a limited number of other places that they might have heard about through political or religious alliances, or even through the stories of travellers.[38] When the authors lived within an empire, they could have had some sense of a larger geographic scale, such as at the height of the Roman Empire (second to third centuries) or the Byzantine Empire (sixth century). This sense of territorial universality, however, was lost in the West as the decline of the Roman Empire led to political fragmentation. The replacement of the Roman Empire by Christendom did create a world ostensibly united by belief, but not one that had defined geographical parameters. By the eleventh century, the ideological split between eastern and western Christianity created a more defined sense of western Christianity's "geographical and ideological units: the papacy and the Holy Roman Empire ... [and] an atmosphere of confident universalism."[39] Universalism in this sense reflected people's sense of belonging to a belief community rather than to a large geographic space; here, local loyalties, identities, and issues took precedence.

Certainly, the efforts and attentions of most fourteenth-century chroniclers focused on local concerns and not on a broader world. Some, such as the Frenchmen Jean de Venette and Jean Froissart or the Englishmen Henry Knighton and Thomas Walsingham, wrote about the universality of the Black Death with the advantage of hindsight, using information collected from the testimonies of authors in other localities.[40] One could thus argue that it mostly was only later, as people had time to reflect upon and share their common experiences, that the universality of the Black Death became common *topos* in plague literature.[41] Some of the early tract authors, though, did make reference to the disease's broad geographical spread. They were writing contemporaneously with the Black Death, and shared their attempts to make sense of plague's cause and origins at the same moment that they witnessed it or awaited its inevitable arrival. News about the many places near and far that plague had already struck spread quickly through correspondence and by word of mouth after 1347.

As concepts and descriptors, then, "universal" or "worldwide" held more than strictly theoretical or rhetorical meanings for treatise writers. These terms implied a physical and metaphorical space that extended beyond their realms of medical knowledge and geographical experience. They also offered a means to communicate the magnitude of the phenomenon. Geoffrey de Meaux certainly believed that a greater part of the earth was affected by the epidemic. Two decades later, Guy de Chauliac reflected on his own Black Death experience, saying "I call the mortality [of 1348–9] great because it overtook the whole world, or nearly all of it ... [Other epidemics have] affected only one area; this one, the whole world."[42]

Explaining such a widespread epidemic, the likes of which did not exist in the medical canon, required an epistemological shift.[43] Treatise writers began by making a clear distinction between the causes of this universal pestilence (*pestilencia universal*) and the more familiar and local pestilence (*pestilencia particular*) that occurred in a defined region, in a city, on a street, or in a specific house. The latter could be rationally explained with reference to traditional medical theory: through the normal or abnormal operation of the four elements (earth, air, fire, and water) in a particular place, through an individual's humoral imbalance, or through tainted food or water.[44] Just as religious writers emphasized universal human sinfulness to make sense of the pandemic, the earliest plague tract writers sought a cause that could affect people in various places at the same time. The most widely accepted answer was a remote celestial or astrological event such as the conjunction of Saturn, Mars, and Jupiter in 1345. As Geoffrey de Meaux explained, it "affected the whole inhabited world between east and north ... because all parts of the world ... shared in the effect of the configuration."[45]

Many subsequent writers invoked the same explanation for the epidemics that followed, although some, such as University of Montpellier Chancellor Johannes Jacobi, rejected universal causation and asserted instead that terrestrial factors were more relevant for explaining the post-Black Death local outbreaks. Underlying the argument about universal versus particular causation was academic disagreement on the nature of the disease itself. Just as critical was a notable shift in how the authors portrayed plague's spatial characteristics. Most new treatises written after 1360 omitted reference to the disease's universality. In contrast to the earlier treatises that continued to circulate, new generations of authors spoke about plague as a local or regional problem that required local or regional solutions. By the later sixteenth century another change took place, as tract authors began to name the specific locations about which they wrote. Plague, in other words, became localized in two different ways.

A Turn to the Local

Almost the mydel part of thy realme [is vexed & trobled] w[ith] the venyms feuer of pestilens.

Thomas le Forestier, London, 1485[46]

Thomas le Forestier, a Norman physician living in London during the first outbreak of the English sweating sickness in 1485, dedicated his tract to the newly crowned English king Henry VII because his kingdom – alone among its neighbours – was suffering from a mysterious and troublesome disease. Le Forestier suggested that Londoners' poor sanitary habits – throwing carrion and other foul things into the streets, leaving privies dirty, and keeping tainted water in their kitchens – had corrupted the air. These things, he said, were the source of putrid odours that caused the disease to break out specifically in London, as opposed to anywhere else in Europe. The printed versions of his tract contained even more pointed geographic notes: by opening with a specific reference to a disease outbreak in London, le Forestier implicitly set all the diseases that he discussed in the English kingdom, if not in London itself.[47]

Although the occasional post-Black Death treatise writer still described subsequent outbreaks as "universal," during the second epidemic most had ceased speaking about plague's especially wide geographical reach.[48] What seemed more relevant was the disease's local appearance and reappearance. In the French treatises (like their Italian and German counterparts), we also clearly see geographic localization already by 1360. Guy de Chauliac spoke directly to his Avignon experience: "We saw this [buboes] clearly in the great and unprecedented mortality which appeared to us in Avignon."[49] Chauliac also mentioned his concern that leaving the city during the outbreak would tarnish his reputation, and so he stayed, contracting plague himself. He furthermore stated that "After [1360] … the mortality revisited us."[50] The relevance of this outbreak was that it was affecting the city of Avignon once again, not that it also affected many other places.

John of Burgundy presented himself as a physician and professor in the art of medicine in the city of Liège; he also made several local references, including to a successful medical recipe that could only be manufactured by a certain apothecary in that city and to a less efficacious one that was originally sent in a letter from Cologne.[51] His primary concern was that the Black Death had, by the 1360s, established itself as a disease with local repercussions. The widespread mid-century epidemic referenced in his introduction quickly gave way to the outbreak that had returned to reinfect the very place in which he was writing.[52] Other writers were even more geographically specific. Jean de Tournemire wrote that he had cured a noble plague victim at his practice in Montpellier.[53] In the early fifteenth century, Jean Piscis, chancellor of the Montpellier medical school, dedicated his tract to "the significant benefit of the whole town of Montpellier" during an outbreak there in 1431.[54]

Coinciding references to plague outbreaks in contemporary French and English chronicles, alongside those written elsewhere in Europe, demonstrate that the later fourteenth-century epidemics were still widespread. Yet both chroniclers and tract writers commented almost exclusively on local outbreaks. The treatise writers may have known or observed that outbreaks were widespread or multi-focal but did not explicitly say so; the genre's primary purpose was to provide prophylactic and treatment advice for local readers. The Black Death had affected everyone everywhere, but as John of Burgundy intimated, it left behind "traces" that subsequently re-emerged locally and did not always spread very far, very quickly, or in predictable patterns.[55] Treatise writers could thus portray the later plague epidemics as being the same disease that had affected them all previously, but as outbreaks that had distinct geographical attributes.

Adaptations made to John of Burgundy's treatise as it moved from France (or Liège) to England in the late fourteenth century, however, suggest that a different kind of shift took place in English terminology. Modern catalogues of English epidemics paint a grim picture of the era: on the heels of the six post-Black Death epidemics of the fourteenth century, outbreaks occurred nationally, regionally, or locally during at least thirty-three separate years in the fifteenth century. Between 1480 and 1580, at least twelve major epidemics are recorded. These later outbreaks were not as geographically extensive as the Black Death but still affected many places simultaneously.[56] The more common shorter English version of John of Burgundy's tract opened with the simple statement that its purpose was to provide readers with guidance "whene pestilens regnes in [the] cuntre."[57] In Middle English, the word "cuntre" referred not to the current notion of country as a nation-state, but most often to a local district or region; in some cases it could refer to the realm.[58] The treatise's advice was designed to be relevant whenever, and wherever, there was a plague outbreak, even though that place was not named. In this version of the tract, the earlier references to plague being a widespread disease and to a succession of epidemics disappear.

The long-term popularity of this treatise should not be taken as evidence that it was sufficiently vague to suit people's needs in different places at different times. Rather, it was its geographic anchoring, and the specific dialects in which it was copied, that contributed to its on-going relevance. One needed to take particular precautions to remain healthy when plague occurred in this particular place, at this particular time.[59] This shorter English version also removed the universal astrological explanation for plague that had marked its original text; reference to widespread disease no longer responded to the interests of the tract's fifteenth-century English readers. Their primary concern was how to address a local outbreak, rather than contemplating where else in the world the disease was currently present or what had caused it.

Two copies of a different version provide more specific geographic references, claiming to have been written in Oxford during an outbreak there in 1407, and then sent to the mayor of London for his use in that city.[60] In the last quarter of the fifteenth century, Thomas Multon produced a new English adaptation and translation of John's treatise that combined aspects of both its longer and shorter versions. From the longer version, Multon reasserted a celestial cause for plague. From the shorter version, he adopted the focus on localized outbreaks. Multon spoke to local spaces by tying his text to an undated current outbreak that appeared "gen[er]alli in this realme."[61]

By the late 1520s, Multon's treatise reappeared in a printed medical miscellany. A new prologue stated that the treatise's purpose was to support the "com[m]onwelthe and helth of the kynges lyege people."[62] Commonwealth or "common weal" is a Middle English term referring to a political community founded for the common good or benefit, loosely based on the Latin concept *res publica*, or public affairs. Multon's use of the term – or rather the printer Robert Wyer's – provides further linguistic and spatial anchoring for an outbreak that was affecting "this realme" and its "commonwelthe."

Many of the English treatises of the first century of print provided no further localization of plague than that seen in the late medieval manuscripts: they spoke to "tymes of pestilens" in broadly defined but unnamed places "where the sayde dysease raygneth." [63] Yet what we can understand from this is perhaps a sense that the broad idea of "cuntre" came to be an important touchstone in the way that English plague tracts evolved: in contrast to their French counterparts, English writers saw their "cuntre," their commonwealth, as a particular place. In his address to the reader, an anonymous late sixteenth-century physician noted that plague "hath heretofore beene too well knowne and felt in sundrie places of this Realme … [especially] in many chiefe Citties."[64] The self-styled Gentleman Simon Kellwaye considered "the great calamitie, miserie, and most distressed state of our Countrie, on which it hath pleased God to inflict the heavie scourge of his wrath, by imposing on them that poysonous infection the plague … [which is] so generally dispersed throughout this land."[65] Even the Aberdeen physician Gilbert Skene, who penned what was the first vernacular medical book of Scottish origin, the first medical book printed in Scotland, and the only known Scottish plague tract, used similar language: "this present plaig and maist detestable diseise of Pest [that] be laitlie enterit in this Realme."[66] Geographical localizations started to appear in English tracts only at the end of the sixteenth century. Even then, French treatise writers were far more place-specific, better attuned perhaps to what was happening in their many plagued cities than the English were, since the latter turned their gaze largely to London.

SPACES OF PLAGUE

Plagued Cities

> God did put in my minde to write a Treatise against the Pestilence …
> I made it especially for the use of the inhabitants of London: both bicause that citie was most commonly, and most greevously visited with that sicknes: and also bicause I my selfe was an inhabitant there.
>
> Thomas Brasbridge, London, 1592[67]

In 1592, clergyman and medical writer Thomas Brasbridge arranged for the second edition of his medical work *The Poore Mans Jewell* to be printed. The book contained a plague tract with remedies "prooved by the practise of the Author, and of many other."[68] Brasbridge had personal experience treating plague: as a medical and divinity student he had tended to the plague-stricken during an epidemic in Oxford in 1563–64, and, as a schoolmaster, preacher, and medical practitioner, he did so again in London in 1578. While he had prepared the first edition of his treatise either during or immediately after his initial encounter with plague in London, the second version was published more as a pre-emptive measure. "[A]lthough the sicknes (thanks be to God) do not at this present raigne among us," he wrote, "yet the Treatise is not in vaine" because it offered treatments to both cure and prevent the disease. Brasbridge seems to have been prescient: an epidemic did in fact break out that year, shortly after his updated treatise appeared.

With its direct mention of Oxford and London, Brasbridge's second edition marked a shift in how English tract authors talked about the places affected by plague. Only the Aberdeen physician Gilbert Skene had written earlier, in 1568, about a specific plague-infected city: he claimed that he wrote his plague tract as a result of what he had witnessed within "the Noble Burgh" of Aberdeen.[69] Some treatises translated into English from Continental sources also added prefatory localizations to make them more relevant to English readers. Thomas Twyne, for example, dedicated his translation of Pierre Drouet's French treatise to Sir James Hawes, the Lord Mayor of London, to assist Hawes with his responsibility for the "government of this Citie of London" as it faced "this greevous plague of Pestilence" in 1578.[70] By the late sixteenth century, though, the city of London was not just the primary place of plague tract writing and printing in England: it was also increasingly both a specifically named place in English treatises and a city that English writers explicitly declared to be diseased.

Over the course of the sixteenth century, the population around London, inside its walls and in the suburbs, increased four-fold while its proportion of the total population more than doubled, dwarfing the next largest cities in the kingdom.[71] Perceptions of the city, of its pre-eminence and of its problems, also shifted noticeably during the sixteenth and seventeenth centuries. Such perceptions were then reflected in the first century of printed English plague treatises. These ideas were fuelled not just by London's rapidly increasing population; they also responded to religious transformation, the city's greatly expanded urban boundaries, its fragmented social, cultural, and economic dynamics, its "new patterns of consumption which ... altered the urban environment," and – particularly after 1578 – renewed and more devastating outbreaks of disease than the city had seen for almost a century.[72] Contrasting a dire and troublesome present against a nostalgically recalled past was a critical component of those perceptions (see figure 4.1).

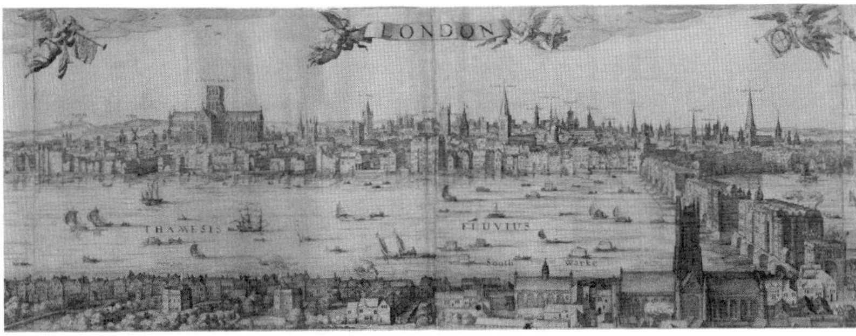

4.1 Plagued London: Visscher's Panoramic View of London, looking across London Bridge from Southwark, 1616.

Before the late 1500s, London was England's primary centre for banking, international trade and commerce, its recognized capital city, and, importantly, its demographic core. The centre of government, and thus of political and royal power, remained in Westminster, but that city was in many ways seen as an extension of London, especially as the suburbs between them expanded. However its own boundaries were defined, London was, according to the sixteenth-century historian and antiquarian John Stow, "the chief and principal city of the land."[73] Thomas Platter the Younger, a Swiss physician and traveller, agreed, writing of his travels through England in the late 1590s that "London is the capital of England and so superior to other English towns that London is not said to be in England, but rather England to be in London."[74]

Recurrent plague epidemics, and the overwhelming number of plague-related deaths in London, prompted contemporaries to assess the changing conditions of the city's topography and its "urban life for sources of divine displeasure" that might explain its apparent link to disease and death.[75] For religious writers, London was also a hotbed of sinful behaviour. Since sin and epidemic disease were bound up with dense populations, these writers described London as being polluted by both spiritual degeneracy and pestilence. In 1603, clergyman Henoch Clapham criticized medically-oriented plague treatises that repeated the ideas of "*Galen* a Greek Heathen Physitian," arguing instead that it was "God [who has] smitten our Citie [London] with the Pestilence."[76]

Indeed, by the later sixteenth century, London *had* become England's foremost site of plague, epidemiologically, metaphorically, and in print.[77] Although epidemics ravaged many towns, the large and devastating outbreaks that hit the city of London in the seventeenth century (1603, 1625, 1636, and 1665) caused treatise writers to concentrate on London's plague experiences. Medical and religious writers alike focused on the disease that was "fearefully over-flowing this famous cittie of London" and sought "to preserve Londoners with their families ... from the ... deluge of the plague."[78] Official proclamations concerning outbreaks in the cities of London and Westminster likewise saw repeated reprinting and distribution throughout the first half of the seventeenth century.

Over the decades that followed the printing of Brasbridge's treatise, London became the *de facto* site of English plague. Dramatist and pamphleteer Thomas Dekker, for example, portrayed London as the vanguard of England's fight against God, a position that left it especially vulnerable to divine wrath and punishment in the form of plague. In 1625, the poet John Taylor authored a pamphlet entitled *The Fearefull Summer: Or, Londons Calamitie.* The pamphlet was updated and reprinted in 1636 with some additional "mention of the grievious and afflicted estate of the famous towne of New-Castle upon Tine, with some other visited townes of this kingdome."[79] Religious works proliferated about London's special level of sin that caused it to be the target of both plague and, in 1666, fire.

Physician and religious writer Francis Herring's plague treatise was "first published [in 1603] for the behoofe of the city of London, and all other parts of the land at this time visited" by the disease.[80] Thomas Thayre provided special "directions for the commons, country-men and strangers that is necessitated to come into the city [of London]"; he sought "likewise to give sufficient instruction and direction unto the Inhabitants of this City, for their preservation in this infectious time."[81] Although an anonymous author claimed in 1625 to have written his treatise in response to the fact that "the disease called the Plague or Pestilence ... now at this time is too fiercely felt in divers Cities, Townes, and other places of this Realme," most writers, like the London medical practitioner Stephen Bradwell, specified that plague was "fearefully over-flowing this famous cittie of London."[82]

A generation later we find much the same construction of London as a plague magnet, sometimes with a focus on particular neighbourhoods within the city suburbs. William Kemp asked in his treatise why the London parish of St Giles in the Fields was more infected than anywhere else in the city.[83] Nathaniel Hodges's treatise is perhaps the most detailed example of a first-hand account of plague in a specific, named English location. He described how plague broke out around the end of 1664 in Westminster, and thereafter moved step by step into London, where it gained strength and spread quickly throughout the entire city. "[M]eerly for Want of confining the Persons first seized with it," he lamented, "the whole City was in a little Time irrecoverably infected."[84]

Several mid-seventeenth century authors even included London in their treatises' titles: a French apothecary working in the city proposed a secret cure for plague in his work entitled *A Mite Cast into the Treasury of the Famous City of London*, while J.V. included the subtitle *A Looking-Glass for London, and the Suburbs Thereof.* The poet John Quarles seems to have taken the further step to make English plague outbreaks specific to London: he titled his 1665 work simply *Londons Disease*. By the end of that outbreak, Quarles was himself dead from plague.[85] Repeatedly reading about the high number of mortalities associated with outbreaks in the city, combined with religious, literary, and medical writers' portrayals of London as the national hotbed of sinful behaviour, reinforced the idea that plague was intimately bound with London's dense population. Everywhere was affected by plague, but London was especially plaguey.

As these examples suggest, localization in English tracts focused almost entirely on London.[86] Even though there were similarly recurrent and devastating outbreaks in many English towns, and even though knowledge of them reached London, these other places were almost never mentioned in the tracts (Brasbridge's recollections of past plagues in Banbury and Oxford being the primary exception). Large and devastating outbreaks in Shrewsbury, Worcester, and Lincoln in 1587, in Reading, Salisbury, and York in 1596–98, in Chester and Leicester in 1613–15, in Newcastle-upon-Tyne in 1636, in Newark and East Stoke in the 1640s – or in numerous other cities in many different years – instigated no printed treatises.[87] Instead, these places were either ignored in the printed works or grouped together into broad discussions of plague outbreaks in "divers Cities, Townes, and other places of this Realme."[88]

Plague's wanderings through the streets and alleys near their shops became profitable for printers and stationers, whose concentration in London helped to shape the treatises' focus on that city and who responded to London's outbreaks, actual or feared, by publishing a steady stream of pamphlets, ballads, sermons, treatises, and other literary and popular works. The vast majority of these works, in turn, addressed the particular relationship that London, its inhabitants, and its political and economic role in the kingdom seemed to have with the disease.[89]

In Oxford, Cambridge, and York, plague orders, sermons, and other religious and political texts addressed plague, but there were very few locally produced tracts. Only one mentioned the city directly: the royalist clergyman Lionel Gatford opened his Oxford-printed treatise by noting "I had not beene long here, but I saw … This unspeakable mercy of God to this *City*, or rather to this whole *Nation* … that formidable judgement of Plague."[90] The sole plague treatise printed in Cambridge reflected that author's experience in London, not in Cambridge.[91] Although printed in London, a tract written by S.M., a "physician in York," in 1721, was meant to be "Sold by Thomas Hammond, Bookseller in York." It too talked more about London's experience of disease than that of any other city, including his own: "I imagine the last Plague at London to have followed upon the City's being so many ways diverted from a Care of it."[92]

In some ways, perhaps, London became a metonym for everywhere else. Certainly, the religious authors of plague treatises advanced such view. Although books produced in London were sold to booksellers in the provincial towns and at markets and fairs, the printers' primary market was always London itself.[93] Thomas Brasbridge may have claimed that he wrote his tract for the inhabitants of London because he lived there and because the city was "greevously visited" by plague, but the reality is that by the late sixteenth century, the printers who could publish his book, the majority of the customers who could purchase and read it, and the worst local sources of disease generation (at least in people's minds) were all concentrated there.

As the imminent danger of plague faded after 1665, London-based printers and authors had little need or desire to continue producing medically oriented treatises that had no ready audience. Religious plague tracts continued to appear, but their numbers also declined considerably after 1665. Overall, England's treatises, and indeed most printed texts about the disease, failed to be geographically representative. This leaves us with a somewhat distorted image of what information might have circulated about plague throughout England more broadly.

The proliferation of larger cities and printing centres across France, by contrast, ensured that many more treatise writers from different places had the opportunity to write about their experiences and see their works published. Plague in Paris never served as metonym for other regional cities. All across the kingdom, plague treatises were written by local authors and printed for local readers. This, in turn, influenced both their discussions of where plague might be found and which cities appeared in them, especially after the turn of the sixteenth century. Instead of simply referring to a location in the preface or address to readers, or speaking to a disease that affected the French people more broadly, authors named the cities about which they wrote, in both in their titles and texts. Figure 4.2 shows some of the cities and regions specifically named by these producers.

Paris had long been the French kingdom's political, economic, religious, intellectual, and cultural capital. But although it was the largest city in the realm – if not the largest city in Europe at the time – it had neither grown as quickly as London, nor did it so completely dominate France's demographic landscape.[94] Several regional cities – such as Lyon, Marseille, and Toulouse – were themselves larger than most other cities in Europe and acted as important centres in their own right. It is primarily these non-Parisian centres of printing, as well as smaller towns such as Poitiers, Douai, Verdun, and Nantes, which are named as places affected by plague. More than half of the French tracts printed between 1644 and 1719 came from outside Paris and responded to outbreaks in other named cities.

The English example suggests that only London's outbreaks prompted the publication of treatises and, once it no longer suffered grievously from the disease, plague treatises in large numbers disappeared from the bookstalls, or at least from printers' shops. Something different was clearly happening in France. Here, printing presses were neither concentrated in one city nor dominated by a single licensing body. Instead, they were located throughout the entire kingdom and were able to respond to the concerns of readers in many different cities and regions. In this environment, authors had much more incentive – and indeed a much greater opportunity – to write and publish accounts of local outbreaks. Already by the early sixteenth century, treatises appeared about specific epidemics that their authors had personally witnessed, survived, or were anxiously awaiting throughout France. In 1520, Nicolas de Houssemaine, medical professor at the University of Angers, wrote a treatise to warn his readers that a plague outbreak was devastating the entire region of Anjou (Angers was the capital).[95] This contrasted with English producers, who at that date still typically copied Continental works

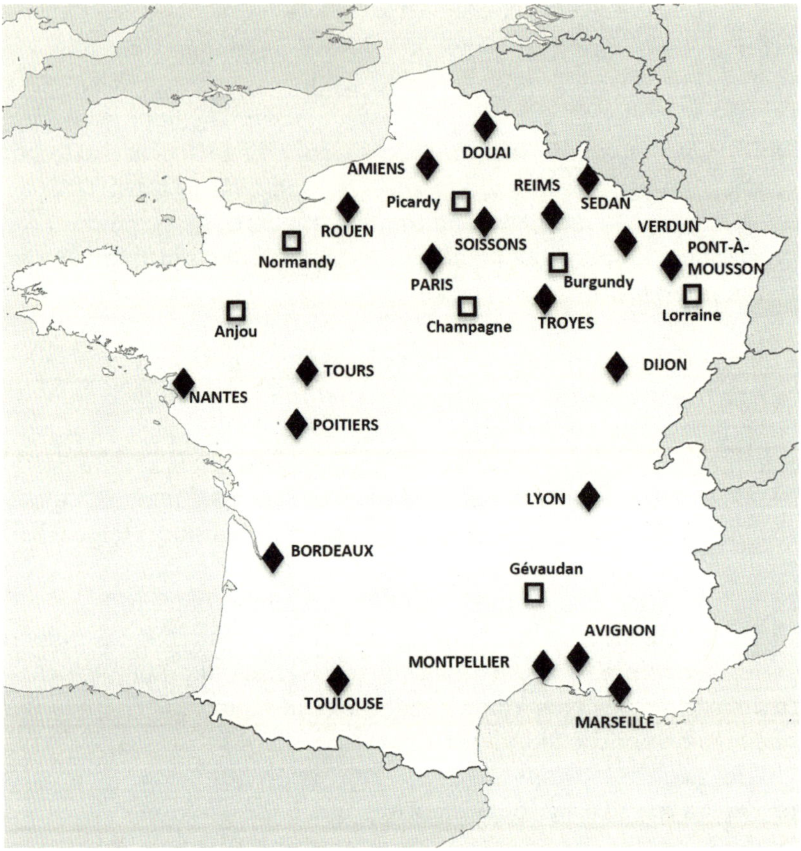

4.2 Cities and regions specifically named in French plague tracts.

and then added subtle local references to ensure that they appealed to an English audience. When he translated Houssemaine's treatise into English some twenty years later, for example, Thomas Phayer removed the opening lines about Anjou and replaced them with a more generic reference.[96]

Before the end of the sixteenth century, an increasing proportion of French tracts spoke of outbreaks in individual cities, directly addressed their readers in named cities, highlighted plague prevention and management practices that had been successfully used in particular places, or even traced plague as it moved from one town to another.[97] In his 1562 treatise, Paris physician Antoine Mizauld evaluated a variety of therapeutic methods used by practitioners across the kingdom, from

Gascony to Provence.[98] Writing to the citizens of Poitiers, surgeon Pierre André promoted his long experience with plague in numerous other cities and regions, all of which he named.[99] Claude de Rubys, an elected official in Lyon, wrote specifically about two epidemics in that city in 1564 and 1576–77.[100]

Geographic specificity continued in French plague tracts into the seventeenth and eighteenth centuries, as authors sought to address and explain the epidemics that they witnessed. Louis du Gardin, medical professor at the University of Douai, offered his advice and services to the people of that city, since people "do not always have the opportunity or the means to use [their own] physicians" during an outbreak.[101] Henry de Rochas d'Ayglun, royal councillor and physician to Louise Marguerite of Guise (Dowager Princess of Conti), wrote his first treatise about "the pestilential disease of this city of Paris"; decades later, he produced another for the city of Toulouse.[102] Royal physician Vincent Robin insisted that an outbreak in Paris had first arisen in the markets of Rouen and spread from there via commercial goods.[103] More importantly, in 1628 an infected person had carried plague from one town to the next, leading to the outbreak in Dijon about which he wrote his tract.[104] Numerous examples can be found for other outbreaks in the first three quarters of the seventeenth century. In most cases, the treatises' titles explicitly mentioned the city or region being discussed, and sometimes the year as well.

These, then, were plague treatises that discussed, reflected, and targeted outbreaks in specific places. Despite widespread concerns about the changing conditions of urban and religious life in Paris and other large cities, however, French tract writers did not typically portray cities *with* the disease as *diseased cities*, in the way that many English writers had come to describe London.[105] This is not to suggest that writers avoided portraying Paris (or any other city) as being disease-ridden: as we'll see shortly, some treatise authors openly argued that the epidemics about which they wrote had come from elsewhere, with Paris and Rouen being the most commonly mentioned origins because of their roles as commercial hubs. On the whole, however, few writers identified any one city as being a particularly diseased place or as the source of their own epidemic. Instead, plague became an ally to the other miseries that a city endured, especially war. French treatises simply did not do what English (often moralizing) treatises did.

As the large epidemic spread through Marseille and southern France in the early 1720s, a flurry of new plague treatises appeared in both England and France. These responded directly to this outbreak and the widespread fear that it engendered; most included the word "Marseille" in their titles, regardless of where they were printed. As Jean Bouillet, a physician in Béziers, noted "Everyone is terrified and trembling, so to speak, at the mere mention of plague: barely does this evil begin to develop somewhere in a town before the nearest neighbours become alarmed and believe themselves to be lost."[106] Although the Provençal outbreak did not spread to England, its sudden and visible reappearance after many years of absence meant that English writers felt compelled to explain once again what caused plague and how readers might protect themselves against it, this time targeting an audience that had no first-hand experience with the disease. In light of the spreading fear, one anonymous English author considered whether previous anti-plague practices would be beneficial or harmful to London if re-enacted in his day.[107]

Although their texts focused on Marseille, for most early eighteenth-century authors the disease's geographic locus lay elsewhere. This perceptual adjustment from local to non-local spaces of plague took place over the sixteenth and seventeenth centuries. It encompassed three discernable shifts in the "un-localizing" of plague. The first shift responded to a sixteenth-century socio-economic reconfiguration of plague-generating places. Such places were still "local" in the sense that they existed in the treatise writers' cities, but they were outside spaces that the authors considered to be their own (and their peers') lived experience. The second change, which I will not examine here in detail, resulted from the rising popularity of chemical and mechanical theories of medicine in the seventeenth century. These theories emphasized the idea that earthquakes and volcanoes released deeply buried plague-causing poisons. Since both the earth and the air were universal, so too must be the origin of plague.[108] The third change was part of a separate "othering" process that relocated plague's locus, both conceptually and geographically, to foreign sites. A key feature of all three shifts was early modern authors' desire, and often ability, to trace plague's movements from one place to another, just as their Black Death-era predecessors had attempted to do centuries earlier.

Plague Made Non-local

Certainly now we see that the eminent peril hounds us so closely, through its occult malignancy the contagion has breached several places in your city (Gentlemen of Tours) & gradually advances to harm more and more people of the city, such as those in the suburbs and neighbouring villages.

Nicolas de Nancel, Tours, 1581[109]

For the humanist physician and man of letters Nicolas de Nancel (from 1587 also physician to Éléonore de Bourbon, the Abbess of Fontevrault), an outbreak of plague in Paris in the early 1580s threatened all nearby towns and villages, including Tours, where he then lived. In a treatise printed in 1581, Nancel described how the disease spread daily, slowly engulfing first the towns and villages closest to Paris, then those further afield, gaining strength as it advanced initially towards and then right into Tours. It was only natural, he argued, that Paris's suffering would be shared by all those living around it; this was, he wrote, "what we expected, it has happened, we see it with our own eyes."[110]

Plague almost always moved towards the west, Nancel pointed out, because it was typically generated in corrupted air and spread by westerly winds. Even though Tours lay to the west of Paris, however, he insisted that this outbreak was different. Rather than spreading through the air, it had been carried to his doorstep by the feet of "poor fleeing Jacobites" who had travelled with the infection from Paris.[111] After walking nearly eighty leagues, he said, two of them had died on the same day; how their illness had remained undetected until then was a mystery. Once they arrived in Tours, these infected people "communicated fraternally with us": worse, some haberdashers and hawkers hoping to make money from the strangers went among them and carried plague out along with their earnings.[112]

Nancel was quite adamant that the disease had not arrived in Tours through the predictable winds; rather, it had come with "showmen and strangers."[113] It was therefore not a natural spread of disease, but a potentially malicious one sent forth from the diseased city of Paris and carried by the religious poor. Tours was, he said, one of the oldest, most famous, and most renowned cities in the French kingdom in terms of its beauty and its convenience of location. It had been one of the centres of the Carolingian renaissance, was the seat of an important archbishopric, and between 1450 and 1550 had become the *de facto* artistic and aristocratic capital of the kingdom.[114] Religious, military, and national mythology surrounding the city ran deep, with links to Charles Martel, the monastery of Saint Martin, and Joan of Arc. Prior to this latest outbreak of plague, however, the city had fallen into a twenty-year-long series of terrible disasters.[115]

Famine and disorder had ripped through the city in 1551–52. During the early years of the Wars of Religion, it had experienced extremely high levels of violence between its Catholic and Huguenot populations. Before the outbreak of 1581 that inspired Nancel's treatise, Tours had also suffered severe plague epidemics in 1546 and 1563. Its status as royal city and residence of the kingdom's financial elite was in decline, as was its economy.[116] Although war, famine, and plague were typically used as biblical analogies (these being three of the four horsemen of the apocalypse), and although Nancel's tract was full of biblical references to plague as a divine punishment, Tours really did face all three disasters over a (more or less) twenty-year period. The latest arrival of plague loaded a further layer of trouble onto the already beleaguered city. For Nancel, Tours by this point had become, paradoxically, both an urban place that demanded honour and reverence for its past greatness and a diseased space that cried out for pity and compassion because of its current plight.

Nancel claimed that the outbreak that he faced in 1581 had begun in – and therefore had come from – Paris, which he called "the head and heart of France."[117] Further on, he emphasized this observation by claiming that he had not heard or read anything from Paris's leading medical authorities to indicate that plague had originated anywhere else before breaking out in the city.[118] It was therefore a disease that not only arose within and belonged to the city of Paris, but one that its poor mendicants had carried forth from there to the rest of the kingdom.

This localization of plague among the poor evolved from longstanding theories that linked disease to certain geographical or topographical features (and hence to the people who lived in them). Drawing on ancient tradition, some of the early treatise writers noted the intrinsic danger posed by these unhealthy spaces and their putrid odours; Jacme d'Agramont, for example, mentioned the filthy streams associated with butcheries and tanneries in Paris, Avignon, and Lérida that contributed to local outbreaks.[119] Some decades later, Johannes Jacobi and Raymond Chalin de Vinario both pointed to the swamps and stagnant waters of Sardinia as sources of plague; Vinario also reiterated Agramont's assessment of Paris and Avignon's uncleanliness. Many authors commented on the southerly winds that invariably spread hot and humid – and therefore unhealthy – air from locations that were already diseased. Reminiscent of the Hippocratic treatise *Airs, Waters, Places*, the Paris Medical Faculty stated that "frequent gusts of wind in the wild southerly gales" had brought "*alien* ... bad, rotten, and poisonous vapours *from elsewhere*: from swamps, lakes and chasms, for instance."[120] The faculty's prophylactic advice to avoid harmful miasma included moving one's house away from putrefied air, such as that found near "marshy, muddy, and stinking places, stagnant waters and ditches," and increasing ventilation through windows open to the north – to avoid the pestilence-ridden southerly winds – "as long as these [northern exposures] did not pass through putrid and infected places."[121]

It was not until later in the fourteenth century, as plague became recast as a recurrent and local problem, that terrestrial arguments gained wider prominence.[122] Johannes Jacobi was one of the first French writers to argue that recurrent outbreaks were better explained by locally specific factors. Drawing from Galenic tradition, he warned that foul standing waters and fields of unburied corpses generated the disease, although he acknowledged that those habituated to living in such unhealthy places were less affected by the resultant diseases than those who were accustomed to healthier environments. While Jacobi echoed some of the claims made by Hippocrates and Galen centuries before – that pestilences particular to one town or region occurred in large part because of local topography – he combined these arguments with his own observations that recurrent plague outbreaks were not as universal as the mid-century epidemic had been. He thus reasoned that a local cause must be responsible. There was no suggestion, as there had been in the Paris Medical Faculty's treatise, that plague-causing corruption was generated elsewhere and then carried to new places on the wind; rather, the stinking ditches and foul streets that Jacobi blamed for plague were a familiar aspect of all late medieval locales.

Many later authors adopted Jacobi's explanatory framework and pointed to aspects of their own environments that might be causing plague. For some, venomous air arose from subterranean caves or crevices, let loose through earthquakes. For others, the culprits were familiar features of rural and urban landscapes. These sites had long been the target of amelioration projects, but recurrent plague outbreaks added urgency to such measures.[123]

While the topography-disease relationship remained largely intact well into the seventeenth and eighteenth centuries, by the sixteenth century English and French treatise writers had begun to reassign the idea of plagued spaces to locations that, while still local, existed outside their own immediate lived experiences. Accounts of the earliest outbreaks had made little socio-economic distinction between plague's victims, noting that it killed indiscriminately. However, prominent citizens who were able to flee during plague outbreaks increasingly noticed upon their return that the poorer districts had faced particularly heavy burdens of mortality. Before the end of the fifteenth century, legislators in northern Italian city-states enacted sanitary legislation that intrinsically linked plague with the poor, and in particular poor migrants and beggars whom they described as disease-carriers. Segregation, isolation, denial of movement/passage/entry, and similar plague-prevention measures were applied disproportionately to the poor, and especially to poor foreigners.[124] Comparable measures appeared in England and France shortly afterwards, as ideas about localized sources of contamination narrowed to areas that the poor inhabited or that they could infect.[125]

In England, poverty levels were quite high before the Black Death, but the sheer amount of poverty, coupled with the significant increase in population, became an especially noticeable and growing political, economic, and social concern to the property-owning and governing classes during the sixteenth and seventeenth centuries. Here, where the shift to Protestantism was more widespread and ultimately mandated by the Crown, the closing of the monasteries also had an immediate and visible effect on poverty rates: not only did lay monastery staff join the ranks of the unemployed, but the alms that larger monasteries had long provided to the poor were also significantly curtailed.[126] The number of beggars on the streets rose as did the level of their hardship, especially in London where people flocked from across the kingdom in search of work. The ongoing enclosure of common lands for pasturage and the termination of long held tenancies likewise pushed more and more people into poverty, forcing them to migrate to the cities, where they joined a growing underclass. The exorbitant cost of war, and the ensuing coinage debasement and extremely high inflation, added to economic misery. By the middle of the sixteenth century, popular revolts against the enclosures and other deprivations – such as Kett's Rebellion in 1549 – simultaneously rendered poverty even more visible and hardened attitudes towards the poor. Poor relief existed in Catholic and Protestant regions alike, but negative perceptions of the poor are more visible in the English plague tracts than in the French ones.[127] Despite the existence of a variety of categories of poor, many authorities (including physicians) perceived the poor as a largely undifferentiated yet distinct threat to public order, morality, and public health.[128] A plague outbreak in Windsor Castle in 1517 was blamed, in part, on beggars.[129]

Deserving of charity or otherwise, in most early modern English cities and towns the overcrowded and filthy living conditions occupied by the poor became closely correlated with plague outbreaks. It was easy to link plague to the poor in medical terms: plague was generated by corrupt or putrefied air and corrupted the bodies of its victims in turn; the poor were believed to be predisposed or susceptible to this putrefaction – or indeed capable of even producing and magnifying it – because they were already corrupted on account of their inferior living and moral conditions.[130]

England's national and municipal plague orders included direct references to the poor and to the spaces they inhabited. To prevent the spread of the disease, the orders specifically banned wandering by vagabonds or beggars, as well as providing lodging to strangers. Central to the orders were clauses related to the rates (i.e., taxes) required to support families forcibly isolated through quarantine and the poor more generally. So too were calls to enforce "the suppressing, punishing, and setling of the sturdy Rogues and Vagabonds."[131]

Also included in England's national plague orders was the College of Physicians' prophylactic and treatment advice that, by 1630, went beyond prescribing plague remedies to include overt descriptions of the overcrowded conditions in which the poor lived. Such conditions, the college proclaimed, endangered public health and had to be rectified. In 1631, Sir Theodore de Mayerne, King Charles I's Huguenot physician, issued a report in which he argued that to protect "the publique health" it was necessary to forcibly expel "the unruly base sort of people" from English towns.[132] He portrayed London as particularly problematic in this regard because of its dirty streets and its large number of beggars. Although these beggars were often local residents, the assumption was that they did not belong and so should be made to leave.

As early as the opening decades of the 1500s, municipal officials had begun to provide information about the number of plague-related deaths and burials to England's royal government. Toward the end of the century, this information was systematized and used in "a publicly available [i.e., privately] printed form," notably the broadsheets known as *Red-Crosses* or *Lord Have Mercy Upon Us.* As I discussed in chapter 3, these weekly broadsheets, which were available for a small cost, reproduced mortality figures by parish during London's major plague outbreaks between 1592 and 1665. Since the poorest parishes were often hit first, and worst, during epidemics, the broadsheets further emphasized the perceived link between plague and poor neighbourhoods.

Before 1563, plague mortality was relatively equal across London's parishes, reflecting the broad intermixture of wealthier and poorer neighbourhoods. By 1665, however, the city's wealthier (and healthier) households were concentrated in the central parishes. This transition, in turn, both shifted the location of the poorest residents from their previous intramural parishes to ones located along or outside the walls, and changed the site of which parishes were first (and/or ultimately worst) affected during outbreaks.[133] Importantly, the first and worst hit parishes were not just poor: none were portside – belying the seventeenth- and eighteenth-century determination (carried over into modern scholarship) that plague was an imported disease. Instead, these parishes had other features that perhaps made them more plague-prone: St Bartholomew's, for example, hosted a hospital where plague victims might have been sent.

Neighbourhoods already associated with poverty, social unrest, and criminality faced still greater stigmatization when they were also characterized as diseased spaces.[134] Together, the broadsheets and the official bills of mortality "inscribed a mental map of the metropolis" by illustrating, in statistical terms, the amount of disease in each parish.[135] In other words, they affected the way that people perceived the relationship between London's layout and the spread of disease through data that established in quasi-official and visual form a direct link between London's poorer parishes and plague. Similar plague mortality tallies appeared in King's Lynn, Norwich, Yarmouth, Bristol, Chester, York, and elsewhere.[136] Even in towns where such printed sheets did not circulate, mortality spikes and rising numbers of burials in particular parishes or wards, as in Allhallow's parish in Newcastle, enabled residents to identify local "epicentre(s) of infection."[137]

For readers in London and elsewhere, these statistical maps tied local geographies to plague's perceived origins. Since the bills of mortality and broadsheets listed plague deaths by parish, and since each parish was contained within a particular and well-defined (and well-known) geographic space, the broadsheets pointed to which areas of the city and its suburbs were most infected and, by extension, most disease-generating. Londoners actively used these bills to determine which parishes to avoid. For their part, merchants and shop owners petitioned to have the death figures further delineated, since being associated with or working near to infected parishes was bad for business.[138] With well-known physicians also claiming in their treatises that poor parishes were diseased, it was difficult to avoid the assumption that poorer, marginalized areas of the city were plague-ridden.

Early tract writers, like John of Burgundy in the fourteenth century, had emphasized humoral predisposition to corruption and plague, but had not pointed a finger at any particular group of people.[139] Yet by the sixteenth and seventeenth centuries, both the largely statistical and image-heavy broadsheets and the narrative plague tracts correlated disease and the poor, warning their readers to avoid both the poor and the places they occupied.[140] These two very different types of document thus worked together to formalize in the city's collective consciousness the idea that London's poor spaces were its local source of plague.

Cambridge-trained physician Francis Herring recognized that the poorer sorts of people were more grievously afflicted during plague outbreaks than their richer neighbours, for the simple reason that they could neither flee nor afford the suggested medicines. Believing that God had "by his wise providence" determined that the poor were "fit objects whereupon [the rich could] exercise their mercy and compassion," Herring's tract included a section comprised entirely of suitable treatments and cures for "the true and honest poore miserable people."[141] The less honest poor, though, he portrayed as indolent drifters who generated and spread plague. These people, he counselled, should be restrained from moving about: "I would intreate the Governours of the Citie of London, and all others in the Country … to restraine the idle Vagabonds, by whose wandring up and downe, the infection may well be spread and increased."[142] For Herring and his contemporaries, the poor were both objects of charity and treacherous sources of infection, "at once most dangerous and in most danger," depending on the degree of their honesty and the nature of their poverty.[143]

English tract authors also made explicit associations between the places the poor occupied and outbreaks of disease. They blamed epidemics directly on the living conditions of the poor. Especially troublesome were their crowded, filthy, and stinking neighbourhoods and their apparent moral shortcomings. In the 1530s, the writer Thomas Elyot had claimed that there were four main causes of the corrupted air that generated plague, one of which was "[m]oche people in a small rome lyvynge unclenly and sluttyshely."[144] By the end of the century, clergyman and medical writer Thomas Brasbridge combined geography and poverty to blame the disease on corrupted air that arose "in a fewe houses, or streetes, through the stenche of chanels, of filthie doung, of carion, of standing pudles and stincking waters, of seeges, or stincking privies … of common pissing places, and such like … [and in] a gret company dwelling or lyving in a small room especially if those roomes be not verie clenlie kept."[145]

Other late sixteenth- and early seventeenth-century writers, like the physicians Thomas Lodge, William Bullein, and Stephen Bradwell, warned against the dangers that arose from poor people and from vagabonds who came from (suspected) infected parishes. Lodge, for example, argued for prohibiting entry to anyone from an infected town, "except they be men of note … [or] men of respect," since men of status could clearly be trusted to not carry the disease around with them.[146] Bullein linked plague to "slotishe beastlie people, that kepe their houses and lodginges unclene, their meate, drincke, and clothyng, moste noisome, their labour and travell immoderate."[147] Bradwell contended that the poor were more subject to plague because of their "living sluttishly, and feeding nastily on offals, or the worst & unholsomest meates … their bodies much corrupted [and] most subject to this Sicknesse."[148] Indeed, he continued, "we see the *Plague* sweeps up such people in greatest heapes." Bradwell complained not just of the culinary choices and homes of the poor, but also their clothing, furniture, habits, and uncleanliness, all of which he contended made them carriers, if not generators, of plague. These writers also (more charitably) offered specific directions for the poor to preserve themselves from plague, but at the same time perceived that the very spaces that the poor occupied were both actually and metaphoricallydiseased.

John Graunt's mid-seventeenth-century *Reflections on the Weekly Bills of Mortality* added to this narrative construction. By revealing and analyzing plague's weekly progress for all of London's outbreaks since 1592, Graunt highlighted those parishes in which plague arose first and which were, by implication, the geographical sources of local epidemics. Like the broadsheets, Graunt's *Reflections* implicated the poorer parishes. Both the poor and the places in which they lived were labeled as stinking, dirty, putrid, and, notably, pestilential. Indeed, by the mid-seventeenth century, plague had become so associated with the poor that Nathaniel Hodges could write in his plague tract that "it is incredible to think how the Plague [of 1665] raged amongst the common People, insomuch that it came by some to be called the *Poors Plague*."[149] William Kemp pointed to the "stinking lanes" of St Sepulchre and the graveyards of St Giles in the Fields as being London's most particularly problematic areas; manufacturing neighbourhoods in all towns that housed both industrial waste and poor labourers were seen in much the same way.[150] English treatise writers continued to point to the poor and the areas in which they lived as the source of local disease outbreaks into the eighteenth century. In 1720, Richard Mead uncontroversially described plague as a disease of the poor "among whom this Evil generally begins."[151] He furthermore called for the sanitary and medical inspection, evacuation, and cleansing of poorer neighbourhoods whenever an epidemic seemed possible. Other physician writers like George Pye, Richard Blackmore, and John Pringle followed suit. The readers of these tracts were unlikely to have missed the descriptions of disease-ridden neighbourhoods and bodies that, even when not linked to a specifically named community, could be identified as the poorer parishes and wards in the city.[152]

French Royal Acts and Orders on plague, in contrast to those produced in England, had little to say explicitly about the poor and their injunctions to limit the movement of goods and people during outbreaks and to enact sanitary measures ostensibly applied to everyone. However, municipal councils passed ordinances designed to combat the disease locally that included, among other measures, temporary bans on begging and the exclusion of poor strangers. In many southern French cities, the poor – and the itinerant poor in particular – became especially associated with filth and illness; as such, they were both targeted for coercive isolation measures and blamed for the spread of disease. Because some socio-economic groups were considered to be more susceptible to the disease, and as poverty became increasingly associated with moral defects, efforts to separate the sick from the healthy focused most heavily on the poor.[153]

As contagion theory gained ground in northern French cities, concentrated efforts there to eliminate or mitigate the natural sources of contaminated air were supplemented by actions designed to separate the sick from the healthy, and by extension the poor from the rest of society. In 1510, the Rouen city council blamed a travelling vagrant for carrying plague from Neufchâtel; in 1534, the Parisian city council blamed the sick poor at the Hôtel-Dieu for infecting those whose job it was to care for them; and in Amiens, foreign (i.e., non-local) vagrants were accused of bringing plague into that city in 1545.[154] In this atmosphere, ordinances against plague quickly became ordinances against the poor. The assumption that poverty and plague were linked led to the implementation of increasingly repressive measures against the itinerant and non-native poor. Just as in England, wealthier itinerant merchants and traders largely escaped censure: they earned a living and were not seen to pose a threat to the well-being of local communities even though they too might have travelled to, and through, infected towns and neighbourhoods.[155]

The perception that the poor died first and more often during plague outbreaks appeared in some of the earliest plague tracts. Few, however, pointed to the poor as the *source* of disease. In the late fourteenth century, Raymond Chalin de Vinario had claimed that the common folk died more regularly from plague in Avignon due to their unclean habits, but did not suggest that the disease originated among them. Even into the mid-sixteenth century, French authors' remarks largely focused either on the types of remedies that the poor used – and specifically the types of popular errors in which they foolishly believed – or on their predisposition to plague due to their habit of eating, as Oger Ferrier remarked: "nasty meats ... rotten grain, and other abominations."[156] A few others made similar comments in their tracts, but did little to suggest directly that the poor or their places of habitation were likely to generate plague. In fact, only a very small number of sixteenth- and seventeenth-century treatise writers, most notably François de Courcelles, Laurent Joubert, Guillaume Potel, and Durand de Montlauseur, actually associated plague with "the putrid exhalations that customarily arise from places that are crowded by the poor," those "common people" who "live in dirty places and who live dirty lives."[157] Both Courcelles and Joubert were Protestant, and their views on the poor reflected sixteenth-century Protestant views that unemployment, poverty, and disease were signs of moral failure.[158] By the Plague of Provence in 1720, more French tract writers pointed to the local slums, especially those near the port, as the place where the outbreak started. The public prosecutor Pichatty de Croissainte, for example, provided a detailed itinerary of the epidemic's movement, beginning in "the Street of *Lescalle*, a Part of the old Town inhabited only by poor People."[159] Few French writers, though, emphasized the role played by the poor in generating the disease, as their English counterparts were doing.

While French Catholic writers did not directly associate the poor with the disease, they did charge Protestants with being plague carriers and spreaders, an accusation that, unlike in England, oftentimes resulted in violence.[160] Religious dissent and heresy persecutions (and prosecutions) rocked the French kingdom during the first half of the sixteenth century, despite (or perhaps due to) the rapid diffusion and acceptance of Calvinism among France's nobility, especially in the south and west. Inflamed by political, aristocratic, and dynastic factionalism, this dissension erupted into a series of massacres of French Protestants by Catholic sympathizers and vice versa, Protestant-led rebellions and attempts to seize power at the local level, and kingdom-wide civic disturbances. Locally, deep religious tension manifested itself in vandalism, riots, and other acts of violence; at the national level, it led to outright warfare fought largely along factionalist lines. These recurrent military battles, interspersed with unsuccessful treaties and edicts, lasted for eight decades.[161] Throughout the period, religion and religious belief "continuously shape[d] a sense of community, of urban solidarity" that was fractured and "in active conflict" with itself at both the local and national levels.[162] Outbreaks of plague further undermined the social, political, and religious fabric of the French kingdom, especially when each faction blamed and attacked the other for intentionally spreading the disease.

Charging "others" with being plague carriers was not new, of course. The Black Death had unleashed mass violence in some places, always against a group deemed to be outsiders who were blamed for generating or disseminating plague. Records survive, for example, of the murder of Catalans in Sicily and of clerics and beggars in Narbonne (France) and elsewhere. Most appalling is evidence of pogroms against Jews. Prominent Jewish leaders were accused of acting as part of a continent-wide Jewish conspiracy to destroy Christendom, using plague as their weapon. Accusations and pogroms commenced first in Switzerland before spreading to France, the Holy Roman Empire, and Italy. Jews were accused of poisoning local wells and using other dark forces to infect people with plague. More than seventy percent of towns hosting a Jewish community in these regions engaged in some sort of retaliatory action, and each followed a typical pattern: the accused were apprehended by local authorities and confessions were extracted by means of torture; the confessions were then used to implicate the wider Jewish community and to give local mobs a justification for violence on a massive scale. Hundreds of Jewish communities in the Rhineland, Spain, France, and Eastern Europe were eradicated, with people locked inside synagogues or rounded up on river islands and burnt to death – men, women, and children. These pogroms devastated the Jewish population and, coupled with the mortality from the plague, to which they obviously were not immune, meant that by the end of the first wave of the plague, as much as half of Europe's Jewish population had been killed.[163]

During later outbreaks, a wide variety of other insiders and outsiders, from high-ranking officers and doctors to the lowest levels of health workers – nurses, plague cleaners, cartmen, and gravediggers – were accused of perpetuating plague for a variety of reasons, including financial gain. Outbreaks were also blamed on people engaged in the secondhand clothing trade, especially those who had violated quarantines by transporting their supposedly infected goods from one town to the next. A renewed rise of plague-spreading (also known as "greasing") conspiracies in the Duchy of Savoy around 1530 typically targeted poor female migrants who worked in plague hospitals.[164] In sixteenth-century France, however, they arose not in the context of anti-Semitism or economic stigmatization, but of anti-Protestantism. Ideological battles between Catholics and Protestants during the Wars of Religion led tract writers to lay the blame for disease outbreaks directly on their religious opponents.[165]

Claude de Rubys, the Lyonnais civic magistrate and a leading member of the Catholic League, provided the longest and most detailed discussion of the opinion that Protestants were directly responsible for spreading plague. In Rubys's opinion, Protestants had also exaggerated the disease's deadly impact in an attempt to destroy the commercial appeal of Catholic cities. Lyon was France's second largest Catholic stronghold, but contained a large number of Huguenots. Some had been burned at the stake as heretics in the 1550s. The Huguenots reacted to their persecution with public processions, civil disobedience, iconoclasm, and in 1562, a successful coup against the city's government (Catholic forces retook control of the city the following year). During a plague outbreak in 1564, local Catholic officials openly accused the Huguenots of having intentionally infected the city's Catholic population.

In his treatise, Rubys described how town officials responded to such threats in 1576–77 by establishing hospitals, enacting quarantines, ensuring that all potentially infected homes were thoroughly cleaned, and holding penitential processions. To protect the wider community against importation of outside infection, they also erected scaffolds at all of the town's crossroads from which they planned to hang and nail Calvinists suspected of spreading plague. By the end of the outbreak, only three hundred Catholics and "good" Frenchmen, women, and children had died, but more than half of the local Protestant "heretics deceived by Calvin's predestination … [had] perished in heaps," their malevolent plague-spreading conspiracies apparently having failed because they had contracted the disease more often than their targets.[166] For Rubys, Protestant bodies were both infected and acted as infective agents: he traced the first sign of plague in 1576 to prostitutes at a local army barracks who had themselves been intentionally infected ("seeded", he said), by Calvinists. He then described how the local official, "no less a wise than faithful and affectionate servant of the King and Crown of France," was obliged to abandon the barracks in order to keep the rest of the city safe.[167] The outbreak thus provided an opportunity for him to engage in virulent anti-Protestantism – and to support violent action against his religious enemies – for the express purpose of re-establishing the city as a Lyonnais Catholic space.[168]

While Rubys's work appears to be unique in directly linking the successful management of plague with the destruction of a religious "other," several treatise writers also commented, at least in passing, on either the "greasing" conspiracies in Lyon or on the religious wars and the threat that they posed to French society.[169] Referring to Thucydides's claim that the Plague of Athens had been spread purposely by the Ethiopians, Oger Ferrier engaged in some of the earliest dialogue in French tracts about religious wickedness and infidelities as causes of plague. Writing in 1548, Ferrier accepted that evil and cruel men often spread plague to harm others.[170] Although his treatise predated the outbreak of open religious hostilities, Ferrier's work is nevertheless notable because of its mention of plague-spreading conspiracies that are otherwise absent from French treatises before this point.

Rubys's case against the Protestants and their threats to Lyon was resurrected in 1629 by the Jesuit Jean Grillot, who claimed that plague-infected grease had been spread on the homes and clothing of wealthy Lyonnais by Calvinists during an outbreak in the city the previous year. Grillot drew from ecclesiastical history to argue that just like all great heresies of the past, "the Heresy of Calvin" was responsible for generating great wars, plagues, and famines. It both began, and would end, with high levels of mortality, he said, because rebellions against the body of the Church "are always followed by rigorous chastisement."[171] In Lyon, such chastisement was meted out, in part, by local officials who sequestered the leaders of the Huguenot population and hanged sixteen of them for allegedly greasing Catholics with plague. Although he admitted that some innocent people might have been massacred in the heat of the moment, for Grillot this was just punishment for heretics who apparently had been caught red-handed trying to take control of the city.[172]

There were, then, two main differences between the English and French authors' efforts to link plague to local outsiders. The first was their discussion of how, and among whom, the disease erupted and moved. The second was the potential, and in some cases actual, violence that surrounded such discussions. For some French Catholic treatise writers, Protestants were inherently wicked and pest-ridden; they deliberately spread plague and needed to be punished. For the English authors, the habits of the poor caused them to be more susceptible to the disease; they needed to be cleaned up or moved out of the city.

But if plague began among the poor or in a particular parish or town, English writers also needed to explain how it got there. In the seventeenth century, some reframed plague as a disease whose actual origin lay elsewhere. Nathaniel Hodges noted that because "plague affects many regions together at the same time," it was necessary to distinguish it from "Endemick diseases, that is, such that are appropriate to one place only."[173] Indeed, recognizing that plague was widespread, Hodge's primary concern was to understand how it operated in climates that were so distant from each other. Since from "Reason [it] is very obvious [that] there is so much Difference between the Diseases of different Climates," Hodges pondered, "how much Alteration [must plague] undergo in such a Travel, from a hot and dry Climate, into a moist and cold one."[174] Such alteration did not and could not, he argued, make the plague endemic in England, not even among its poor. Although Hodges believed that plague could reignite in the same place "from the original Cause that as yet hath never been extinguished" – a reflection reminiscent of John of Burgundy's earlier claim that the Black Death had left behind relics of itself – he argued that it was erroneous to assume that plague was "co-æval with the World" since its continued reappearance necessarily relied on "external Circumstances."[175] Plague was not, in other words, a local or endemic disease in England: it came from elsewhere and then first affected the most susceptible and undesirable parts of a town before engulfing neighbouring districts. It did not take long for this idea to become entrenched.

PLAGUE REUNIVERSALIZED

Plague Made Non-national

> The causes of malignant fevers and common diseases originate in the country in which they produce their effects, and in no way pass into other countries, neither close-by nor distant ones. The cause of the Plague [by contrast] is foreign.
>
> Jean-Baptiste Goiffon, Lyon, 1722[176]

Writing in 1722 as the outbreak in Marseille came to an end, former military physician Jean-Baptiste Goiffon sought to distinguish between plague, which he considered to be both epidemic and contagious, and other malignant fevers and common maladies, which could be epidemic but were never contagious. Plague, he argued, had only a "moderate and small origin," while the non-contagious epidemic diseases came from "abundant, extensive, and general" sources.[177] In other words, plague began in one specific place and then spread through contagion. Other epidemic diseases, by contrast, could erupt simultaneously at many places in the same country without multiplying or reproducing. "These types of diseases," he said, referring to the latter, "always have a vast source and rely [for their eruption] on a vast quantity of spoiled and corrupted matter … and not on being transferred" from one person or object to another.[178]

More importantly, Goiffon asserted that outbreaks of non-contagious epidemic diseases in a new country or location should not be attributed to any kind of reproduction or multiplication; rather, the source of the disease must have been there all along. Outbreaks of plague, by contrast, could be tracked because they originated in one location and then were transferred from that place to another. "There can be no doubt," he stated, "that the origin [of plague] is very limited."[179] Unlike many of the earlier treatise writers who had identified a plethora of local spaces capable of generating the disease, however, Goiffon insisted that plague's primary locus was foreign.

Municipal and regional authorities tasked with protecting their towns had long recognized the potential spread of disease from one location to another. Ordinances that established *cordons sanitaires* and that excluded or quarantined travellers and goods from known or suspected infected regions were in place in some Continental cities by the early fifteenth century.[180] English plague orders were not enacted kingdom-wide until the later sixteenth century, but local surveillance and quarantine measures appeared much earlier.[181] Advice from London's College of Physicians accompanying the national orders called for restrictions on "men or goods from foreign infected places."[182] Writers like Samuel Collins emphasized the propensity of infected, pestilential air to travel not just from house to house, but also from country to country. By the later seventeenth century, information about both local and foreign disease outbreaks moved not just by word of mouth or letter, but also in increasingly popular printed newsheets.[183]

Writing about London's epidemic of 1665, some English treatise authors reflected on its connection to outbreaks elsewhere. Less than ten years earlier, an especially devastating outbreak had decimated the city of Naples; now, in the midst of London's epidemic, an English translation of a short Italian treatise about the Neapolitan crisis appeared.[184] This translation stands as a turning point, whereby a direct link was made between England's outbreaks and epidemics elsewhere in the world; until then, English plague-tract producers had focused almost exclusively on outbreaks that arose, lived, and waned locally (except, of course, for their discussion of historical outbreaks). This also marked the first time that a treatise appeared in English print that solely addressed an outbreak somewhere else. Unlike previous translated tracts, the Italian work was not Englished by having foreign identifiers removed and local ones inserted. Rather, the purpose of translating this treatise was to inform English readers about a plague outbreak that *was* foreign. This cast the English experience as part of a larger, geographically broad phenomenon.

The change in the places that treatise writers blamed for spawning local outbreaks went further. Antoine Davin, a French physician and royal councillor, noted in 1629 that plague began in large and dense cities "such as Grand Cairo, Constantinople, Paris, Toulouse, and Lyons ... where the nature of the place has something to do" with generating the disease.[185] In 1721, a York physician went so far as to calculate mathematically "How this Infection exerts itself mostly upon great Cities and populous Towns."[186] Those who lived in such places were, he estimated, already tainted on account of breathing the same air over and over again. "'Twould be too long to make the Calculation here," he contended, "but observe, that a Man sitting in a Room, into, and from which, no Air can come or go; I say, a Man sitting in such a Room, containing a hundred Gallons of Air, and supposing him to breathe four times in a Minute, and allowing him to take in each time four Ounces of Air, he would breathe over all that Air in thirteen Hours two Minutes." The unwholesomeness of recycled urban air he left to his readers to ascertain; the implication, though, was that living in crowded cities exposed people more often and more regularly to plague than living in rural locations.

If, for their predecessors, disease-generating environmental features were to be found locally, for Davin and the York Physician they were particular to the world's cities. For others, geographic explanations of plague shifted almost entirely to foreign places. While Hodges contested whether plague could be endemic to England, George Thomson pointed a suspicious finger, in 1666, to plague being the product of foreign places whose airs "are observed to produce the Pest Periodically (as in *Gran Cairo* in *Aegypt*)."[187] Very quickly thereafter, while still acknowledging that plague could arise from unhealthy local places – especially urban spaces dominated by the poor – seventeenth-century writers' associations between local outbreaks and epidemics in other places meant locating the local outbreak's origin elsewhere. By the eighteenth century, such thinking was commonplace, and most writers accepted French abbé Martin Gaudereau's claim that "during the eighteen years that I served [as French consul] in Turkey, Armenia, Persia, Arabia, and India, I found myself in an infinite number of towns afflicted by plague."[188]

Although the Marseille outbreak of 1720 did not spread to England, "the dismal prospect of a destroying Disease in a Foreign Neighbouring Country" after many years of absence raised considerable alarm.[189] For many English writers, reflecting upon the "Sickness now in France" meant that they were responding to an outbreak that that had once again become universal.[190] As English naturalist and botanist Richard Bradley observed, "all the Trading Ports of Europe are now in [danger] of being infected by the Plague which rages in the South parts of France and every day spreads itself more and more over the neighbouring Countries."[191] English tract writers were now deliberately constructing plague as a transnational threat.

For Richard Mead, fellow of the Royal College of Physicians and of the Royal Society, suggestions found in earlier tracts that plague was or had become endemic were incorrect, it being "a satisfaction to know that the Plague is not a native of our country."[192] Philip Rose assigned two types of causes to plague: "Domestick and Foreign" – the foreign causes being responsible for disease outbreaks that spread from one country to another.[193] Since everyone believed that plague had arrived in Marseille from somewhere else, and did not simultaneously break out in England, it was clearly and obviously foreign.

French writers also spoke of "the plague that causes alarm throughout all of Europe."[194] Both they and local administrators were quick to claim that plague had arrived in Marseille through maritime commerce. Jean-Baptiste Bertrand argued that the outbreak could not have possibly originated in Marseille itself, because neither the city nor its surrounding countryside had the kind of environment to generate corrupted air; simply put, "Marseille is exempt from all these infections."[195] By the early eighteenth century, both English and French writers almost uniformly portrayed plague as a disease that was natural to some other part of the world and then made universal through various means, including commerce, the winds, or the movement of sick travellers. How tract writers perceived the geography of disease likely also reflected visible patterns in the circulation or recurrence of plague itself, given the waning of outbreaks in both England and France, yet there was more at play here than simple epidemiology.

This shift to the foreign is examined in more detail in chapter 5. First, though, it is important to step back to the Black Death to determine how the places and movements of plague were traced across the centuries. Early modern writers were not the only ones who tracked the movement of plague from one place another.

Lands of Darkness

> We have not said that the future pestilence will be exceptionally dangerous, for we do not wish to give the impression that it will be as dangerous here as [it has been] in southern and eastern regions.
>
> Paris Medical Faculty, Paris, 1348[196]

The Paris Medical Faculty's allusion in 1348 to southern and eastern regions being more heavily impacted by plague echoed other contemporary writers' descriptions of the disease's geographic trajectory.[197] Gabriele de' Mussis traced plague's steps from east to west, from the lands of the "Tartars" and "Saracens" to Caffa (modern Feodosia, in Crimea) and thence on Genoese ships to various Mediterranean port cities.[198] When speaking of plague's purported roots, many writers relied heavily on first- and second- (or even third- or fourth-) hand reports of merchants, pilgrims, courtiers, and other travellers who, in passing through already infected areas, could provide some sense of plague's path. The general perception, as Boccaccio wrote, was that plague "had originated some years earlier in the East, where it had claimed countless lives before it unhappily spread westward, growing in strength as it swept relentlessly from one place to the next."[199]

European writers were generally vague about the actual location of plague's eastern origins. In his *Historia de Morbo*, Mussis claimed that plague had begun in "countries of the east" before infecting "almost everyone who had been in the East, or in the regions to the south and north [of Caffa, including] Chinese, Indians, Persians, Medes, Kurds, Armenians, Cilicians, Georgians, Mesopotamians, Nubians, Ethiopians, Turks, Egyptians, Arabs, Saracens and Greeks (for almost all the East has been affected)."[200] For Mussis, the epidemic was synonymous with the easterly-dwelling "heathen Tartar races," whose "broad regions, far-spreading provinces, magnificent kingdoms, cities, towns and settlements [were] ground down by illness" before they laid siege to Caffa. Eventually he said, the Tartars threw their disease-ridden corpses into the city. Although Mussis claimed to find it "extraordinarily difficult" to give an accurate picture of the devastation caused by plague in the regions immediately surrounding him, he confidently reported on "trustworthy accounts" of death tolls among the Saracens and those living in "other countries of the East, which are so vast that it takes three years to ride across them." Giovanni Villani, a Florentine banker and local official, likewise commented that "there were uncountable deaths in Turkey [that is, Anatolia] and other countries overseas ... These pestilences occurred as far away as Turkey and Greece, having come from the area of the rising sun."[201]

Greek and Islamicate writers living in the eastern Mediterranean concurred that plague came from the east. Some placed its origins in an area not far from Crimea. Byzantine historian and scholar Nicephorus Gregoras, writing in the late 1350s, claimed that the disease had begun in "Scythia and Maeotis and the mouth of the Tanais [Don River, in central Russia]."[202] Byzantine Emperor John VI Kantakouzenos (r. 1347–54), wrote that the epidemic had started "first [among] the Hyperborean Scythians." Abū Hafs ᶜUmar Ibn al-Wardī, who witnessed the plague outbreak in Aleppo in 1348, provided a more comprehensive itinerary. He was, however, as vague as his European counterparts in defining the disease's eastern roots. Basing his report on what he had learned from Muslim merchants returning from Crimea, al-Wardī claimed that the disease had begun some fifteen years earlier in a distant "land of darkness" before moving through India, Uzbek lands, Crimea, Byzantium, and across the eastern Mediterranean.[203]

Modern scientific and historical studies place the biological origins of the Black Death at the eastern edge of Central Asia and offer convincing possibilities for a Mongolian role in its spread.[204] However, the contemporary accounts noted above also raise important cautions about how mid-fourteenth-century discussions of plague's emergence and progression were linked to the actions and/or lands of specific peoples. Such reports were presented as fact, yet the further removed from the original source of information they were, the more embellished they became. To a large extent, the perceived trajectory of plague mirrored the spread of information, news, and rumour, and not necessarily the path taken by the disease itself.

Mussis's claim that infected Genoese sailors carried plague from Crimea and into Italy as a result of the Tartars catapulting plague-infected corpses over the walls of a besieged Caffa is no longer accepted as truthful. Instead, it is a "great refugee odyssey ... best understood as the path of rumours rather than [of] pestilence itself."[205] The clearest debunking of Mussis's narrative demonstrates both that no plague-infected corpses flew over Caffa's walls at all, and that grain exports, not diseased sailors, played the most significant role in transmitting the disease into the Mediterranean: "overreliance on Mussi's treatise has misled scholars about the geography, chronology, and human intentions behind early plague transmission. [Mussis's] *Historia de morbo* directed attention to Caffa, the Crimean Peninsula, connections with Genoa, fast transmission, and intentional bioterrorism rather than Tana, the Sea of Azov, connections with Venice, delayed transmission, and the unintended consequences of long-distance grain shipment."[206] European writers reflecting on the Black Death also relied on narratives like Mussis's because such accounts suited their political purposes, yet records left by those in Caffa made no connection between the city, the siege, and the outbreak of plague.

The terminology that Black Death-era writers relied on to describe plague's origins point more to contemporary worldviews and geopolitical biases than to verifiable, observed fact. It was also steeped in legend. Just as the Ancient Greeks disputed the location of the mythical land of Hyperborea – placing it anywhere from the Arctic to Celtic lands to northeast Asia – and as hints of barbarism underlaid the Byzantine term "Scythian,"[207] Europeans' historical use of the vague labels such as "Tartars" and "Saracens" oversimplify a complex reality. The broader context – geographic, commercial, political, and religious – in which these terms were used involved different branches of the Mongols, different Muslim caliphates, different European powers, and the constantly shifting alliances between them. Separate branches of the Mongols arrived in the Middle East after the 1250s. The branch that took over the Abbasid Caliphate eventually became the Ilkhanids; at their peak, they dominated a region that stretched from southwestern Pakistan to Turkmenistan and westward through the Caucasus and Anatolia. Both before and after the Ilkhanids' conversion to Islam in the late thirteenth century, Western European rulers made many (ultimately unsuccessful) attempts to form alliances with them against their mutual enemy, the Mamluk Sultanate. After the mid-1330s, the Ilkhanate ceased to exist as a unified dynasty, and a separate Mongol branch ruled over Crimea and much of modern-day Eastern Europe. This branch, known as the Golden Horde, developed trading relationships with the Mamluks, Venetians, and Genoans.

Troubled relationships between the Golden Horde, the Genoese, the Venetians, and the Byzantines – and ongoing disputes between Christian and Muslim communities in Crimea – may well have helped spark the original story about the siege at Caffa and the catapulting of plague-infested corpses over the walls.[208] Blaming the Tartars and Saracens for instigating the epidemic would have appealed to Christians who typically saw little distinction between the Mongols, the Muslims, and the wide ethnic, linguistic, and religious variety of people who lived under their rule (somewhat similar to the way medieval Muslims referred to Europeans by the generic term "Frank"). Non-Christians were deemed to be infidels and it was therefore conceivable that the plague pandemic had originated in their lands.[209]

Each subsequent narrative about the Black Death – whether written in Avignon or Venette (France), or in London or St Albans (England) – built upon those that preceded it. Most repeated, sometimes verbatim, the story of how the disease had first begun in the East. For Europeans writers, plague began specifically "among the Saracens and other unbelievers" before it progressed westward to engulf the Christians.[210] That subsequent writers more readily repeated the Caffa-specific portions of Mussis's account than his allusions that plague first emerged further east suggests the influence of cultural and religious biases on the interpretation of events. The end of the Pax Mongolica by 1360 witnessed a considerable decline in the Golden Horde's power and a subsequent retraction of European commercial and territorial interests around and beyond the Black Sea, as access to trans-Eurasian continental trade and communication routes declined. The coincidental timing of the Black Death and the end of the Pax Mongolica could have served to entrench the idea among later Christian writers that the Tartars had initiated the Black Death in Caffa.[211] For Muslim writers living in the eastern Mediterranean, too, locating plague's origins among political and economic rivals or threats, or among threats to one's allies, also made sense. Ibn al-Wardī's claim that plague had begun in the "land of darkness," for example, could be interpreted as an effort to move its locus further from the Mamluks' trading partners.[212]

Although many chronicles and other contemporary texts spoke about plague's supposed geographical origins, few of the early tracts did so. The most detailed report comes from Andalusi physician Ibn Khātimah. He noted in 1349 that while many Christian merchants claimed plague emerged from "'Hata,' which is called China in Persian speech … [and which] is the limit of the inhabited earth to the east," others had told him of reports suggesting its origin lay in Abyssinia (Ethiopia), from whence it had spread to neighbouring lands before reaching Egypt and Syria.[213] He also repeated reports from "many sides" that the outbreak had begun in Caffa during the siege of that town by "an army of Mohammedan Turks and Romans" before spreading through the Mediterranean. These different opinions, he suggested, "show that the catastrophe has visited universally all lands and zones. The reason for the difference of the reports is that when it appears in lands laying at the edge of the world, its inhabitants think that the disease originated there; and from there this view spreads."

Of the French tracts, only Alfonso de Córdoba suggested a possible locus for the disease; he claimed that the "pestilence was naturally located in regions of Italy and in parts overseas."[214] Most early treatise authors who wrote about the disease's reach addressed either its widespread nature or its approach from nearby regions, not where it had begun. Pierre de Damouzy felt compelled to write his work once plague came close to his doorstep: "this pestilence has increased, it has extended near to us, as may be seen in many places, from Rheims to other neighbouring areas."[215]

If Ibn Khātimah perceived that plague's purported origin depended on a writer's location, contemporary vagueness about the pandemic's starting point is perhaps unsurprising, even though geographical knowledge among Europeans was not lacking. Centuries of interaction between Europeans, Asians, and North Africans meant that much of the Eurasian world was linked directly or indirectly through trade, diplomacy, war, and religion. Recent work on Sub-Saharan Africa is adding that region to the network as well.[216] Long before the Black Death, Europe was well integrated into global trade networks that reached as far east as China, India, and Malaysia, as well as into Africa south of the Sahara. Its rising urban populations, growing markets and production capacity, and expanding taste for luxury trade goods fuelled Europe's "eastward enterprise."[217]

At the same time, reports from travellers circulated widely and contained detailed information about parts of the world largely unknown to the Greeks and Romans. Franciscan and Dominican orders had been active in Central Asia for one hundred years before the mid-fourteenth century. Pilgrims to Jerusalem met like-minded travellers from Ethiopia and beyond. Political and religious envoys moved between various Mongolian, Papal, and European courts throughout the second half of the thirteenth century. Compendia of geographical information expanded as new knowledge accumulated. Isidore of Seville's *Etymologies* and Vincent of Beauvais's *Speculum Naturale,* for example, provided medieval scholars accessible sources of information. Travel itineraries, such as those written by Matthew of Paris, and *mappae mundi* (world maps) created both textual and visual frames of reference of the world's territorial limits and its spatial configuration, as it was socially constructed at the time. Ethnographies – variously called "'descriptio' (description), 'itinerarium' (journey), and 'travels'" – likewise provided detailed descriptions of the manners and customs of other peoples.[218] Dismissing such works is anachronistic, and misses the spatial story they tell.[219]

Nevertheless, contemporary scholarly and popular geographical awareness was predicated largely on classical Greek and Roman sources. Even learned medieval scholars such as Roger Bacon "described [and located with precision] places and even whole regions of the earth's surface ... which did not exist at all."[220] Medieval European views of space and place were profoundly influenced by theological beliefs and relied to a large extent on biblical accounts of faraway places. This worldview was not meant to accurately portray contemporary spatial knowledge or observed reality; rather, it represented a common narrative that drew Christendom together. For most fourteenth-century Western Europeans, the East beyond Constantinople and Jerusalem was a large, vaguely defined, and rumoured space that was associated, at once, with the earthly paradise, traditionally-defined "marvelous lands, peoples, and events," and the terrors of Gog and Magog.[221] Popular travel writing, including Marco Polo's accounts and John Mandeville's fantastical stories, emphasized marvels and monsters, divine miracles and apocryphal threats, and strange and unusual customs, beliefs, and laws at the same time that they accurately described geographical and natural observations. In short, contemporary travel writing – a form of medieval Orientalism – informed its readers while simultaneously supporting and reflecting "the fertile ground of an imagined community's noblest hopes, wildest dreams, and worst fears."[222]

Existing "textual geographies" thus combined with "visual geographies" (*mappae mundi* and other iconographic depictions of terrestrial and celestial worlds and their inhabitants) to both blend and distort "geographical traditions" and "geographical imaginings."[223] The great commercial integration between West and East that had characterized the twelfth and thirteenth centuries was in severe decline before the mid-fourteenth century, with long-used land and sea trade routes effectively closed to Europeans (and to the Genoese and Venetians in particular) as power struggles redrew boundaries within the Middle East.[224] In this context, a new, mysterious, and devastating disease could simultaneously be traced through its observed movements from east to west *and* have its imagined point of origin set figuratively and symbolically into a distant and mysterious "East."

If few of the earliest writers commented on plague's easterly origins, after the Black Death such ideas disappeared almost entirely from the treatises. Aside from Guy de Chauliac's description of the second wave of plague being a revisitation of a disease that came "back from Germany and northern regions," little more was said about the disease's purported geographic roots.[225] Most writers discussed plague as a local problem, not a universal one. Neither its origins nor the other more distant places that it was affecting were important enough, or perhaps evident enough, to mention.

Silence about plague's origins after the 1360s was not unfounded. Contemporary records show little indication that post-Black Death outbreaks followed the same traceable paths that the Black Death seemed to have taken. Nor did the outbreaks appear in obvious geographic succession. In many localities, once it arrived, plague established itself in a local reservoir and reappeared as an epidemic every six to eight years; not every place experienced renewed outbreaks at the same time. The full extent of plague's concurrent or near-concurrent outbreaks was likely not evident to the treatise authors as they wrote their texts. Writers did not track plague because there was nothing to track.

Efforts to map plague were almost entirely absent from French and English tracts until the later sixteenth century. Despite widespread knowledge about significant new geographic realities – Europeans had begun to establish colonies in the Americas, opened the sea route to India, explored the Sub-Saharan African coast, and devised new cartographic maps and navigational aids – this information had little immediate impact on geographic and medical discussions about plague.[226] It remained primarily a local disease, even though treatise writers sometimes did not hesitate to point to the origins of other epidemic diseases like the French Pox that they argued were generated in specific places.

Throughout the fifteenth and sixteenth centuries, tract producers concentrated either explicitly (in France) or implicitly (in England) on explaining and providing advice about local outbreaks. For that concern, quarantine and isolation recommendations sufficed. Even though the English plague orders of 1625 specified that local justices "shall inquire, and presently informe themselves by all good meanes, what Townes and Villages are ... infected within every [one of] their Counties," administrative efforts to track plague were still primarily local and remained largely absent from the plague treatises.[227]

During the last quarter of the sixteenth century, writers in France started to trace plague's movement across a larger area once again and, often pointing to the disease's contagiousness, reconsidered its geographical origins. For the most part, they looked either inside their own borders or to neighbouring regions. Claude de Rubys discussed the local route by which he believed that the disease had arrived recently in Lyon through the malevolent actions of Calvinist "greasers" who already had actively spread the disease in Basle, Venice, Milan, and Lombardy.[228] Guillaume Briet, Bordeaux's municipal physician, claimed that plague affecting that city in 1599 was not locally generated but had "arrived with a stranger from Spain."[229] An anonymous treatise written after the mid-seventeenth century about a plague outbreak in Rouen argued that the disease must have come from Flanders, because Rouen itself had been so "perfectly purged of the disease for many years ... that it had almost forgotten" about plague.[230]

In each of these cases and many more, the treatise writers pinpointed a place, usually not too far away, in which their local outbreaks had begun. They typically blamed either strangers or travellers for carrying plague with them, or infected merchandise that arrived through trading channels from infected ports or cities. Centuries-long medical and administrative discussions about whether epidemic diseases were transmitted by corrupted air (miasma) or by contagion had shown that the two explanations were not mutually exclusive, and many writers used both to explain how plague in one place could also erupt in or be transported to another.[231] Being able to trace outbreaks made the concept of movement-by-contagion appear more likely; it also underlay administrative measures to stop plague from entering or spreading through cities, such as quarantines, *cordons sanitaires*, and the isolation and removal of suspected cases to plague hospitals. Similar measures were implemented, or at least recommended, in England, but English writers did not begin to actively trace the source of their outbreaks until the seventeenth century. Then, rather than describing plague's routes within their own country, these writers pointed blame at the Ottoman Empire.

For French writers who claimed to have traced plague's arrival in Marseille in 1720 to a ship recently arrived from the Levant, there was little question that the outbreak had come from the eastern Mediterranean. For English writers, it was an outbreak that, should it arrive in England, would most definitely have come from somewhere else. Fears about the outbreak in Provence spreading further also sustained a relatively new interest in the broader geography of plague, one that contextualized local epidemics with similar outbreaks happening elsewhere at the same time. In other words, the later outbreaks of the seventeenth and eighteenth centuries reignited a sense that plague was, once again, a universal phenomenon, but one whose source was definitively foreign, in general, and Turkish more specifically.

CONCLUSION

People's ability to visualize disease in spatial terms did not emerge only after the production of Andreas Vesalius's 1543 *De humani corporis fabrica*, as has been argued elsewhere.[232] This anatomical work included a large number of intricately detailed, three-dimensional drawings of human dissections that revealed how each body part functioned in relation to all the others. It offered "a new way of seeing and of verifying as real these epistemic things, the body and the environment, in which health and disease would be located."[233] Although Hippocratic treatises such as *Airs, Waters, Places* had long insisted that disease and place were linked, Vesalius's work was the first to provide a full illustration of how that spatial relationship played out in the human body. Twenty years later, in 1564, the anatomist Bartolomeo Eustachi published his *Tabulae anatomicae*, which included images of dissected bodies arranged inside a set of framed coordinates resembling contemporary maps. Even so, it has been argued that as late as "the seventeenth century, a map of the plague [from Bari, on the Adriatic coast] suggested a radical idea – that the disease was carried and spread by humans"; any possibility that this idea might have been recognized earlier, or that disease maps could have existed before then, was extremely unlikely, "because of the many things that [first] had to come together to *create the idea of disease as a thing that could be visualised in space.*"[234]

As I have shown here, however, people recognized that plague could be transmitted by humans and that the disease had a spatial component long before the seventeenth century. Medical writers located buboes on specific parts of the human body before Vesalius's anatomical book was published; although they were not as lifelike as Vesalius's drawings, such sketches demonstrated an awareness of the spatial relationship that existed between the body and the tell-tale symptoms of plague (see figure 2.15). Disease maps were unknown before at least the mid-sixteenth century, and thus were not used to create or to share knowledge about plague's geographic movements. However, tract authors did *write* about plague as a contagious disease that had spatial and geographical attributes, one that moved from one person and place to another. Understanding this process of spatial movement and geographical spread was integral to contemporary understanding of plague, including how it could affect so many different places at the same time, how it could keep returning, and who might be blamed for carrying it. Disease chronologies and geographies anchored plague outbreaks in both time and place. Treatise writers' discussions about the types of places that generated disease, where such places were located, and how to mitigate their harmful effects also point to a spatial construction of disease emergence, spread, and management.

All of the precepts on which contemporaries constructed their portrayals of the spaces occupied by plague – and thus their very understanding of the disease – evolved over time, responding not only to epidemiological observations of outbreak patterns, but also to emerging intellectual trends, available information, and new domestic and geopolitical realities. They also differed by location: discussions about the places that plague occupied did not emerge at the same time or in the same ways in England and in France. Writers' geographical locations and political/cultural backgrounds necessarily influenced their views of disease outbreaks. The notable shift in sixteenth-century English treatises towards blaming plague outbreaks on the living conditions and neighbourhoods of the poor was not replicated in France. Instead, the French tracts were more concerned with tracing the movement of plague from one city to another, especially when religious rivalries were in play. One treatise writer went so far as to propose regionally-specific therapies on the assumption that customs and practices differed throughout the kingdom. The emergence of the "*successo della Peste*" narrative in Italian plague tracts in the 1570s, which included "plott[ing] statistically" each individual outbreak, has already been noted.[235] This, in turn, generated a sequential chronology and geography for the larger epidemic and made it easier to understand plague's spatial parameters. Such practices were replicated in numerous French treatises.

Plague treatise writers did more than simply notice that outbreak patterns had changed from widespread to local (in fact, this is the making of the early modern origins of epidemiology). They discussed their ideas about where plague was generated and the spaces that it occupied. Initially conceived of as a universal disease that affected most of the known world, from some (often vaguely) defined eastern realm all the way to the place where each writer sat, plague was subsequently recast in local terms. Over the sixteenth century, first French and then English authors started to name the places about whose outbreaks they wrote. This was not the only aspect of localization that distinguished the French treatises from their English counterparts. Certainly, the distinct patterns of population growth and urban development in the two kingdoms, with many more large cities and towns in France than in England, played a key role in fostering discussion about plague in multiple sites. The dispersed nature of the French printing industry also meant that details about and reflections on outbreaks in many different cities appeared in print. England's centralized print industry and the overarching dominance of London limited the localization of narratives to that city. Here, one could read in the treatises only about London; all other affected places were de-individualized through vague phrases like "diverse cities and towns."

Plague's geographical narrative was not static. Although later fourteenth-century writers had already accepted the idea that the disease was both recurrent and local, subsequent generations of authors incrementally shifted its locus further away from the places that they inhabited. In England, this shift involved blaming the poor, while some French tracts targeted Protestants. Eventually, writers in both kingdoms no longer argued that the disease was just the product of unhealthy local environments. Beginning in the later sixteenth century, English treatise writers began to reuniversalize plague by linking local outbreaks to others both nearby and further away. Then, even before the last great epidemics devastated London (1665) and Marseille (1720), writers in both England and France pointed to plague being *imported* from foreign lands.

Over time, the geographic origin of plague was increasingly politicized, influenced by local socio-economic concerns, by travel accounts, and, as the next chapter will show, by distant colonial projects and the availability of new historical texts that revealed the wide geographical reach of the First Pandemic. As new information changed the visual map of the world and as political realities on the ground shifted, a disease once perceived to be universal became increasingly local, before the local disease in turn acquired a new universality, albeit one that had become foreign.

Plague tracts allow us to see, at one level, how the perceived links between humans, diseases, and place were continuously reconstructed over time. In the fourteenth century, Raymond Chalin de Vinario noted that Avignon, where he lived and worked, was an unclean place; it was no wonder, then, that plague, which purportedly arose from unhealthy landscapes, was a frequent visitor. By 1720, the English physician John Quincy claimed that "The Histories of Physick abound with Relations of Pestilences from no other Cause than what arises from the Importation of the Disease ... from distant Countries."[236] Writers' portrayals of plague's geography were not simply influenced by intellectual currents or contemporary medical theories; they also reflected other social concerns and are thus tied to national, or even local, environments.

Other factors were simultaneously at work in efforts to locate the source of plague. Humanist reception of and interest in Greek works offered more than just access to new information about the historical past; it also provided new information about the geographical past. The geographies of Ptolemy and Strabo, for example, were acquired in the West and translated for the first time only in the fifteenth century; they proved to be very popular throughout Western Europe and contributed both to new conceptions of geography and to the early development of the emerging discipline of geography.[237] As one historian has argued, "[n]o single event so mobilized and reoriented this new [geographical] learning as the recovery and translation into Latin of Ptolemy's *Geographia.*"[238] It also likely contributed, at least to some extent, to the push for travel and exploration in the fifteenth and sixteenth centuries by opening up the possible expanse of the world in new ways. It certainly influenced the way in which Europeans measured and calculated their place – and understood the events that they experienced locally – in a much larger world that they now travelled more frequently. Yet, geography was also distorted for economic and political ends. Determining where plague's initial source was to be placed on a map was therefore "a politically and commercially charged" action.[239] As we will see in the next chapter, it also served to influence how the disease itself was understood.

5

Imagining the Oriental Plague

From Us to Them, from Fearsome Disease to Turkish Threat

It has been frequently experienc'd, that of all the Goods, which harbour Infection, Cotton in particular is the most dangerous, and Turkey is almost a perpetual Seminary of the Plague.

Richard Mead, London, 1720[1]

WRITING THE PLAGUED OTHER

Writing from the safety of London as the latest major plague outbreak engulfed Marseille in the early 1720s, English physician Richard Mead sought to explain what caused this still fearsome disease. Proclaiming that plague was contagious, Mead described how it was transmitted: via corrupted air, by contact with infected persons through their touch and breath, and in commercial goods transported from contaminated ports. He claimed, based on what he called the evidence of "the Natural History of several Countries" and the observations of "the ancientist and best Authors of Physick," that underlying the outbreak were specific topographical and environmental features.[2] In Mead's view, it was the particular combination of stagnant bodies of water, deep crevices, poorly managed burial practices, and weather patterns that gave rise to plague. Most especially, it was the very hot, moist, and invariable climate found in the eastern and southern parts of the world that was to blame. Furthermore, because the disease was contagious, it stood to reason that plague originated in foreign places characterized by these features. Only then would it move into France and possibly threaten England. The most obvious place for plague's origin, Mead asserted, was Turkey, which he deemed to be almost "a perpetual *Seminary*" of the disease.

By the nineteenth century, the notion that plague was a specifically Oriental disease, both geographically and historically, was well entrenched. When the French, under Napoleon's rule, invaded Egypt and Syria in 1798, they immediately encountered a series of plague epidemics (see figure 5.1). Despite its attempts to control the outbreaks, the French army was ultimately forced to withdraw, the number of its plague-sufferers mounting, the unconquered region deemed pestilential. European narratives, medical literature, and public imagination concurred. Historians and travel writers like Alexander William Kinglake emphasized that it was "Plague, and the dread of the Plague" that both distinguished and spatially demarcated civilized Europeans from sickly Ottomans.[3] Physicians and medical writers like William Brownrigg, when faced with news of an outbreak in Eastern Europe in 1770–71 that had begun during a war between the Russian and Ottoman Empires, pointed to "universally known" facts – purportedly based on the experiences and records of "ambassadors, consuls, merchants, of the several European nations, residing at Constantinople, and in other great cities of the Turkish empire" – that Ottoman epidemics were inherently more common and more severe than anything experienced in Europe.[4]

Following his experiences with plague in Egypt, including the outbreak of 1834–35, Antoine Barthélemy Clot, the first director of Cairo's medical school and Egypt's chief medical officer, considered the disease – which he had never witnessed before his arrival in the city – to be non-contagious and endemic throughout the region.[5] The International Sanitary Conferences initiated in 1851 to standardize global quarantine regulations against the spread of cholera, plague, and yellow fever disagreed on the issue of contagion and pointed to the need to block diseases ostensibly still (or newly) entering Europe from eastern Mediterranean ports.[6] Even cartoons in popular magazines like *Punch* depicted Turkey as the "sick man of Europe."[7] This "orientalist" conception of plague, embedded within "the new [nineteenth-century] science of epidemiology and [the] border control policies that it informed," significantly influenced modern disease historiography, creating and then perpetuating the myth that plague was eternally tied to the East and to the Ottoman Empire in particular.[8]

The assignation of plague to the eastern Mediterranean was not new. By the later seventeenth century, the number and severity of plague outbreaks was waning considerably in Western Europe at

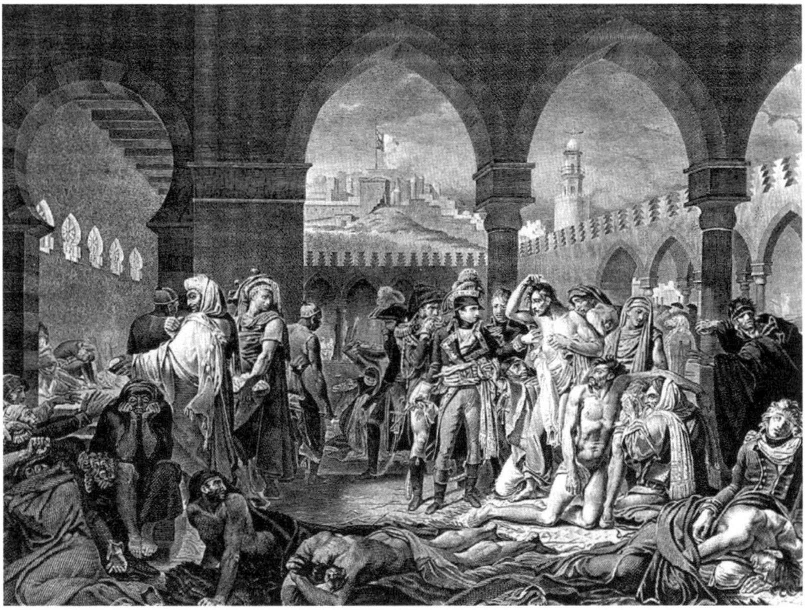

5.1 Napoleon Bonaparte visiting plague-stricken soldiers at Jaffa in 1799. Engraving by François Pigeot after Antoine-Jean Gros, 1804

the same time that the disease was starting to become a "permanent presence" in the Ottoman Empire.[9] This epidemiological shift – measurable as it is by modern standards – accounts for only part of the relocation of plague to the eastern Mediterranean. Richard Mead's assertions about the unhealthiness of the eastern and southern parts of the world had long been commonplace in English travel writing, and were already being broached by tract writers during London's devastating 1665 outbreak. Similar allegations became mainstream in French plague texts and travel accounts only in the 1700s, in stark contrast to the observations of some earlier French writers who had pointed with envy to the apparent healthiness of Ottoman territories. Pierre Belon du Mans, a mid-sixteenth-century physician and naturalist, for example, admired the Turkish landscape because "among other things," he said, "it is *free* of the plague and all other fluxes."[10] To understand the forces that contributed to the creation of the Oriental plague episteme, then, it is necessary to look to early modern European discussions about which landscapes, and which peoples, were said to give rise to plague.

This chapter investigates how, and why, Western European assessments of the apparent healthiness or unhealthiness of the eastern Mediterranean generally, and of the Ottoman Empire specifically, changed between the sixteenth and early eighteenth centuries. First, it continues chapter 4's themes and explores how the reuniversalization of plague ultimately settled on the lands of the Ottoman Turks. It asks how efforts to track plague's movement within kingdoms or across Europe gave way to seeing the disease as a Levantine import. It is important to note here that when early modern Western Europeans used the term "Turk," they typically meant the Ottoman Empire's Muslim subjects; regardless of their actual ethnicity, language, or culture, all people were categorized together, their individualities collapsed into a single religious identity. For example, the European phrase "turning Turk" meant converting to Islam. It was even claimed that Christians living in oriental lands were not affected by plague as much as Muslims because they knew how to protect themselves.

This chapter then reconnects with chapter 3 to consider how a new historical narrative for plague took shape during the later sixteenth century. The attribution of the disease's origin to the Ottoman Empire was not just geographical but also historical. Although a small Ottoman polity existed already in 1348, the larger empire did not; nevertheless, shifting blame from the place or landscape to the people themselves allowed this sleight of hand to work. The chapter also considers how the rediscovery and reuse of older written references to plague recreated a past for the disease, one that not only stretched back almost to times immemorial but that also implicated the eastern Mediterranean. These two aspects together – plague's new geography and its new history – fostered the beginnings of the Oriental plague myth. And, as explored in earlier chapters, the process of orientalizing plague differed between English and French treatise writers.

Perhaps more important than a shift in perceived disease patterns, which is often noticeable only in hindsight, was a shift in attitudes. Europeans' attempts to create and maintain healthy local environments and to export their ideas about what such healthscapes looked like to their colonial spaces emphasized the otherness of those regions. The promotion of the European imperial project, which relied in part on emphasizing the idea of healthy landscapes to encourage settlers, made distinctions between those sites under the control of European powers and those that remained uncolonized, foreign, and unhealthy. Increasing emphasis on, and debate about, the role of contagion in the spread of plague further spurred efforts to identify its source. The expansion of the Ottoman Empire into southeastern and central Europe between the fourteenth and seventeenth centuries generated fear alongside commercial opportunity but, by the mid-seventeenth century, the Empire's importance to Western Europeans as a military and economic partner had diminished.

A nascent interest in the history of epidemics in the sixteenth century, linked in part to a return to mid-fourteenth-century descriptions of the Black Death and to the rediscovery of writing about the disease from the East, also fostered a desire to locate plague both geographically and historically. Not only did the prominence of *historia* in medical and scientific writing stimulate the creation of a history of plague, but prominent new disease threats such as syphilis and typhus were also attributed to other lands and places, to other people and their customs. Underlying all these factors was a significant increase in European travel for diplomacy, commerce, missionary work, pilgrimage, and pleasure, and in the resultant production of popular travelogues and narratives. Witnessing – or at least reading about – regular outbreaks of disease in the faraway Levant must have given Europeans with decreasing plague experience at home (and often little tangible knowledge of the region itself) the sense that the entire eastern Mediterranean under Ottoman rule was, and always had been, disease-ridden. In other words, as European plague became anchored in time, plague of the Ottoman "Other" became timeless: it had always been there and was thus de-historicized.

Observations that linked the Ottoman Empire and plague were repeated in contemporary medical literature, giving them further credibility and authority. Richard Mead's early eighteenth-century assertion that Turkey was the source of Europe's plague outbreaks was part of an existing trend based on inherited tradition, (purported) observation, assumption, and identity politics. His ideas reflected the still-influential Hippocratic *Airs, Waters, and Places* tradition that suggested a relationship between particular geographies, topographies, climates, and their diseases (see chapter 4) but, unlike earlier tract writers, who had interpreted this tradition to identify local spaces of plague, Mead used Hippocratic arguments to support his belief that plague could not possibly be endemic in England. Instead, plague always arrived in the kingdom from elsewhere, most commonly through commerce; in fact, he argued, "in this *Island* there is [not] any one Instance of a *Pestilential* Disease among us of great Consequence, which we did not receive from other *Infected* Places."[11] In England, he claimed in a later edition of his treatise, the cool climate and changing seasons mitigated the negative effects of any potentially unhealthy landscapes, making the "Air of our climate ... so far from being ever the Original of the true plague."[12] Even the mysterious sweating sickness, "commonly thought to have taken its Rise here [i.e., in England]," was, Mead suggested, "most probably of a foreign Original ... very probably from a Turkish Infection."[13] He extended his argument by insisting that "the *Contagion* [of the 1665 outbreak] came by *Cotton* imported from *Turkey*."[14] Not only were the Ottoman region and its landscape disease-ridden then, but anyone and anything coming from it also carried the dreaded disease. "I cannot but think it highly reasonable," Mead continued, "that whatever Cotton is imported from that Part of the World, should at all Times be kept in *Quarantine*."[15]

It was not just current and recent plagues that came from Turkey. For Mead, "the History of the most terrible of all the Plagues, that ever were in these Parts of the World, which was that in the Year 1349, gives a manifest Proof from whence all *Europe* may trace the Origine of these Evils, viz. from *Asia*."[16] Relying on the fourteenth-century account of the Florentine chronicler Matteo Villani, Mead noted that the disease had first arisen in China and then spread westward through Syria, Turkey, Egypt, Greece, and North Africa. Its entry into mainland Europe had begun in the Levant, from whence ships carried plague into Sicily, Pisa, and Genoa. The Levantine region of the Ottoman Empire he especially linked to plagues both past and present, not only because of its climate, but also because the contagious poison of the disease "maintains it self there by circulating from *Infected* Persons to Goods; which is chiefly owing to the Negligence of the People ... who are stupidly Careless in this Affair."[17] In the Ottoman Empire, then, one could find the perfect combination of precipitating factors: a consistently hot and sultry climate, a stagnant landscape, and a population that apparently had little sense of how to maintain a healthscape or to contain disease outbreaks.

In the sixteenth century, Calvinists had been French Catholics' diseased "Other," blamed and persecuted for generating and spreading plague. In England, Catholics were blamed to some extent, but more especially it was the poor, regardless of their religious affiliation, who were scapegoated. Blaming social outcasts, heretics, vagabonds, beggars, the infirm, and other strangers within European communities had enabled tract writers to move plague's origins from the sins of the people to the margins of their local communities (see chapter 4). By the eighteenth century, perhaps as national religious identities became somewhat more secure and as a way to shift attention from domestic concerns, writers in both kingdoms defined the Other more distantly. To Richard Mead, the Ottomans represented the quintessential Other. The East had long figured as the Other in Europeans' constructions of their own identity: its religious difference, its cultural difference, and even its climatic and topographical differences all marked it out as not just foreign, but alien. Mead harnessed the apparent exoticism of the Ottoman Empire's "perilous landscape and iniquitous people" to facilitate its identification as the original source of disease. Eyewitness accounts of early modern travellers in the empire, and especially of medically trained travellers, had bolstered this identity, shifting the region from a curiosity-cum-ally (and sometimes military foe) into a distinct, biological threat.[18] The docking of the ship *Grand Saint Antoine* at the port of Marseille in 1720, after its arrival from the eastern Mediterranean with a purportedly plague-infected cargo, eerily replicated the entrance of plague-infested ships into Sicily, Pisa, and Genoa from the Levant centuries earlier. Of this, numerous early eighteenth-century tract writers were wholeheartedly convinced.[19]

THE OTTOMAN THREAT: PRESENT AND PAST

Plagued Orient

> And for what concerns that Pestilence now under Enquiry, this we have as to its Origin, from the most irrefrigable Authority ... it came tither from *Turkey* in Bails of Cotton ... For that Part of the World is seldom free from such Infections.
>
> Nathaniel Hodges, London, 1672[20]

Richard Mead was not the first English medical writer to claim that a plague outbreak had originated in the eastern Mediterranean: such assertions had become commonplace in that kingdom's treatises more than half a century before. As early as its 1636 *Certain Necessary Directions* for plague, London's College of Physicians had noted a concern about "Men or goods from forreigne infected places."[21] In particular, it emphasized the necessity of ensuring that "neither men nor goods may come [to London] from any suspected places beyond the seas." The college did not name which places it suspected of being infected, but it is clear that perceptions about plague's origin were already changing and were being tied to sea travel. Although it often first emerged among the poor, to London's top medical authorities plague no longer arose within the kingdom but came from beyond: *foreign* goods and *foreign* people brought the disease to England. All ships or persons arriving without clean health certificates were to be either "sent suddenly away" or quarantined "according to the custome of Italy" until their healthiness could be confirmed.[22] Similar policies had been in place for some time for domestic foreigners, that is, anyone arriving from a different city or shire; now, the gaze shifted outward, across the sea.

For English plague writers just a few decades later, the vaguely "foreign" sources of plague were more specific. William Kemp, for example, considered the Ottoman Empire, and especially its territories in the eastern Mediterranean, to be a hotbed of infection. This was so especially because the "*Turks* are perswaded that every one's fate is written in his fore-head, and hath a fatal destiny appointed by God, which it is impossible for any to avoid; so that they … slight and neglect all care of avoiding the infection."[23] Despite having no personal knowledge of Turks, of the Ottoman Empire, or of Islam, Kemp felt it entirely unnecessary to question whether this rumour – commonly accepted among Europeans for a century already – was in fact true: it was obvious that "at *Grand Cayre* [Cairo] and *Constantinople* there have been thousands that have suffered death, and multitudes that have been executed by the Plague for this Heresie." The Turks' purported lack of care exacerbated outbreaks there, he suggested, and enabled them to spread. Astrologers such as John Gadbury argued that the disease had come "out of Turky, into Germany, out of Germany into Italy, out of Italy into Holland, and out of Holland into England."[24] For Gadbury, while a heavenly apparition had portended the 1665 outbreak, there was no doubt that the disease had arisen first in "Turky." Even the English practice of shutting up individuals and families suspected of having plague was blamed on the Ottomans: an anonymous author decried the practice, claiming that "this inhumane forsaking took its rise from the *Turks* and Infidels."[25]

Nathaniel Hodges's *Historical Account of the Plague in London in 1665* provided its readers with a retrospective, step-by-step examination of how the plague outbreak had begun and its after-effects. Hodges had remained in the city during the epidemic and his account, initially published in Latin in 1672, presented details about his treatments for plague victims and his observations of a city devastated by disease. As Hodges's account demonstrated, by the second half of the seventeenth century, treatise writers felt competent to state, quite categorically in some cases, that plague had arrived from elsewhere. No longer pointing to the poor and their "sluttish" living habits, but insisting instead that pestilential diseases like plague reign most commonly in maritime regions because of their landscape's – and hence their population's – "saline constitution," Hodges considered the Mediterranean coastal cities and ports ruled by the Ottomans to be the most likely origin of plague. That part of the world, he argued, "is seldom free" from disease.[26] Like Mead some years later, Hodges acknowledged that the "Maritime Parts of our own Country [i.e., England] do by sad experience too much testifie" to port cities being plague's points of entry – despite the fact that the first cases typically erupted in parishes located some distance from the ports.[27] Yet he too was confident that England's seacoast exposure and its population's constitution were categorically different from those found in the consistently hot, moist climates of the eastern Mediterranean. England's coastal populations may have been more susceptible to the disease, and the great outbreak of 1665 may have begun (according to his account) among "two or three Persons [who] died suddenly in one Family at *Westminster*" at the end of 1664 (i.e., March 1665), but plague did not arise initially among them. Instead, it came from the Turks, by way of "Holland, in Packs of [Turkish] Merchandize."[28]

The European belief in Turkish fatalism appears to stem from letters written by Ogier Ghiselin de Busbeq, the Habsburg ambassador to the Ottoman Empire in the mid-sixteenth century. Busbeq later transcribed his letters and notes into a memoir, which was then translated and published repeatedly in several European languages. His claims about Turkish fatalism are "possibly among the most influential passages to shape European perceptions of the Ottomans' attitudes in the face of plague," even though archival records show them to have been entirely false.[29] His commentary about Turks and their reaction to plague was regularly repeated in early modern travel narratives, alongside other disparaging observations about Ottoman lifestyles and medical practices; they even continue to be repeated in scholarship to this day.

Like their medieval predecessors, sixteenth- and seventeenth-century travel writers appeared to their readers to be authoritative, not only because they had (they claimed) personally witnessed the places about which they wrote, but also because many of them held high positions as physicians, diplomats, royal geographers, and so on. Many travel narratives became bestsellers, less because of the veracity or practical utility of their contents than because they gave readers what they wanted: an adventure in an exotic land written in a particular narrative style.[30] Later writers did much to shape their readers' ideas about the places in which the Ottomans lived and over which they ruled, largely by focusing less on their military might – as earlier travel accounts had done – and more on their social customs, their health status, and their local environments (see figures 5.2 and 5.3). The image of the Ottomans, and of the Ottoman Empire as a whole, that these travel accounts portrayed was mixed and rather paradoxical. It also changed over time, since the accounts reflected their authors' different religious, economic, political, and national interests and prejudices.[31] Many of these writers, regardless of their backgrounds, characterized the Ottomans as cruel, tyrannical, and ignorant Others who nevertheless were religiously tolerant and politically enlightened (because their governance was based on merit rather than hereditary rights). While the points of view expressed by the writers were as varied as their motivations and backgrounds, it is nevertheless possible to tease out some of the specific impressions held by French and English writers about the nature of the Ottoman healthscape, ideas that only coalesced in the eighteenth century during the outbreak in Marseille. These perspectives were then carried into explanations of plague's origins in French and English plague treatises.

Some of the early French travellers appeared to envy what they saw in the Ottoman Empire and painted a positive picture as a result. Nicolas de Nicolay, a mid-sixteenth-century soldier and royal geographer, spent several pages in the account of his travels describing the vast number and style of Turkish public baths that he witnessed. Like many of his contemporaries, Nicolay returned to Europe full of wonder at and praise for Turkish cleanliness and public amenities. Although the Turks' apparent devotion to regular bathing was portrayed by the artist Guillaume-Joseph Grelot as an unhealthy practice because it "overmoistened" the Turk's brains and caused "continual Rheume in their eyes," in general their hygiene practices were seen in a positive light when compared to those of Europeans.[32] While he found their dedication to cleanliness extraordinary – or perhaps extraordinarily strange – Grelot nevertheless concluded that Ottoman cities

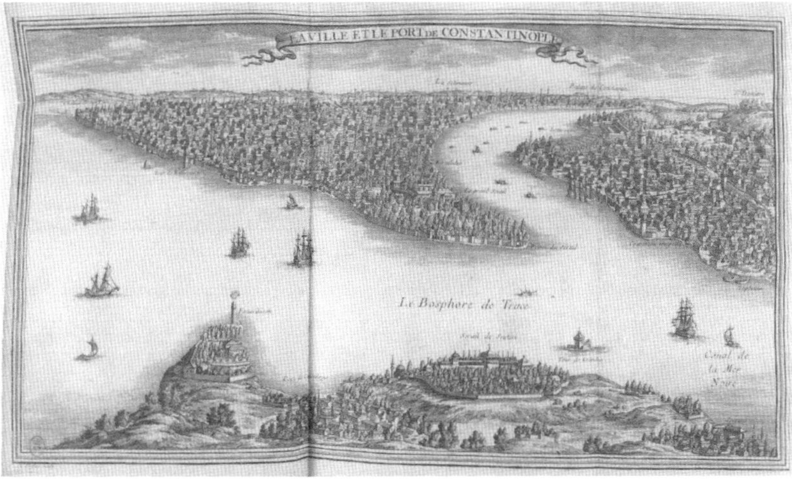

5.2 The plagued Eastern Mediterranean: view of Constantinople from Asia, engraving by C. Duflos in Jean-Antoine Guer, *Moeurs et usages des Turcs, leur religion, leur gouvernement civil, militaire et politique*, 1746.

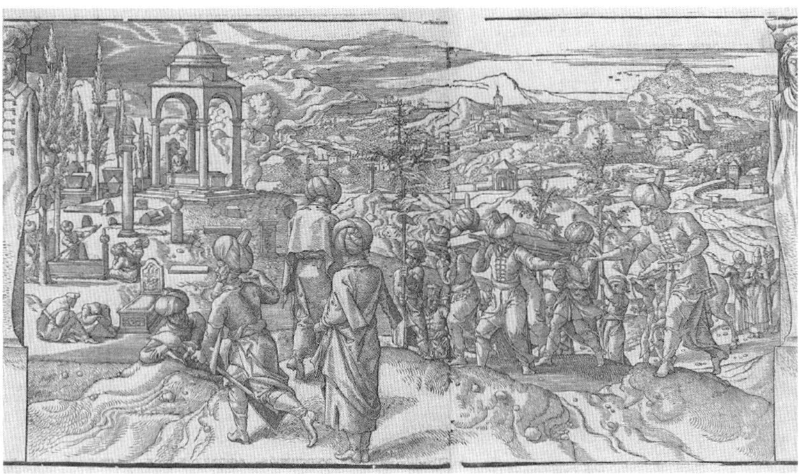

5.3 Western perceptions of Ottomans: a Turkish funeral from the frieze *Ces Moeurs et fachons de faire de Turcz*, woodcut after Pieter Coecke van Aelst, 1553.

and people were far healthier than those in Europe. "You shall never see in Travelling all over the East," he asserted, "what is dayly obser'd and suffer'd in our Cities, the Walls of our Churches stain'd with Urine, and bedeck'd at the bottom with the excrements of those" who approached those places with little respect.[33] Mid-seventeenth-century botanist Jean de Thévenot further claimed that Turks "live for a long time, and are not often sick; we [Europeans] suffer from many dangerous diseases that they do not know at all ... I believe that their good health results partly from the baths that they use so often."[34] The Turks were so healthy, Thévenot claimed, that physicians could make no money there. Thévenot actually fled Constantinople during an outbreak of plague, reported that there were outbreaks of the disease in Egypt every seven years, and repeated the well-rehearsed story of Turkish fatalism in the face of contagious disease. Yet he did not make any direct association between the Ottoman Empire's geography or culture and the origins of plague.

Other sixteenth- and seventeenth-century French travellers spoke of witnessing famine, plague, and war-engendered desolation throughout their journeys across the Ottoman Empire but, like Thévenot, did not portray it as a particularly plagued environment. Although the diamond merchant and explorer Jean-Baptiste Tavernier claimed of Smyrna in the seventeenth century that "hardly a year goes by that this city is not attacked by the plague," he believed that the outbreaks were not as bad as they were in Christian Europe.[35] French travellers' ubiquitous references to the high levels of charity that Ottoman administrators and citizens provided to the sick and the poor throughout the empire also shone a positive light on the region while simultaneously pointing out the failures of Christian kingdoms for not doing the same.

Some of the earliest English accounts of the Ottoman Empire were, like their French counterparts, full of praise for the wealth and splendour they contrasted to the dreariness of life at home. But in English travel accounts we also find vivid condemnation of Ottoman cities, despite little real difference between them and the cities of Europe. Here the English observations are similar in spirit to contemporary English plague treatises, finding Ottoman cities immoral and thus plague-ridden. The sixteenth-century merchant trader Peter Mundy criticized places like Scanderone (İskenderun), describing the city as "very unwholesome by reason of the hugh high hills hindringe the approach of the Sunne Beames ... [and the] greate Marshe full of boggs, foggs, and Froggs."[36] Perceived as particularly problematic were the urban streets, which some English writers described as being narrow, crooked, filthy, stench-ridden, and pestilential. Travel writer Fynes Moryson wrote in the early seventeenth century that the "streetes of this Citie [Constantinople] are narrow ... In many places of the streetes lye carcases, yea sometimes the bodies of dead men, even till they be putrified, and I thinke this uncleanlinesse of the Turks is the chiefe cause that this Citie ... is continually more or lesse infected with the plague."[37] Curiously, Moryson noted that Christians in the area regularly fell ill and died; he did not comment on the health of the Muslim inhabitants.

The preacher Charles Robson, reflecting on his visit to "*Alexandretta alias Scanderone*," called it "[t]he unwholesomest place in the world to live in, by reason of the grosse fogges that both discend from the high mountains, and ascend from the moorish valleys."[38] Robson then praised the city of Aleppo, which he found to be much more salubrious; however, here too the place was being ruined by "these usurpers" – the Turks – whom Robson called slothful and stupid. The insinuation was that although (Robson claimed) Aleppo suffered from plague only once every ten years and each outbreak "never endureth longer then the Twelfth of *July*," it was inevitable that the situation would get worse unless the Turks were cast out and Aleppo was "restore[d] ... to the true owners, the Christians."[39] English diplomat Sir Paul Rycaut complained that the "great number of diseased Curs [dogs] in all streets ... are mangy and foul, and no small causes of breeding the plague, so frequent [are they] in all the Cities of the *Turks*."[40] A number of travel writers also pointed to local graveyards and secondhand markets as sources of disease.

Such references to the Ottoman Empire's rural swamps, bogs, fens, and stagnant waters, to its crowded and filthy urban streets and markets, and to its foul-smelling air reinforced contemporary English beliefs that the entire region was disease-ridden and to be avoided. Emphasizing their perceptions that not only were the Ottoman Empire's cities foul but also that the Ottomans failed to implement public health measures, such as quarantines or burning the belongings of plague victims, enabled travel writers to highlight the contrast between a healthy Western Europe and an unhealthy eastern Mediterranean.[41]

Alongside developments in geographic knowledge and the increasing publication of travel narratives, contemporary physicians and chorographers – those who described and/or mapped particular regions or countries – were expanding their application of the Hippocratic *Airs, Waters, Places* tradition by examining why some places were healthier than others. By the late sixteenth century, chorography emerged as a new genre in English writing that blended geographic, climatic, and cultural descriptions of local places with expressions of local pride, sentiment, or nationalism. Although some chorographers mentioned the unhealthy features of regions in England, such as William Lambarde's description of Romney Marsh as "Evill in winter, grevious in Sommer and never good," or William Camden's statement that parts of Essex suffered from "unwholesome vapours [which] very much impair the health of the adjacent inhabitants," more often these chorographers did *not* discuss disease-generating places in their descriptions of their homeland.[42] Instead, they painted a picture of overall healthiness.

Beginning in the fourteenth-century, plague tracts often pointed to stinking, marshy, stagnant areas as sites of disease. Early modern treatises continued to make the same connections, but now emphasizing the preponderance of such features in the Ottoman Empire rather than in England or France. Fynes Moryson's description of the "Fenny Plaine," "ill vapours," "boggy earth," and "perpetuall heat" of the eastern Mediterranean helped writers of different ilks to direct attention away from local sites and reinforce biases against foreign places, especially those deemed exotic in landscape, custom, and religion. It also fostered a growing perception of a West-East geographical divide of healthy versus unhealthy. Richard Mead's early eighteenth-century comparison of England's "*Northern Air*" and changing seasons with the sultry heats and stagnant waters of Egypt, Turkey, and other southern regions was simply another step in this process.

In the early modern era of increasingly long-distance exploration, trade, and colonial settlement, the relationship between a place, its landscape, and the health of its inhabitants (and newcomers) took on added importance. Colonial promoters found it necessary to assess and market new settlements in terms of their environmental healthiness, and to do so in a familiar way that reflected "an Old World framework of medical and environmental knowledge."[43] Overwhelmed by malaria, smallpox, dysentery, and, later, yellow fever, for example, the American colonies were nevertheless considered to be, and continuously promoted as, healthy places to live because their physical environments were much like, or even better than, what potential colonists experienced in England. Explaining large-scale deaths among settlers sometimes relied on the *Airs, Waters, and Places* tradition to minimize obvious problems with the settlements. English writer William Strachy deemed the site of Jamestown in the colony of Virginia, for example, to have been poorly selected since it "appears to be unwholesome and subject to many ill ayres, which accompany the like marish places."[44] Yet despite evidence to the contrary, promotional material for the Carolina colonies put special emphasis on the region's salubrity and downplayed high mortality rates among newcomers. Writing of New France, the Jesuit missionary Pierre Biard sought to lure settlers by declaring that the colony was "a twin land to ours, subject to the same influences, lying in the same latitude, and having the same climate."[45] Presumably, he believed that it enjoyed the same level of healthiness too, although the frigid winter temperatures soon discouraged colonists. Although fear of plague travelled across the Atlantic, there were no outbreaks of that disease in the Americas; thus there was little need to consider whether its origin lay there.

Plague *was*, however, an ongoing concern in India, where European ambassadors had established diplomatic and commercial relations with the Mughal Empire and where traders set up trading and manufacturing sites. European travellers to the region in the late sixteenth century provided accounts of various types of fevers, bloody fluxes, and venereal diseases, but not plague. One Dutch traveller, Jan Huyghen van Linschoten, who was in Goa in the 1580s, claimed that plague "hath never been in India, neither is it known unto the Indians."[46] Within a few short decades, however, the *Memoirs* of the early seventeenth-century emperor Jahangir spoke about the new problem of plague in northern India, recounting a widespread outbreak in 1615–17 centred in the Punjab region. The disease became a very serious problem later in the century. Even so, Europeans did not discuss it openly as much as they did other diseases. In the context of European physicians who worked in India being "sought and pampered by" India's ruling class, one might consider that these doctors were able to "translate [their] professional goodwill into concrete commercial concessions" for European companies.[47] Speaking openly about plague outbreaks, or tracing plague to India, was not good for business.

As a result, even though Europeans often viewed all foreign spaces and foreign bodies as sites of disease, it made economic and political sense to locate the origins of plague in a place that would remain foreign, not in one already or soon to be inhabited by the English or the French.[48] Relocating plague among geographic and cultural Others – like the Turks – likewise helped bolster suggestions that outbreaks in Europe were imported from or carried by peoples who were themselves diseased or otherwise undesirable. By the mid-seventeenth century, the source of plague had moved from marginalized persons and groups to a new and distinctly defined kind of Other. This shift from one type of religious and cultural Other to another also made sense in the context of the 1648 Peace of Westphalia, through which Calvinists and other Protestant groups "were being re-integrated into Continental networks of communications" following decades of destructive and bloody religious warfare.[49]

If their colonial and imperialist projects required the English and the French to find a place outside of their control (or desired control) in which to locate plague, the economic and political decline of the Ottoman Empire over the seventeenth century provided them with a suitable location. By the sixteenth century, the Ottoman Empire was becoming established as Western Europe's most visible competitor, military threat, and cultural and religious Other. It was also an important economic and diplomatic partner, a paradox that generated a complex image of the Turks among Europeans, as seen in travellers' accounts.

Aside from Venice, France was the first Western power to establish diplomatic and commercial relations with the Ottoman Empire. King François I and his successors, in fact, engaged in a purposeful pro-Ottoman policy beginning in the early sixteenth century against their mutual enemy, the Holy Roman Emperor Charles V. The French monarch even allowed the Ottoman naval fleet to overwinter in the Mediterranean port city of Toulon in 1543–44.[50] This may have contributed to the more positive assessments of the Ottomans among French writers than one finds in English texts. Commercial trade did flourish between England and the Ottoman Empire in the later sixteenth, seventeenth, and eighteenth centuries, initiated, in part, by "Tudor fascination with the Islamic World."[51] Even so, numerous Elizabethan attempts to establish diplomatic and military alliances with the Ottomans against Europe's Catholic powers had been largely unsuccessful. For both the English and the French during the sixteenth and seventeenth centuries, then, commercial and political pragmatism had generally taken precedence over religious or military qualms about being too closely allied with a visibly foreign power.

The defeat of Ottoman forces at Lepanto in 1571 by the Holy League marked the beginning of the end not only of Ottoman military expansion across the Mediterranean, but also of the Ottoman Empire's relevance to Western Europeans. By the later seventeenth century, it held much less importance for either England or France. Although a century later both kingdoms tried to keep the Ottoman Empire alive against the threat of the growing Russian Empire, the Turkish military presence in southeastern Europe was nevertheless perceived as a serious religious and political threat that outweighed any diplomatic benefit from ongoing commercial interests.[52]

The late sixteenth to mid-seventeenth century thus marks a crucial period during which a variety of factors combined to foster a shift in English (especially) and French (later) perceptions of the healthiness, or lack thereof, of the Ottoman Empire. The region provided the perfect combination of unhealthy environment, foreignness, and plague persistence. While many Black Death-era writers had placed the initial outbreak among the Tatars (Tartars) and the Saracens, the early modern addition of the Turks as a specifically named people reflected the geopolitical reality of the Ottoman Empire. For English and French tract writers, adding plague to the list of threats posed by the Turks was neither difficult nor unreasonable.

An anonymous commentary on the weekly bills of mortality in 1665 emphasized "Forreign Visitations by the Plague," pointing in particular to "the city called the Grand Caire ...where the plague cometh with such fierceness, that the most part of the people there do die thereof: and divers of them that remain alive lose their eye-sight with the vapours and great heat which cometh from the ground."[53] The physician George Thomson likewise argued that it was in Cairo "where the beginning and end of raging Plagues may punctually be foretold."[54] Very quickly thereafter, associating local outbreaks with outbreaks occurring in other places came to mean locating the origin of one's own outbreak elsewhere. Other English treatise writers agreed that the London outbreak of 1665 had come through Holland from the Ottoman Empire, with Cairo and Constantinople being particularly troublesome places.

By the early eighteenth century, this idea was well entrenched: Philip Rose, another physician and member of the College of Physicians, argued that plague spread through the importation of goods, "especially from ... *Turkish* Dominions."[55] In observing that "the Contagion [is] now spreading it self in Foreign Parts," that is, in Provence, Richard Bradley considered whether the "destruction of the City [of London] by fire in 1666" had forestalled any further outbreaks there.[56] During London's plague outbreak in 1665, he said, the city had been full of the kind of crowded, narrow, unpaved, and suffocating streets that generated the disease. Now, however, it was much airier and more salubrious, unlike the plague-ridden cities that travellers described in the Ottoman Empire.

The physician John Quincy suggested that unhealthy places, such as those containing stagnant rivers, could be improved by redirecting cleaner waters to flush out the sluggish ones. Such efforts, he noted, had already been made in Oxford and, along with enlarging the city boundaries to ease overcrowding and keeping the streets clean and empty of dung and offal, this had freed the city from further outbreaks. The implication was that foreign places where this had not been done, such as "*Grand Cairo* in *Egypt* … are [therefore] hardly ever free from *Pestilential Disease*."[57] And Richard Mead noted, "in these latter Ages, since our Trade with Turkey has been pretty constant, the Plagues in these Parts of Europe have evidently been brought from thence … [and] the late *Plague* in *France* [in 1720–21] came indisputably from Turkey."[58]

Mead's idea that plague outbreaks were generated in unhealthy places, and that such places were more likely foreign, was relatively uncontroversial. Even those who disputed his assessment of how plague was transmitted agreed that the disease could arise only in particular places – like Turkey – that generated plague-corrupted air. There were only a few voices of opposition to the idea that plague spread from Turkey: the physician Joseph Browne reasoned that, since the Turks regularly suffered from the disease, and since Europeans traded heavily with them, if plague was indeed contagious then Europe's port cities would likewise be constantly infected. This was not the case, and so the disease could not be contagious and could not come from the Turks. Instead, Browne argued, plague came from further afield; Tartary was his choice, "for the Plague has ravaged that country in all ages."[59]

French authors soon began to make similar arguments about the origin of the Marseille outbreak.[60] Many pointed to a specific ship – the *Grand Saint Antoine* – that had recently arrived from "the countries of the Levant that are often wasted by the plague."[61] The Abbé Martin Gaudereau claimed, based on almost thirty years of personal observation while travelling on diplomatic business throughout the Ottoman region, that "an infinite number of places in Asia are infected by the plague."[62] The physician and medical writer Jean-Jacques Manget concurred, pointing out that while plague had become relatively rare in Europe by the early eighteenth century, it nevertheless was brought in from time to time from "oriental" countries where it occurred regularly, "particularly among the Turks."[63] For Manget, it was primarily the Ottoman climate, rather than its customs, that generated plague.

Blaming the Turks was also projected backwards onto the mid-fourteenth century. By the time plague had disappeared from British records (and as it was disappearing from France), the disease was being used for nationalistic and ethnocentric propaganda. Although the writers disagreed, often vehemently, about how the disease was generated and the means by which it spread, they agreed almost unanimously that it came from the Levant, or at the least from some part of the Ottoman Empire. Indeed, the fact that outbreaks continued to occur in Ottoman lands long after they had slowed down in Western Europe served only to validate the growing belief among French and English writers that the Ottoman Empire was – in both popular and medical imaginaries – the ultimate source of the disease. Plague became "the marker of spatial demarcation" between two perceived geographic and historical realities: a healthy Europe whose plagues had always arrived from foreign lands, and an unhealthy, perpetually plague-ridden Orient – a "plaguescape" *par excellence.*[64]

Historically Plagued Geographies

> We see the plague enter France; we see it moving from town to town, from province to province. We find, moreover, that the authoritative history of so many plagues that have been brought into Europe and communicated from one kingdom to another makes it reasonable to believe that this disease is foreign.
>
> Pierre Baux, Nîmes, 1722[65]

In 1722, Pierre Baux argued that it stood to reason that plague was a foreign disease that had emerged in some other part of the world before spreading globally. Historians too had shown that plague had always been a foreign disease imported from elsewhere, especially from places around "Africa" where it still recurred regularly. Baux extrapolated from historical accounts of numerous outbreaks to demonstrate that all of them had come from Africa or the Levant. Not only did Thucydides's fifth-century BCE Plague of Athens come from Ethiopia, he argued, but also Procopius's sixth-century bubonic plague, Cedrenus's great outbreak in eighth-century Constantinople, and St Augustine's devastating mortality in Africa had all emerged from the same general region. We find, he said, "in searching through the Histories" many cases of disease coming from "some part of Africa."

In addition, he claimed, one could find in the histories "without doubt ... a great number of other plagues coming from the Levant."[66]

Citing *Les Visites charitables* by the seventeenth-century Protestant pastor Charles Drelincourt, Baux explained the link between these regions: "This disease is normally in Egypt but not dangerous" and had spread through regular commerce to Constantinople.[67] Due to the Turks' "predestination" that prevented them from establishing any semblance of order, plague then ravaged all of "Turquie." Ongoing trade with the Levant then communicated the disease to Europe. Furthermore, Baux contended, Guy de Chauliac had stated that bubonic plague came from the Levant in 1348, making it reasonable to believe that the same disease had continued to come from there repeatedly over time. More recent outbreaks, such as the great epidemics that began in Marseille in 1649 or in Neuhäusel (Germany) in 1679, likewise could be linked directly to Turkish trade and military activities. Implicit in Baux's argument was the assumption that plague outbreaks separated by great distances of time – those from the distant past just as much as the one that had recently shocked Marseille – were one and the same disease. By extension, they had all come from the same geographical source.

Baux's early eighteenth-century references to what historians had written about the geography of previous plagues, and his recasting of geography onto his current outbreak, reflects a further trend in tract writing that had begun in the late sixteenth century. As they interpreted what they read from earlier accounts, authors began to recount – and, importantly, revise – the geographic origins of the Black Death. In many ways, these treatise writers were the forerunners of the nineteenth-century historiographers of the Black Death who created the concept of the "Oriental plague" and projected it backwards to the fourteenth-century.

As early as 1577, Claude de Rubys extrapolated from Matteo Villani's chronicle and Boccaccio's novella to point specifically to the Levant as the source of plague, noting that "this sickness had long reigned" there.[68] A short time earlier, Laurent Joubert had incorporated Guy de Chauliac's comments about the origins of the Black Death into his own work and, in so doing, refamiliarized treatise readers with Chauliac's assertion that plague had come from (a somewhat less definitively explained) East: "Sometimes the plague is universal, such as the one described by Guy de Chauliac in the year 1348, which had initially begun in the East before spreading over almost the entire world."[69] Efforts to recount historical plagues in the seventeenth and eighteenth centuries (see chapter 3) also sought to associate these outbreaks with an eastern locus. Just what exactly was meant by this "east," however, remained subject to each author's interpretation. In 1665, John Graunt described the Black Death's trajectory as beginning "in the East part of the world towards *Cataya*, the higher *India*," before it spread throughout the world.[70] An anonymous commentary on London's *Bills of Mortality* proposed that the Black Death had begun "in the East Indies, among the Tartarians, Saracens, and Turks, [where it] lasted the space of seven years ... [before it] was dispersed in many *Christian* kingdoms."[71]

The geographically imprecise terms "East," "Asia," and "Orient" were all broadly construed as areas somewhere east of ancient Greece, the western half of the Roman Empire and, later, Latin Christendom. Their cultural meanings and physical locations changed over time as Western Europe's interactions with the broader world expanded. In agreeing that Asia, broadly speaking, was the origin of plagues, most early modern English writers considered that Asia began in or near the eastern Mediterranean, that is, around the Ottoman Empire.[72] Joseph Browne was nearly alone in denying that the "Turks" were responsible for spreading the disease, preferring instead to argue that plague "proceeded from the great Quantities of Horse-Flesh eaten by the Inhabitants" of Tartary, which nevertheless lay just beyond the Ottoman borders.[73]

Richard Mead continued his discussion of the Marseille outbreak by mapping the Black Death across the Eurasian continent, beginning in China in 1346, and then progressing through the East Indies, Turkey, Syria, Greece, and Africa in 1347 before passing into Europe. "The ancientist and best Authors of Physick" he argued, referring to the ancient medical authorities of the eastern Mediterranean, "lived in a country more exposed to these Calamities than ours."[74] By the 1740s, however, he had changed his mind about the source of the Black Death, removing China from consideration. Mead came to regard Matteo Villani's history of the great plague as "so very incredible, that I cannot think we ought at all to rely upon it." Villani's accounts of plague arising from a "great *Ball* of *Fire*," that is, a comet, were simply beyond belief. Furthermore, Mead argued, there were no historical accounts of plague in China. Instead, the "the most accurate Accounts in all Times of this Disease ... bring it from Africa."[75] To Mead, Africa meant North Africa or Ethiopia, regions that were part of or bordered on the Ottoman Empire.

When writing the ninth edition of his treatise, Mead reconsidered the origin of plague according to accounts culled from antiquity, not from the time of the Black Death. Among those texts he now found to be the "most accurate accounts," Mead included Pliny's first-century AD *Natural History* and Thucydides's description of the Plague of Athens. Using these ancient sources, he argued for a locus in the eastern Mediterranean. Even if its ultimate source was the north coast of Africa, Mead nevertheless insisted that plague had long ago found a home in "*Turky*," and it was from there that it had historically spread into Europe. This other "East" – and especially "*Turky*"– became the site that English writers most commonly cited as the historical home of plague.

Aside from Pierre Baux, few of the later French treatise writers spoke directly about the geographic origins of historical plagues. Abbé Martin Gaudereau's tract focused on the widespread occurrence of plague throughout the Middle East, and on the various types of the disease that were engendered there; for him, it was obvious that "since the earliest times" this region had been "regarded as the source of pestilential illnesses."[76] He argued that in creating their empire over the previous four centuries, the Turks had made the disease situation there worse. By not maintaining the ancient works already in place throughout the region – works that had in previous times mitigated disease outbreaks – and by not taking appropriate precautions during outbreaks, he said, the Turks had allowed the conditions that generated plague to become widespread and entrenched. In other words, he claimed, the Turks themselves had caused the region to become the locus of the disease. Although Gaudereau did not specifically mention historical epidemics, by pointing to four hundred years of Turkish mismanagement he made it clear that the Black Death and all subsequent outbreaks of plague originated in the lands ruled by the Ottomans.

While Gaudereau claimed that his accusations were based on personal observation, they reflected more than a century of European writing about Turks. Although the Ottoman Turks had conquered the Balkans and established a transcontinental empire by the mid-fourteenth century, it was not really until the fall of Constantinople in 1453 that Western Europeans really started to pay attention to the changes that were taking place in the eastern Mediterranean. The flight of Byzantine *emigrés* and their manuscripts to the West after 1453 intersected with the nascent humanist movement, ultimately generating an interest in the history of the Byzantine Empire that the Ottomans were now replacing. This new awareness of the deeper history of the eastern Mediterranean included a growing recognition in Western Europe of the extent of the First Plague Pandemic (sixth through eighth centuries) and its impact on the lands now controlled by the Ottomans.

Like the travel writers, early modern historians adopted and reflected a Christian viewpoint about the Ottoman Empire's inhabitants and their religious beliefs, sometimes embedding into their accounts negative attitudes about the eastern Mediterranean as a historical place of disease. While Richard Knolles's extensive English-language history of the empire (printed in 1603) is largely a political and dynastic narrative that speaks of plague and other diseases only in passing, it does include numerous references to what Knolles calls plague outbreaks. His view of the Ottomans – which he claimed was based on "the very truth" that he had "Faithfullie collected out of the best Histories, both auntient and moderne, and digested into one continuat Historie" – was that "the glorious Empire of the Turkes [is] the present terrour of the world."[77] The plagues that Knolles highlighted primarily coincided with military sieges and battles during the Crusades, long before the Black Death. Calling such outbreaks "plague," which most contemporary writers would not have done – since fevers, dysenteries, fluxes, and other diseases were known to accompany military activity and were often labeled as such – promoted the idea that plague was both a natural and historical part of the Ottoman landscape. Indeed, in the majority of plague outbreaks that Knolles mentioned, both pre-Black Death and up to the end of the sixteenth century, it was Christian warriors who suffered most grievously, either in the Levant or in south-eastern Europe. Knolles's audience would not have missed allusions that placed plague not in Europe proper, but in the lands of Ottomans who had perhaps become acclimatized to it.

Knolles's history was one in a very long list of works produced in England and France (and elsewhere in Western Europe) between the fifteenth and early eighteenth centuries that discussed the Turks, their history, their manners and customs, their military strength, their system of governance, their religion, and their aggressive expansion.[78] Most, but not all, were based solely on Western sources and espoused a Christian point of view. Knolles's *Generall Historie*, by contrast, purportedly drew from Latin translations of Eastern histories that he then "'digested' (to use his term) … and assimilated … to a Protestant, providential framework."[79] Like most contemporary histories of

England and France, few of these works had much to say directly about plague; what they did say, however, suggested that the historical home of the disease lay in the Ottoman Empire.

Early modern Western historians of the Ottoman Empire made plague an essential part of the region's history in order to advance claims about the region's backwardness. Writing during the London outbreak in 1665, English diplomat and historian Sir Paul Rycaut contended that replenishment of the Turkish population had historically been threatened by, among other things, the regular "Summer-slaughters of the Plague"; only the importation of slaves had kept the Ottoman Empire from collapsing.[80] French historian François Eudes de Mézeray likewise situated the disease in Ottoman lands: a great outbreak in 1637 in Istanbul was not unexpected, since "the plague is an ordinary scourge in the land of the Turks."[81] In this light, since Europe's still-ongoing outbreaks were to be viewed as extraordinary events while those in the Ottoman Empire were simply "ordinary," the authoritative histories suggested – and numerous plague tracts concurred – that the same must have been true in the past.

CONCLUSION

While the majority of early modern English and French tract authors acknowledged that plague arose from specifically unhealthy landscapes, by the mid-seventeenth century their thinking was moving away from local spaces. Some decades earlier, English treatise writers had begun to reuniversalize plague by linking local outbreaks to epidemics in other regions, notably among trading partners such as Holland. Then, before the last great epidemics devastated London (1665) and Marseille (1720), writers in both England and France began to argue that plague was *imported* from foreign lands, meaning in most cases the Ottoman Empire. The geographic and historical origins of plague were politicized increasingly over time, influenced by local socioeconomic and environmental concerns, by travel accounts, by distant colonial projects, and by the availability of new historical texts that revealed the path purportedly taken by the First Pandemic. As new information changed the physical map of the world and as political realities on the ground shifted, plague ultimately became foreign in every way.

Tract writers specifically pointed to the Ottoman Empire, both in the eastern Mediterranean and in northern Africa, as the source of plague. Their purposeful insertion of "Turks" and "*Turky*" into their historical narratives of the disease – when such terms rarely existed in the original sources – also demonstrates that contemporary concerns about and opinions of the Ottoman Empire influenced how these writers read and interpreted their sources. This enabled them to assemble plague's historical narrative in a way that both made sense of the present and privileged geopolitical imperatives. In other words, treatise writers culturally constructed plague's history and its geography. In many respects, doing so reflected broader historiographical practices in which the truth of the past mattered less than the legitimation of contemporary propagandist and political goals. Indeed, within a few short decades of the Marseille outbreak, the contemporary and historical reassignment of plague to the Ottoman Empire was complete.

In his contribution to Diderot and d'Alembert's mid-eighteenth-century *Encyclopédie, ou dictionnaire raisonné des sciences, des arts et des métiers,* Louis de Jaucourt wrote the following entry on *Peste*: "the plague comes from Asia, and for two thousand years all the plagues that have appeared in Europe have been transmitted to us by the Saracens, Arabs, Moors, or Turks; all of our plagues had no other source."[82] In the early 1770s, English physician William Brownrigg took the argument even further, (erroneously) attributing the creation of quarantines solely to the Venetians' attempts to stave off diseased Ottomans: "the Venetians seem to have been the first who established Quarantines in their dominions, about the year 1484, soon after the Turks became their neighbours in Europe: the constant intercourse which they maintained with those powerful neighbours, either in war, or by commerce, rendering it necessary for them to take this, and other precautions, against the introduction of this contagion into their country."[83]

Jaucourt had used the term *peste d'Orient* only in relation to the First Plague Pandemic of the sixth century. Nevertheless, as plague historiography started to be written in earnest in the early nineteenth century, the term was applied more broadly to outbreaks of bubonic plague across time. In his history of the Black Death in 1832, Justus Hecker wrote that the "great pestilence of the fourteenth century … was an oriental plague … [marked by] buboes … [which] are the infallible signs of the oriental plague."[84] In his tract of 1840, Antoine Barthélemy Clot provided many pages of plague definitions and etymologies; citing numerous authorities, he defined plague as a fever that "comes from the oriental countries … [it] always has its origin in the Levant … [and] is endemic in Egypt."[85] Many other medical writers followed suit. This "oriental" plague, in turn, meant both historical outbreaks of plague and those outbreaks of the disease that were still occurring in the eastern Russian and Ottoman Empires. Hecker's use of the term for the Black Death was thereafter entrenched in the historiography. Along with the association that Hecker's history intrinsically created between buboes and the Orient came the attendant assumption that plague had originated, both historically and geographically, among "the Turks."

Plague treatises demonstrate how the links between humans, diseases, and places were continuously reconstructed over time. The treatise writers' contentions about the source of plague, however, were the products of particular places and times. Recent scholarship is only now beginning to dismantle the influence that the narratives created by Mead, Brownrigg, and others have had on the historiography of the Second Plague Pandemic.

CONCLUSION

Rewriting Patterns of Plague

Were it possible to represent those Times exactly to those that did not see them, and give the Reader due Ideas of the Horror that every where presented it self, it must make just Impressions upon their Minds, and fill them with Surprize. *London* might well be said to be all in Tears.

"H.F.," London, 1665/1722[1]

H.F.'s recollections of his plague-besieged city were intended to strike a chord with London's residents as they once again faced the dreaded disease, this time from afar. Through H.F.'s fictional narrative, Daniel Defoe encapsulated contemporary thinking about plague's power to decimate communities, alongside its likely causes and suitable treatments and cures. His references to "those Times" and to the weekly Bills of Mortality set plague into a clear historical context: facing the threat of disease from Marseille in the early eighteenth century, Defoe's readers were transported back to their own "last past plagues" sixty years and more earlier.[2] The majority of London's population in 1722 had no direct experience with the disease, but *A Journal of the Plague Year* offered a "dynamic history" that "harness[ed] the past in order to confront the anxieties and mediate and shape the debates" of the present.[3] It certainly did so, bringing long dormant, and perhaps purposefully supressed, community memories to the surface.

H.F.'s meanderings through the near-empty streets of London imitate the unpredictable mobility of plague itself. His detailed topographies inform readers not only about his walks – during which he encounters "many dismal Scenes before my Eyes" – but also of the archaeological remnants of the plague pits to which he is repeatedly drawn: "the Mark of it was also many Years to be seen in the Church-Yard on the Surface lying in Length, Parallel with the Passage which goes by the West Wall of the Church-Yard, out of *Houndsditch*, and turns East again into *White-Chappel*, coming out near the three Nuns Inn."[4] Although plague had spread far and wide across the city, H.F. "perceiv'd the Infection keept chiefly in the out-Parishes, which being very populous, and fuller also of Poor."[5] Here, he says, "the Distemper found more to prey upon than in the City." Not only are more deaths noted in the poorer areas of town, but the bodies of those who live in these areas are also more likely to be diseased: "So it drew by Consequence, a great Number of Workmen, Manufacturers, and the like, being mostly poor People, who depended upon their Labour."[6] The purported arrival of plague from Holland in a parcel of Levantine silks, followed by that country's refusal (along with France, Spain, and Italy) to accept trade from London once the outbreak was recorded, contrasts with the "not so very rigid" attitude of the "*Turks*" and their propensity to both export and import the disease without concern or precaution.[7]

In H.F.'s narrative, plague is temporal and spatial: it is both modern and historical, both local and foreign. The plague tracts of Defoe's day were much the same: many of them also considered the disease's location in time and space, even blaming the "*Turks*" for the disease's emergence and continued circulation. The overlap between these two contemporary forms of plague literature – fiction and medical – is not surprising, since Defoe drew some of his content directly from the plague treatises of Richard Mead and Nathaniel Hodges. Defoe's *Journal* was also advertised as "This Day is Publish'd" in the same London periodicals such as *Post Boy* and the *Evening Post* that announced both plague news out of Marseille and the printing of new and reissued tracts, such as those by Richard Bradley and Thomas Phayer.[8] Plague treatises were thus associated with Defoe's book "in the popular press and also, presumably, in the booksellers' shops," both types of publication offering advice about precautions to take should plague arrive on England's shores.[9] Just as importantly, the *Journal* was presented as a piece of historical writing and then used as a reliable source of information in the ninth edition of Mead's treatise in 1744.

The close relationship that existed between the *Journal* and eighteenth-century plague tracts accentuates the evolution in those treatises' contents over time, but only when we look beyond them solely as texts that offered formulaic medical explanations and advice. Identifying and unpacking the ways in which social changes, both incremental and transformative, influenced and are reflected in the treatises lies at the heart of this book. A short examination of tracts written by John of Burgundy, Nicolas de Nancel, and Richard Mead both provides evidence of the formulaic responses and medical continuity long recognized in the historiography and highlights many of the key findings presented here.

These physicians' treatises spanned some three and one half centuries and came from three separate cities. They appeared in three different languages.[10] All followed the genre's formulaic arrangement of explanation, prevention, and treatment. Each author also touted his medical credentials, proclaimed his humility, insisted that he was writing for public good rather than for individual gain, and inserted personal vignettes. In all three instances, the authors drew explanations and advice from longstanding medical tradition and practice. Yet each also claimed to provide the most up-to-date evidence of successful plague prevention and management, confident that *his* treatment and preventive recommendations were effective and practical, and thus more likely to succeed than those of his predecessors.

Writing in the mid-1360s in Liège, at the time of the first severe reappearance of plague after the Black Death (*the pestis secunda*), John of Burgundy argued that since some physicians had gained direct experience with plague, there now existed a set of specialized medical skills and knowledge unknown to ancient authorities: "the masters of the present day rely more on experience [for treating and preventing plague] than did their predecessors. And so it is said ... that experience makes talent."[11] In Tours in the early 1580s, Nicolas de Nancel downplayed physicians' *lack* of success in actually treating plague victims, and advanced the recommendation of late sixteenth-century humanists: return to the traditional sources. For Nancel, closely following the ancient masters was more beneficial than relying on the trials and errors of modern apothecaries who "muddle innumerable Arabic words, and pervert in a number of places the intent of the good Greek authors whom [they] neither read, nor followed, nor understood."[12] In early eighteenth-century London, Richard Mead contended that he needed to promote current knowledge rather than old errors and misunderstandings: "proper Directions should be drawn up to defend our selves from such a Calamity ... [including] some new Regulations ... [which] I persuade my Self, will be found agreable to Reason."[13] Despite his appeal to the evolution and advancement of medical theory and practice over the centuries, though, many of Mead's proposed treatments would not have seemed entirely foreign to those who read John of Burgundy or Nancel's tracts centuries earlier. In fact, the three writers offered the same basic recommendations: manage the six non-naturals, use plasters, specially-prepared powders, theriac, and herbs mixed with wine, and rely on phlebotomy.[14] Their temporal and geographical distance, then, had little impact on the treatises' medical-therapeutic contents, despite their authors' fervent claims to the contrary.

Although each author offered much the same medical advice as his predecessors, a closer look reveals that ideas about when and where plague arose did change over time. John of Burgundy's tract discussed, in hindsight, his belief that the Black Death had been caused by the relics of a malevolent astrological conjunction that were likely to re-erupt: "in fact, it was chiefly due to the influence of the celestial bodies [in 1345] that the air became corrupted and the pestilential effects appeared … [and] infected many."[15] The next outbreak of the early 1360s thus occupied a place on a short timeline that he expected would continue into the future. In modern terminology, he spoke of endemicity.

Nicolas de Nancel wrote his work specifically for the people of Tours to explain an outbreak in the midst of France's Wars of Religion. For Nancel, plague was both a human disease and a sign of the declining health of his kingdom. It had emerged from the disordered heart of the city of Paris and then spread throughout the kingdom by human endeavour, much like everything else did at the time. "It was only right that since Paris, the head and heart of France, was suffering, all of the other members and dependencies [of the kingdom] should also suffer. Being the centre, it distributes its misfortune to the whole circumference; this is just like in times past when it was flourishing and sent forth its goods, gifts, and favours both for the proper regulation of justice, and also for all the good arts, sciences, and disciplines and for trade."[16]

Nancel drew from descriptions of past epidemics found in manuscripts carried to Western Europe by *émigrés* after the fall of Constantinople in 1453 and compared his own outbreak to them. He tentatively interpreted the origins of Tours's outbreak in a way that differed considerably from the explanations used by earlier writers.[17] His successors then built upon, expanded, and extrapolated from his chronology, ultimately feeding into the construction of narratives about plague's long history and broad geography.

When Richard Mead penned his treatise in 1720, plague was raging in Marseille but had been absent from London for almost sixty years. This suggested to him that plague could not have ever been endemic in England, despite the kingdom's centuries-long history with the disease. Rather, he argued, it had always been imported from overseas. Turkey was the most likely original source of plague because its climate, its landscape, its foreignness, its cotton exports, its ongoing epidemics, and its inhabitants' perceived fatalism and lack of public health measures contrasted so sharply (in Mead's mind) with the healthiness, hardiness, orderliness, and rationality of England and its people. Like Nancel, Mead situated the origin of plague among dangerous Others; to Mead, though, these Others now lay outside rather than inside his own homeland: "From all that has been said, it appears, I think, very plainly that the *Plague* is a real Poison, which being bred in the Eastern or Southern Parts of the World, maintains itself there ... chiefly owing to the Negligence of the People in those Countries, who are stupidly Careless in this affair."[18]

Digging deeper into the particular contexts in which English and French tract writers lived, and into the divergent production practices through which they disseminated their works, reveals the many important local differences that exist in these works. These differences reflect allusions to events, persons, or belief systems that might have been comprehensible only to a specific audience at a particular moment in time. This is not to suggest that all treatises included insightful comments about their authors' beliefs concerning plague. Nevertheless, the majority of authors that I examined did step outside, or around, this formulaic structure to address other issues, demonstrating the great value that can be gained with close reading, historical context, and material analysis. The tracts are, in short, "emphatically more interesting and revealing than [their] innocent, arid, infra-literary text character appears to suggest."[19]

The ways in which local knowledge is generated is contingent upon time and place. Just as the accumulation and evolution of plague experiences reshaped national literary cultures, so too did the evolution of socio-religious, technological, intellectual, and geopolitical experiences reshape plague treatises.[20] Broader societal-level changes influenced how people perceived the world around them and directly shaped the dialogues that authors were having with their readers. Whereas the earliest writers blamed universal disorder for the Black Death, local (national) disorder – and especially poverty and religious dissidence – had become the culprit by the late fifteenth and early sixteenth centuries.[21] In the latter case, plague arose in and was spread through those people whose bodies and behaviours ran contrary to what was perceived to be the appropriate local identity. After the mid-seventeenth century and into the eighteenth, blame shifted yet again, and plague was carried on and within persons and commodities imported from elsewhere. This time, it was the eastern Mediterranean that was to blame, where religious, political, and epidemiological differences set the Ottoman Empire clearly apart from nascent European imperial projects. The spaces onto which writers wrote the disorder on which they blamed plague – universal, local/national, foreign – thus corresponded, albeit in a somewhat delayed fashion, with the evolution in thinking about the communities to which they belonged: a universal Christendom, an emerging state, a trans-polity empire.

Greater attention to the role of religion lies outside the scope of this book, but it is important to recognize that the Reformation and Counter-Reformation were widespread, regional movements that had local implications on the development of plague tracts. Reformation and Counter-Reformation ideology and rhetoric, heated and often violent debate, and decidedly religious explanations for plague appear in plague treatises during the more tumultuous years of the sixteenth century, before largely disappearing again in the second half of the seventeenth century. The appearance of new and radical changes in medical theory and practice during the same turbulent era likewise brought change – and again heated debate – even to the apparently stable prevention and cure sections of plague tracts.

The rise of humanist natural philosophy and science generated a new esteem for both history and geography as branches of learning and of knowledge that had a longer-term influence on plague tracts. The significant increase in published works on *historia* and *geographia* after the fifteenth century, and the increased production of narratives based on travel abroad, are a testament to growing interest in these topics not only among erudite readers, but also among the broader public. Treatise writers were slow in their uptake of humanist principles but by the later sixteenth century, significant changes began to appear in both the contents and style of plague treatises. The inclusion of ancient sources enabled authors to talk about recorded outbreaks of the past. Consideration of other places also facilitated comparisons of outbreaks from one city or country to another, and the turn to a more narrative style of writing allowed for longer discussions of (and digressions about) issues of local interest and concern that had little, on the surface, to do with disease epidemics.

I also have drawn attention to important phenomena in the evolution of plague epistemology. As the target audience became increasingly familiar with the disease, historically specific information about it became less necessary and plague knowledge became both vernacularized and localized. Historical knowledge was an integral part of medieval medicine: treatise authors had attempted, and some openly remarked on their failure, to link the Black Death to historically-known medical facts. Yet already by the fifteenth century, the recently acquired historical references about a universal plague were, in a sense, stripped out of the plague treatises because recurrent, localized outbreaks made them increasingly less relevant.

By the early fifteenth century, people's participation in and shared experience of a world with plague also meant that some of the body of accumulated knowledge about the disease could be excluded from the tracts because both writers and their audiences were sufficiently familiar with contextual references to "the mortality" or "the pestilence" to know what was being discussed. This is evidence of "residual orality" and suggests that the oral transmission of plague knowledge far exceeded its textual counterpart.[22]

Further, increased familiarity with the disease and its symptoms, coupled with the at-most cursory mentions of later outbreaks in lay sources, points to an emerging recognition that plague had become what is now known as endemic (or, more properly, enzootic, because humans are not long-term carriers or hosts of the disease). Guy de Chauliac wrote his work in the early 1360s "in case" the disease returned; by the end of the century, writers commonly used the phrase "when pestilence reigns." Textual references like these, and to the disease's "traces" (as noted by John of Burgundy), indicate recognition that this disease was both different from other epidemics and that it returned with regularity.

Finally, evolving concepts and use of space, place, mapping, and geographical imagination – including in relation to nature, the environment, landscape, and geographical Otherness – influenced contemporary perceptions of the source and spread of disease. These perceptions transformed in step with evolutions in geographic imagination, the map of the world, and territorial expansion/colonization. Together, they contributed to the shift of plague's origins from local to foreign. All of these phenomena are based, in part, on historical and geographical realities, but they also reflect changing political contexts from which the evolution of plague epistemology cannot be separated.

Two observations become immediately clear. First, the pace and direction of change differed between English and French treatises. Most of the trends related to authorship, printing, historical timelines, and the naming of plagued places began in the French tracts long before they took hold in the English ones. The main content change that appeared first in English tracts was the identification of "Turkey" as the source of plague in the mid-seventeenth.

Second, the period covering approximately the last quarter of the sixteenth century to the Great Plague of London in 1665 saw the most transformative sets of changes in tract contents in both kingdoms. This era witnessed the turn to history and the first renewed recollections of the Black Death and, eventually, of the First Pandemic. Plague had for centuries been domesticated. Then, relatively suddenly, it was not. This period observed authors' early attempts to trace epidemic outbreaks as they advanced from one place to another, both domestic and foreign. The period also marked the emerging tendency to blame the Ottoman Empire for both historical and modern outbreaks. Finally, it was also in this era that London became the site of disease in English treatises. While some scholars herald the last quarter of the fifteenth century as a key point of historical change because of the transition from manuscript to print, print technology had a less significant impact on plague tract contents than the spread of humanist ideas and modes of writing and the slow decline of the Ottoman Empire. These changes in thinking and writing appeared across Western Europe around the same time, albeit in noticeably localized ways.

By shifting the focus from the plague treatises' medical contents to the people who produced them, I suggest that the tracts can be recast as cultural works. Such treatises are not simply containers of medical knowledge; rather, they act as witnesses to their authors' specific times and places and capture changing ideas about the world. They offer, for example, the nascent beginnings of the Oriental plague myth. Between the last great outbreaks in London in 1665 and in Marseille in 1720–22, a newly constructed plague mythology took hold that focused on the eastern Mediterranean as the disease's ancestral locus. This story then became an integral component of all subsequent discussions about the disease. Plague, as later treatise authors portrayed it, was no longer just a disease; it was also a manifestation of disorder and Otherness in the contemporary world. These primary sources offer a window into how people perceived the world around them and where they believed that disease fit into that world.

Such observations are not, of course, limited to England and France. Ongoing comparative studies will bring into the mix tracts produced in the Holy Roman Empire, the Italian republics, Iberia, the Byzantine Empire, the Islamic polities, the Ottoman Empire, and elsewhere – as well as the treatises written by Jewish and Muslim authors in Europe. This work will further elucidate the ways in which the trends noted here intersected with purely local contexts to inform discussions of plague that were at once universal and particular. A more comprehensive comparison of plague tracts with other types of medical writing would also elucidate whether the evolutions noted in the plague texts are unique.

Additional questions may also be asked of the treatises studied here: Is it possible to identify who read and/or used these treatises and, if so, to what effect? Did the status of the printer – royal, guild-registered, or unregistered – affect the tracts' contents and/or circulation? What role did censorship and patronage play on treatise contents? In what ways did changing understanding of plague impact local actions taken to manage it? These questions are especially relevant because local places of disease were conceived of differently in England and in France.

Two decades ago, one scholar observed that the "proliferation of experts' plague treatises in the sixteenth and seventeenth centuries [in Italy] ... occurred partly because one set of experiences about plague was not transferable to another locale. However generic medical and public health understanding might have been, plague's causes and meanings were attached to place, person, and the particular."[23] Through its detailed exploration of some two hundred treatises from England and France, my book has reinforced this observation. Whether he wrote his own tract in anticipation of a universal outbreak, or penned one in the midst of a local epidemic, or copied and adapted a much older treatise to suit new historical and geographical contexts, each French and English writer represented a singular intersection of knowledge, belief, practice, experience, and context. I have teased apart some of these factors across linguistic, historical, and geographical boundaries to demonstrate continuity and change, evolution and revision, in a long-lived genre of medical literature. Together, these tracts provide personal stories of plague and the ways in which writers, copiers, translators, and printers attempted to set the disease into a framework of the world – local, national, universal – that was itself constantly evolving.

To this cause I have endeavoured to write this little regimen to aid, to succour, and to provide for everyone who is or may be taken and touched by pestilence. And whoever would like to read and understand without being bored of what I have composed, would benefit more from doing so than they would from [reading] romances and chronicles where many often pass their time. And thus I put an end to this present regimen made and composed by Master Thomas le Forestier, medical doctor.[24]

Notes

INTRODUCTION

1 Defoe, *Journal*, 1. Candia was the Venetian Republic's colony on Crete (c. 1212–1669). It was surrendered to the Ottomans in 1669, after several years of siege.
2 Ibid.
3 Ibid., 73.
4 Ibid., 89. By "invisible Creatures," H.F./Defoe referred to theories proposed in Kircher, *Scrutinium Physico-Medicum Contagiosae Luis*. Kircher had used a microscope to investigate the blood of plague victims and claimed to have seen little worms or animalcules that he argued had infected that blood with plague.
5 Ibid., 14.
6 On newly-discovered contemporary medical writing about the First Plague Pandemic, see Mulhall, "Confronting Pandemic." I address this point -further in the chapters that follow.
7 This discontinuity in plague memory among Western European scholars stands in stark contrast to the Islamic Mediterranean, where there was unbroken learned and historical knowledge of the disease between the First and Second Pandemics. See more on this topic in chapter 3.
8 Silva, *Miraculous Plagues*. Silva's work focuses on early New England, but his observation that recurrent disease experiences caused deep social and religious turbulence applies well to late medieval and early modern "Old World" societies.
9 On different types of plague writing in England, see, among others, Totaro and Gilman, ed., *Representing Plague*; Totaro, trans. and ed., *Plague in Print*; Gilman, *Plague Writing*; Healy, *Fictions of Disease*; and Achinstein,

"Plagues and Publication." For France, see Slerca, "Guillaume de Machaut et Boccace"; Hobart, "L'Imaginaire de la Peste" and *La Peste à la Renaissance.*

10 Varlık, "Between Local and Universal," 177.

11 Ibid.

12 Cummins, Kelly, and Ó Gráda, "Living Standards," 5.

13 Siena, *Rotten Bodies*, 49–51; and Slack, *Impact of Plague*, 245.

14 Jones, "Plague and Its Metaphors," 99. On the peril of relying on unverified historical assumptions about plague outbreaks and mortality in any location, see Roosen and Curtis, "Dangers."

15 Plague tracts continued to react to large outbreaks in Russia and the Middle East, and to smaller outbreaks around the Adriatic, in the later eighteenth and nineteenth centuries. These later outbreaks are beyond the scope of this book, but their long-term effect on Western Europeans' plague *mentalités* are explored persuasively in Varlık, "Oriental Plague."

16 On the influence of early modern foreign-origin assumptions on plague historiography and epidemiology, see Varlık, "Oriental Plague," and chapter 5. This assumption has also appeared in the scientific literature, as I discuss below.

17 The phrase comes from Morsel, "Traces? Quelles traces?" 858.

18 Cavallo and Storey seek to overturn long-standing historiographical portrayals of health regimens as static, uninteresting, and unworthy of detailed analysis in *Healthy Living.*

19 Fissell, "Making Meaning," 365.

20 An outsider's (*etic*) approach does not fully consider contemporary personal experiences and mind-sets (*emic*) or the historical context in which they existed. For a theoretical discussion, see Jardine, "Etics and Emics." On the importance of using both approaches for plague studies see Green, "Editor's Introduction."

21 Thomas, *Religion and the Decline of Magic*, 219.

22 Jenner, "Plague on a Page," 261. Jenner was writing about plague broadsheets when he made this observation, but the point is equally valid for the treatises.

23 Siraisi, *History, Medicine, and Traditions*. Eggert's recent work points to a decline in the pre-eminence of humanism, and indeed a growing disdain for it, before the early seventeenth century due to "a number of sixteenth-century sea changes in intellectual culture" and to humanism's inadequate response to "the religious, intellectual, and political challenges of the day." Even so, she notes, humanist education persisted, leading to "a complex and often fraught interchange between a humanistic reverence for classical

learning and empirical demonstrations of how Galen, Aristotle, and other paradigmatic classical authors on medicine" had been incorrect. *Disknowledge*, 15–16, 159. Some of the same complex and fraught interchanges can be viewed in the later plague tracts, but the point here is that the innovations in writing style, the integration of different disciplines, and the availability of new (old) source materials that marked humanist medicine brought about a permanent change in the tracts and their contents. I discuss this in more detail in chapters 3 and 4.

24 Several excellent studies examine visions of religious/social disorder through plague tracts, especially during the Reformation/Counter Reformation. See, for example, Healy, *Fictions of Disease* and "Discourses of Plague"; Semmens, "Plague, Propaganda and Prophetic Violence"; and Harris, *Foreign Bodies*. I explore some of these ideas in the chapters below.

25 Leong, "Transformative Itineraries."

26 Spyrou et al., "Analysis of 3800-Year-Old *Yersinia pestis* Genomes"; Rascovan et al., "Emergence and Spread"; and Spyrou et al., "Ancient Pathogen Genomics."

27 The possibility of a Bronze Age pandemic has also been raised in Brooke, "Thinking Big," drawing on Valtueña et al., "Stone Age Plague"; Rasmussen et al., "Early Divergent Strains"; and Furholt, "Massive Migrations?" There is, however, no clear evidence to support this suggestion. Historical and scientific literature on the effects of the First Pandemic throughout the Mediterranean and across Europe has expanded recently; see especially Little, ed., *Plague and the End of Antiquity*; Gruber, "Indirect Evidence"; and Keller et al., "Ancient *Yersinia pestis* Genomes." For a contrary (but at points problematic) consideration of its social and demographic effects, see Eisenberg and Mordechai, "Justinianic Plague," and Mordechai and Eisenberg, "Rejecting Catastrophe." Rebuttals of their arguments can be found in McCormick, "Gregory of Tours," and Meier, "Justinianic Plague." On the possibility of plague in medieval Sub-Saharan Africa, see the special 2018 volume of *Afriques*, which examines historical, archaeological, literary, and genetic evidence. The large regional outbreak in Central Europe implicated the Balkans, the Habsburg territories, Poland, the Baltic State, Brandenburg–East Prussia, Denmark, and Sweden. On late Russian and Ottoman outbreaks, see Mikhail, "Nature of Plague"; Alexander, *Bubonic Plague*; and Panzac, *La peste dans l'empire ottoman*. On the Third Pandemic, see Echenberg, *Plague Ports*.

28 Green, "Climate and Disease," 14; Gage and Kosoy, "Natural History of Plague"; and Poinar, "Synergies."

29 Green, "Putting Africa on the Black Death Map."

30 Thus, multiple strains of *Y. pestis* from the same lineage are now known to have existed during the First Pandemic, "demonstrating the geographic range of plague [during the pandemic] and showing microdiversity in the Early Medieval Period." Keller et al., "Ancient *Yersinia pestis* Genomes," 12363.

31 Varlık, "New Science and Old Sources," 198. See Varlık's longer discussion, 196–201. Fancy's current work on pre–Black Death Islamic writings about plague also emphasizes this point. Fancy, "Knowing the Signs of Disease." On the earlier beginnings of the Second and Third Pandemics, see also Green, "Putting Africa on the Black Death Map."

32 Ziegler, "Black Death," 266.

33 For excellent summaries of both the debates and the microbiological studies that ended them, see Green, "Taking 'Pandemic' Seriously," and Little, "Plague Historians in Lab Coats."

34 On the establishment of European plague reservoirs, see Carmichael, "Plague Persistence"; Slavin, "Out of the West"; Seifert et al., "Genotyping"; Bos et al., "Eighteenth Century *Yersinia pestis* Genomes"; Spyrou et al., "Phylogeography"; Giffin et al., "Treponemal Genome"; and Morozova et al., "New Ancient Eastern European *Yersinia pestis* Genomes." In *Plague and Empire*, Varlık demonstrates how, for at least the period 1453–1517, the Ottoman Empire was in fact infected from the West, rather than the other way around. On the archaeological presence of rats, see Orton, "The Long Black Rat," and McCormick, "Rats, Communications, and Plague."

35 For a thorough assessment and summary of palaeogenetic studies of *Yersinia pestis* and their implications for a new understanding of the history and geography of plague, see Green, "Putting Africa on the Black Death Map" and "The Historian, the Archaeologist, and the Geneticist"; as well as Green and Jones, "Evolution and Spread."

36 Before the Late Bronze Age, the bacteria had not yet acquired the virulence factors associated with epidemic spread. The evidence at this point also suggests that "multiple forms of the bacterium were circulating in Eurasia between five thousand and three thousand years ago that may have had different transmission cycles and produced different disease phenotypes." Spyrou et al., "Ancient Pathogen Genomics," 334–5. On the challenge of tracing origins, see Poinar, "Synergies."

37 The first modelling suggested c. 1268 CE for the polytomy; subsequent modelling puts it around the year 1196 (Cui et al., "Historical Variations"; and Spyrou et al., "Analysis of 3800-Year-Old *Yersinia pestis* Genomes") or

c. 1300 (Spyrou, "Towards an Understanding"). For the broader significance of this polytomy, see Green, "Four Black Deaths."

38 Recent research also points to the "pandemic-like" behaviour of strains in Branch 2, which are widely spread throughout Eurasia and have been associated with high mortality epidemics. Eroshenko et al., "Evolution and Circulation of *Yersinia pestis*." I thank Hendrik Poinar for bringing this research to my attention.

39 Using contemporary chronicles and references to them, Barker provides a very insightful overview of the emergence and spread of plague around the Caspian and Black Seas before it was transmitted into the Mediterranean and thence into Europe in "Laying the Corpses to Rest." I am grateful to Hannah Barker for allowing me to see a pre-publication version of her article.

40 Among many other sources, see on climate: Green, "Climate and Disease"; on regular versus mass graves: Kacki, "Black Death," and Cressford et al., "Beyond Plague Pits"; on plague selectivity: DeWitte and Kowaleski, "Black Death Bodies," and DeWitte and Wood, "Selectivity"; on immunology and syndemics: Crespo, "Leprosy in Medieval Europe." For the ways that new scientific studies are informing historical studies of plague, see also Poinar, "Synergies."

41 Later, their theoretical conceptions of human illness also left little room to consider the possibility that long-lasting local plague reservoirs had established themselves in Europe and around the Mediterranean. Modern historians and scientists have had difficulty considering that same possibility until recently. Schmid et al., "Climate-Driven Introductions"; Spyrou et al., "Ancient Pathogen Genomics"; Bos et al., "Eighteenth Century *Yersinia pestis* Genomes."

42 Varlık, "Oriental Plague."

CHAPTER ONE

1 "*timentes de corrupcione propter vicinitatem sicut illi de Parisius, et nos et multi alii.*" Paris, Bibliothèque nationale de France (BnF), Latin MS 11227, cited in Coville, "Écrits contemporains," 329.

2 Ibid.

3 "*et teneo firmiter quod cum bono regimine illud sufficeret pro remedio epidemie vel pro resistendo.*" Ibid., 329–30.

4 Boccaccio, *Decameron*, 7. Other contemporaries were even less generous in their assessments. The Florentine chronicler Matteo Villani complained that "doctors from every part of the world had no good remedy or

effective cure ... To gain money some went visiting and dispensing their remedies, but these only demonstrated through their patients' death that their art was nonsense and false." Quoted in Aberth, *Black Death*, 37. Others blamed physicians for refusing to treat the ill or for running away. Tract writers also frequently condemned the theories and techniques of their colleagues and of non-university-trained practitioners. Even when not so viscerally criticizing physicians, chroniclers were quick to notice their apparent inability (or unwillingness) to treat or heal plague victims. The fourteenth-century Florentine chronicler Marchionne di Coppo Stefani thus noted "neither physician, nor medicine sufficed, either because the disease was not yet understood or because the physicians had never encountered this disease in their studies and no remedy applied was of value ... either one could find no doctor, because they had died alongside plague's other victims, or those who could be found wanted a huge sum of money before agreeing to enter the house" ["*non valeva né medico, né medicina, o che non fosse ancora conosciuta quella malattia o che i medici non avessero sopra quella mai studiato e non parca che rimedio vi fosse ... i meilici non si trovavano perché morivano come gli altri e quelli che si trovavano volevano smisurato prezzo innanzi che entrassero nella casa*"]. Crisciani, "Città e medici," 12. I thank Ann Carmichael for both bringing this article to my attention and her translation of Crisciani's work.

5 For a detailed review of the broad literature on both *consilia* and *regimina* in the Christian European medical tradition, and a troubling of the distinction between the two genres, see Hardingham, "Regimen in Late Medieval England," especially 1–8. See also Agrimi and Crisciani, "Consilia medicaux"; Cavallo and Storey, *Healthy Living*; and Nicoud, *Les régimes de santé*. On the *consilium* and *regimen* in Islamicate and Jewish cultures, see Bos, *Maimonides, On the Regimen of Health* and *Maimonides, On the Elucidation of Some Symptoms*.

6 This overview belies a rather more complicated situation. Medical texts on plague appeared with a largely similar formulaic structure across the Mediterranean world (and beyond) in several languages within a very short period of time, making it difficult to determine exactly how and when the genre coalesced. When we examine the contents of different tracts in more detail, it also becomes evident that not all included the three main components noted here. In the Christian and Jewish traditions, some writers focused on one component over the others, often with great elaboration, and even neglected some parts altogether. In the Arabic tradition as well, the tripartite structure is neither a given nor necessary for a text to be considered a plague treatise. Many of the latter do incorporate the

causation, treatment, and prophylaxis elements, but within a larger narrative framework that, unlike the Christian and Hebrew texts, also engages directly with prayer, ḥadīth, and additional elements. Others are a blend of chronologies, medical explanations, religious responses, and even poetic laments. The tripartite structure too was the standard formula for discussing disease in Arabic medical texts in general, such as Avicenna's *Canon of Medicine,* a traditional authority in Latin medical education. Perhaps what best distinguishes the plague tract genre from earlier texts about the disease was that before the Black Death, few if any individual (i.e., monographical) works were devoted specifically to plague. I discuss the absence of this tradition in the Christian European world in chapter 3. I thank Susan Einbinder, Nahyan Fancy, Monica H. Green, Justin Stearns, and Nükhet Varlık for discussing these points with me. On early Islamic plague writing, see Conrad, "Arabic Plague Chronologies and Treatises"; Fancy, "Knowing the Signs of Disease"; Fancy and Green, "Plague and the Fall of Baghdad"; and Stearns, *Infectious Ideas.* On Hebrew plague tract writing, see Bos and Mensching, "The Black Death in Hebrew Literature," and Einbinder, *After the Black Death.*

7 "Treatise of John of Burgundy," in Horrox, *Black Death*, 186.

8 For a detailed discussion of the earliest tracts written by university-trained physicians around the Mediterranean, see Arrizabalaga, "Facing the Black Death." On Agramont, see "Regiment de Preservacio," 57–89. Agramont has been called the first plague tract author in Winslow and Duran-Reynals, "Jacme d'Agramont," although his work also speaks to other diseases.

9 On Foligno, see Campbell, *Black Death*, 9–10; on Ibn Khātimah, see Stearns, *Infectious Ideas*, 82–5; for the argument that the Paris Medical Faculty requested Damouzy's tract, see Jacquart, "La perception par les contemporains," 240; on Caslari, see Einbinder, *After the Black Death*, 57–87.

10 The term "Islamicate" refers to regions in which Muslims were culturally dominant, but the person in question may not have been Muslim him/herself. The term is increasingly preferred over "Islamic," which ignores the many different cultures and religions present in Muslim-dominated territories.

11 I thank Susan Einbinder and Justin Stearns for discussing these cases with me. See also García-Ballester, Ferre, and Feliu, "Jewish Appreciation." Even among Christians, university physicians were not the only healers who discussed or treated plague, but they were much more likely to record their opinions in these early decades of the Second Plague Pandemic.

12 Research on early Arabic treatises from the eastern Mediterranean is still in its early stages, and new treatises are being discovered and studied as this book is being written. Given the broader definition of plague tract in the Arabic tradition, it is likely that this number will grow.

13 Ḥadīth are reports about or records of what the prophet Muhammad is believed to have said and done. Since the First Plague Pandemic coincided with the emergence of Islam, Muhammad's actions and directives about how to address and cope with the disease were an important consideration in Arabic treatises.

14 Totaro and Gilman, eds., *Representing Plague*; Totaro, trans. and ed., *Plague in Print*; Gilman, *Plague Writing*; Healy, *Fictions of Disease*; Achinstein, "Plagues and Publication"; Slerca, "Guillaume de Machaut et Boccace"; and Hobart, "L'Imaginaire de la Peste" and *La Peşte à la Renaissance*.

15 "Astrological Causes of the Plague, Geoffrey de Meaux," in Horrox, *Black Death*, 167.

16 See, for example, Fabbri, "Continuity and Change."

17 Such personal interjections and the repetitive elements of the early treatises might be seen as an effort to counter popular notions that elite practitioners had no effective responses to plague and to impress upon plague sufferers that they did not need alternative medicines or groups of practitioners. Crisciani, "Città e medici."

18 See Rawcliffe, *Medicine and Society*, 30–9; and Nutton, "Humoralism."

19 "Astrological Causes of the Plague," in Horrox, *Black Death*, 167.

20 Abraham Caslari, the Jewish physician in Catalonia, stands as a marked contrast here. Einbinder has demonstrated clearly how Caslari's tract is imbued with confidence, both of his conviction that this epidemic was *not* abnormal (and not a true pestilence), and that he could (and did) properly and successfully diagnose and treat those stricken by the illness. Einbinder attributes this to the fact that the disease only (relatively) lightly touched Besalú, where Caslari was living. His experience with plague was thus much different than that of most of his peers. See *After the Black Death*, 58, 62, 71.

21 A similar method of rethinking traditional theory has recently been uncovered in the writings of the sixth- and seventh-century physicians John of Alexandria, Stephanus of Athens, and Paul of Aegina, for whom plague was likewise unknown. These authors not only described the symptoms of plague, but also developed a medical understanding of the disease that required them to adapt what they had learned in light of their hands-on experience during the First Plague Pandemic. In so doing, they

constructed innovative responses to an unprecedented pandemic. Much of their thinking about and explanations of what caused plague was replicated anew during the Black Death, even though their writing on the subject was unknown to mid-fourteenth century physicians. See Mulhall, "Confronting Pandemic." I thank John Mulhall for sharing his article with me before its publication.

22 One obvious exception to this is Jacme d'Agramont, who claimed that plague was God's punishment for human sin. For an exemplary comparison of the religious contents of two contemporary tracts written in Catalonia by Agramont and Abraham Caslari, a Jewish physician, see Einbinder, *After the Black Death*, 57–87.

23 The malignant temperaments of Saturn (bad luck/misfortune) and Mars (war/anger/violence) were believed to dominate Jupiter's more benign temperament (prosperity/good fortune), with predictably catastrophic results. These theories evolved from the thirteenth-century philosopher Albertus Magnus's *De effectibus planetarum in elementis*. Since the universe acted as an integrated system, planetary conjunctions had the power to influence the state and health of people and everything else on earth. Some medical practitioners offered astrological predictions along with remedial therapies, and all good physicians took astral influences into account when making diagnoses and prescribing treatments. Medieval physicians who neglected astronomy appeared to their peers as incompetent or negligent. The Alpine earthquake caused massive damage and was one of the most devastating earthquakes in the eastern Alps in some two thousand years. Its occurrence just before the arrival of plague in Venice made the link between the two disasters appear obvious to some tract writers. The September 1349 earthquake in central Italy was comprised of four separate, related quakes and is still seen to be one of the most catastrophic natural events in the region.

24 London, British Library (BL), Cotton Caligula MS AII, f. 65v. A similar explanation appears in the writings of medical writers during the First Plague Pandemic. See Mulhall, "Confronting Pandemic."

25 Oxford, Bodleian Library (Bodl.), Ashmole MS 1443, f. 376v.

26 Einbinder, *After the Black Death*, 76. As Einbinder notes, Caslari was well aware that his views were in the minority, and he felt the need to ensure that they were heard and disseminated. They are worth noting here because they point to the lack of agreement among tract writers about what ultimately caused the Black Death as well as the need to read each of the texts on its own terms.

27 "*Et fuit tante contagiositatis, specialiter que fuit cum sputo sanguinis, quod non solum morando sed eciam inspiciendo unus recipiebat de alio.*" Chauliac, *Inventarium sive chirurgia magna*, 118.

28 Arrizabalaga emphasizes this point for the earliest tract writers in "Facing the Black Death," while Kinzelbach makes it for later authors in "Infection, Contagion, and Public Health." See also Jacquart, "Theory."

29 Even centuries later, the distinction between contagion and miasma remained murky, and became a hot topic of debate among medical writers. DeLacy, *Germ of an Idea.*

30 On Agramont and Cordoba's references to manufactured plague and their possible links to attacks on Jewish populations, see Einbinder, *After the Black Death*, 64–6; and Arrizabalaga, "*Pestis Manufacta.*"

31 Arrizabalaga, "Facing the Black Death," 262–87. Similar ideas can be seen among Muslim medical practitioners. Stearns, *Infectious Ideas*, 69.

32 For a more detailed discussion of this disconnect between medical training and hands-on plague experience, see Jones, "Experience over Education."

33 Mussis, "The Arrival of the Plague," in Horrox, *Black Death*, 24.

34 Agramont, "Jacme d'Agramont," 57, 62.

35 "*ex quibus humoribus sit dispositus causabuntur bubones, herisipili, carbunculi, et alia diversa genera apostematum.*" Bernard Alberti, quoted in Chase, "Fevers, Poisons, and Apostemes," 165, fn. 21. Erysipelas is an infection marked by a fiery red rash with raised edges, while a carbuncle is a cluster of boils.

36 Leipzig, Universitätsbibliothek (UB Leipzig), MS 1178, cited in Sudhoff, "Pestschriften" (17), 37–8.

37 For a longer discussion of plague descriptions in the treatises, see Jones, "'Apostumes, Carbuncles, and Botches.'"

38 On medieval phlebotomy, see Voigts and McVaugh, "Latin Technical Phlebotomy," and Gil-Sotres, "Derivation and Revulsion."

39 Cambridge, Trinity College (TCC), MS R.14.52, ff. 156v–7r.

40 London, Wellcome Collection (Wellcome), MS 674, 32. This part of the manuscript is paginated, rather than foliated.

41 A pomander is a ball or perforated container of sweet-smelling substances, often carried or worn on the clothing to protect against infection.

42 TCC MS R.14.52, ff. 155v–6r.

43 Fabbri, "Treating Medieval Plague."

44 Chauliac, cited in Grant, *Source Book*, 774.

45 "*premierement escrit en langue syrienne par Rasès … interprété en grec par Alexandre Traillian et nouvellement traduit de grec en françois par M. Sebastien Colin Medicin a Fontenay.*" Colin, *Traicté de la peste*, title page.

46 Drouet, *Consilium novum de pestilentia*, translated as Twyne, *New counsell against the pestilence*, n.p.

47 Ibid.

48 Occult sciences also appeared in Islamicate and Jewish tracts, as discussed in Melvin-Koushki, "Taşköprīzāde," and Einbinder, *Writing Plague*.

49 Drouet, *Consilium novum*, n.p.

50 Aberth provides an excellent analysis of early tract writer Gentile da Foligno's discussion of poison in *Doctoring the Black Death*, chapter 1.

51 Miller provides a good overview of the vociferousness of some of these debates in *Literary Culture of Plague*, especially in chapter 3.

52 Thomson, *Loimotomia*, A3, 174, A3–4. On the rise of alternative medical theories and practices in England, see Webster, *Great Instauration*; and Wear, *Knowledge & Practice*, 353–443. On the link between the new medicine and civil unrest in England, see Webster, "Paracelsus."

53 Thomson, *Loimotomia*, 20.

54 Brockliss and Jones, *Medical World*, 119–28, 138–9; and Debus, *French Paracelsians*.

55 Fabre, *Traicté de la Peste*.

56 "*Les Impostures Spagyriques, & plusieurs abus de la Médecine, Chirurgie & Pharmacie*." Suau, *Traitez contenans la pure et vraye doctrine*, title page. A spagyrist is an alchemist.

57 On the shift to empiricism and experimentation, see Jones, "Experience over Education"; Stolberg, "The Student Perspective"; Cook, *Decline of the Old Medical Regime*; Carvallo, "Empirical Turn of Medicine"; and Barry, "'Compleat Physician' and Experimentation."

58 Coste (*Représentations et comportements*) has explored changes in medical discourse in printed French plague tracts vis a vis evolving attitudes towards the disease, while Heinrichs's work on early modern printed German tracts (*Plague, Print, and the Reformation*) traces German reforms of healing.

59 This differs sharply from Islamicate plague treatises. The First Plague Pandemic overlapped with the emergence of Islam, and the disease's impact on the bourgeoning Islamic polity in Western Asia and North Africa, as well as on Islamic religious thought over the subsequent centuries, meant that plague could not be discussed without also discussing issues of theodicy. See Fancy, "Knowing the Signs of Disease." Thyr's examination of high medieval ecclesiastical/hagiographical/*historia* sources from Ireland and Wales reveals that memory of the First Pandemic also survived there, albeit curiously labelled as "yellow" plague. In Ireland, these memories faltered after the Norman invasion, while in Wales they

escaped into secular poetry; mentions of yellow plague lingered in Welsh secular poetry into the fifteenth and sixteenth centuries, although by that time it had come to be understood as a sort of predatory monster, not a disease. In both instances, no contemporary writing linked the First and Second Pandemics. Thyr, "End of an Era." I thank Nicholas Thyr for discussing his work with me.

60 This story recounts King David's divine punishment for census taking and his need to choose between three retributions: seven years of famine, three months of being pursued by enemies, or three days and three nights of plague. David chose the latter, since he felt that it was the punishment most likely to affect him as much as his subjects. In the end, he watched helplessly as seventy thousand of his subjects died.

61 Keiser provides a detailed analysis of Multon's religious reworking of John of Burgundy's late fourteenth-century tract in "Two Medieval Plague Treatises."

62 Heinrichs, *Plague, Print, and the Reformation*, 1–3.

63 "*Peste proprement est une verge de Dieu envoyee sur la terre, & sur l'iniquité du monde pour punir les pecheurs, les admonestans de delaisser leur mauvaise vie, & se retourner à nostre Sauveur & Redempteur Jesus Christ.*" Ydeley, *Des secrets souverains*, 17.

64 "*La peste n'est pas une maladie, mais une verge de Dieu*"; "*je prie tous ceux qui se trouveront entachez de la dite maladie de peste … ils ayant recourse au medecin spirituel.*" Ibid., title page, 71.

65 Slack has traced the shift toward religious explanations in England after 1563 in *Impact of Plague*, 228–47. He points to the creation of a separate genre of plague literature written by the growing number of divines and other religious men and differentiates these works from medically-focused tracts that typically included little more than "a final caveat or an introductory formality" dealing with divine providence. *Impact of Plague*, 38. Coste has done the same analysis for French tracts in *Représentations et comportements*, 353–414. See also Jones, "Plague and Its Metaphors," and Fabbri, "Continuity and Change," 182–96, which calls these "hybrid" works. Heinrichs, *Plague, Print, and the Reformation* offers a useful comparison with German tracts.

66 Keiser, "Two Medieval Plague Treatises," 294.

67 Coste's analysis, for example, suggests that professional religious authors wrote no more than about 13 per cent of all printed French plague treatises. Coste, *Représentations et comportements*, 49.

68 I thank an anonymous reviewer for pointing to this example. For a longer discussion of Clapham and Balmford's debate, see Gilman, *Plague Writing*,

143–5. Miller provides an extensive discussion of nonconformist writing about plague in seventeenth-century England in *Literary Plague*, 95–129.

69 Jones, "Plague and Its Metaphors," 109. Jones offers a compelling discussion of the religious plague script of early modern France.

70 Skene, *Ane breve descriptioun of the pest*, 3.

71 André, *Traite de la peste*, 3.

72 Healy, *Fictions of Disease*, 16, 43.

73 Phayer, *Regiment of Life*, 10, 11. Phayer is sometimes spelled "Phaer." For this analysis, see Healy, *Fictions of Disease*, 69.

74 "*aussi peult une haleine ou vapeur venimeuse infectez toute une region.*" De Houssemaine, *Ung regime singulier*, 60. De Houssemaine also wrote that the principal plague preservative was to live in a state of grace, an idea that appeared commonly in the tracts.

75 Wellcome MS 674, 37. I discuss this revision in more detail in "Itineraries and Transformations."

76 Calamy, *Englands Antidote*, and Brough, *Preservative*. Slack discusses the Puritan interpretation of plague in more detail in *Impact of Plague*, 243. For the spread of plague during the Civil War, see Jennings, "Anatomy of a Civil War Plague," and "'A Stinking, Miserable, Infected Town.'"

77 Gatford, *Logos alexipharmakos*, 7–8. In a nice twist, Gatford opens the tract by comparing Puritans to "*Mountebancks* [who] poyson the People"; he had been imprisoned by Cromwell and the Long Parliament for seventeen months for his pro-royalist writings. Gatford died of plague in 1665.

78 Cook, *Decline of the Old Medical Regime*.

79 Hodges, *Loimologia*, 30.

80 Quincy, *Different Causes of Pestilential Diseases*, 5.

81 Ranchin, *Opuscules*, 5.

82 Baux, *Traité de la peste*, 10. Emphasis added.

83 Girolamo Fracastoro's mid-sixteenth century writings on contagion were not original; rather, they reformulated Galen's earlier, lesser known, writings. Nutton, "Reception," and "Seeds of Disease."

84 I discuss this in more detail in "Experience over Education."

85 Drouet, *Consilium novum*, 14.

86 Herring, *Certaine Rules*, 1.

87 Thayre, *Excellent and Best Approoved*, title page. Emphasis added.

88 Bradwell, *Physick for the Sicknesse*, ii.

89 Bradwell, *Watch-man for the Pest*, title page, ii.

90 Bradwell, *Physick for the Sicknesse*, iv, title page, 5.

91 Physician in York, *Treatise of the Plague*, 1–2. The physician then proceeded to offer his own assessment, concluding that "this sad Disease" resulted from great unusual heat or drought that caused the in-air suspension of "a vast quantity of Volatile Salts, not much unlike the Salts to be discovered in the Juice of the Viper, taken from the Bag under its Tooth, tho much nicelier divided" (2–3). While he likened the signs and symptoms of plague to those caused by viper bites ("livid Spots, Buboes, Tumours, and the Vomitings and Loosenesses"), his proffered remedies remained much the same as those suggested in other tracts – except for his suggestion that the land in and around London should be plowed up so that each householder could have a package of fresh turf to smell. For an especially detailed attack on Richard Mead's ideas of contagion and the arrival of epidemic diseases from elsewhere, see Pye, *Discourse of the Plague*.

92 Crisciani's discussion of pharmacological experimentation (especially with alchemical recipes) and incentivization as early as the 1350s is useful here, though, as it points to ongoing attempts to repackage old ingredients and to find new ones that could make plague remedies more effective, especially when traditional humoral-based therapies seemed ineffective. Crisciani, "Città e medici," 18.

93 "*C'est la doctrine qu'on nous a enseignée à Montpellier en 1688. 1689. 1690. & 1691. pendant que j'y faisois mes études … Mais cette doctrine n'etoit fondée que sur la simple presomption, Mrs. les Professeurs de ce tems là n'ayant jamais vû de Peste.*" Pons in Boecler, *Recueil des observations*, 15.

94 "*la Maladie dont cette Ville est affligée, étoit la veritable Peste, décrite par tous les Autheurs qui en ont traité, & accompagnée de tous les Symptomes les plus essentiels; en sorte qu'il n'y a plus lieu de douter, que la Peste ne soit une Maladie réelle & existente.*" Ibid. Pons's comment here brings to mind Cunningham's epistemological argument that the definition and identity, and thus understanding and recognition, of a disease like plague changes over time depending on the dominant knowledge system in play. Cunningham, "Transforming Plague."

95 "*Les experiences réiterées que nous avons eu occasion de faire, dans l'espace de neuf mois, pendant lesquels nous avons traité journellement un grand nombre de Pestiferez, ouvert plusieurs cadavres, & fait des dissections … certain nombre de faits évidens & incontestables.*" Chicoyneau, Verny, and Soulier, *Observations et reflexions*, 6, 26.

96 Baux, *Traité de la peste*, 10.

97 Brookes, *History*, title page.

98 Browne, *Practical Treatise*, title page.

99 Brookes, *History*, 5, 7.

100 For a good overview of these debates, which involved poison, minute insects and worms, bad food, and a variety of other ideas, see DeLacy, *Germ of an Idea*, especially chapter 9.

101 See, for example, Sudhoff, "Pestschriften" (1–19); Klebs and Droz, *Remèdes contre la peste*; Klebs and Sudhoff, *Die Ersten Gedruckten Pestschriften*; Singer, "Some Plague Tractates," and "Survey of Medical Manuscripts"; Singer and Anderson, *Catalogue of Latin and Vernacular Plague Texts*; and Campbell, *Black Death*.

102 A number of works are particularly noteworthy here, some already mentioned above: Arrizabalaga's detailed analysis of the earliest tracts produced by university-trained physicians ("Facing the Black Death"); Chase's exploration of plague disease classification debates among Montpellier tract writers ("Fevers, Poisons, and Apostemes"); Fabbri's study of the evolution of European plague medicine up to 1599 ("Continuity and Change"); Coste's diachronic analysis of the causal explanations and treatment recommendations found in French printed tracts (*Représentations et comportements*); Jones's elucidation of French plague scripts ("Plague and Its Metaphors" and "Languages of Plague"); Cohn's work on Italian tracts (*Cultures of Plague*); Heinrich's exploration of early modern German treatises (*Plague, Print, and the Reformation*); Matheson's work on John of Burgundy ("John of Burgundy: Treatises on Plague" and "Médecin sans Frontières?"); Keiser's examination of Thomas Multon's tract ("Two Medieval Plague Treatises"); Einbinder's work on Abraham Caslari (*After the Black Death*), and Sublet's on Ibn Hagar al-ʿAsqalanı ("La peste prise aux rêts de la jurisprudence"); Conrad's study of early Islamic plague writing ("Arabic Plague Chronologies and Treatises") and Dols's detailed follow-up work ("Al-Manbijī's 'Report of the Plague'" and "Ibn al-Wardi's *Risalah al-Naba'ʿAn al-Waba*'"); Barkai's preliminary examination of Jewish tracts on the Black Death ("Jewish Treatises on the Black Death") and Bos's subsequent work on them ("The Black Death in Hebrew Literature" and, with Mensching, "The Black Death in Hebrew Literature") as well as similar work by Barroso ("Un *Regimen sanitatis* contra la peste"). A plethora of literature scholars have also engaged with the tracts.

103 Taavitsainen, et al., "Medical Texts," 13; and Slack, *Impact of Plague*, 329.

CHAPTER TWO

1 "*quod quondam fuit pestilencia in Montepessulano et ego non potui vitare communitatem, quia transivi de domo in domum ad curandum infirmos causa paupertatis ... Socii autem mei, non credentes me vitam retinere.*" Erfurt, Universitätsbibliothek (UB Erfurt), Amplonian MS Q.192, cited in Sudhoff, "Pestshriften" (17), 31.

2 On Jacobi, see Wickersheimer, *Dictionnaire*, 422–3. See also Dumas, *Santé et société*, especially 314–15 where she corrects the long-mistaken notion that Jacobi stayed to treat the sick because of his own poverty. Dumas notes that it was Karl Sudhoff who added the word *mea* after *paupertatis* in the early twentieth century. Curiously, though, early modern printed adaptations of this tract also use the phrase "by cause of my poverte," so the error must have been introduced into a manuscript copy of the tract at some point (i.e., possibly the one consulted by Sudhoff) and was then carried over into print. Alternatively, perhaps Jacobi meant "poverty" in a completely different context than financial.

3 Wickersheimer, *Dictionnaire*, 423; and Dumas, *Santé et société*, 196.

4 Klebs and Droz, *Remèdes contre la peste*, 5. See also Winslow and Duran-Reynals, "Jacme d'Agramont," 751. Singer dates the tract to 1364, while Sudoff suggests 1373. It is possible that they are referring, respectively, to the French and Latin prose versions. Singer, "Some Plague Tractates," 179; and Sudhoff, "Pestshriften" (17), 30.

5 Wickersheimer, "Jehan Jacme," 109.

6 Some definitions of the history of the book field note specifically that it encompasses the material aspect of texts: "all aspects of the history of production, publication, and distribution [of books], from the initial stages of authorship to the impacts of books on their readers and society." Adams and Barker, "New Model," 7. See also Chartier, *Order of Books*, and McKenzie, *Bibliography*.

7 Scase, "Introduction," 2.

8 Boffey's work on book manufacture in London likewise emphasizes the influence of location on a book's relationship with its readers. Boffey, *Manuscript and Print*, 17.

9 Scase, "Introduction," 2.

10 On the mobility of books, see Shep, "Books in Global Perspective."

11 Schurink, "Introduction," 2, 5. On the role of translators, see also Barker and Hosington, eds., *Renaissance Cultural Crossroads*.

12 Among a great many examples, see in Horobin and Nafde, eds., *Pursuing Middle English Manuscripts*: Pearsall, "Tribulations," and Mooney,

"Scribe of Lydgate's"; in Connolly and Mooney, eds., *Design and Distribution*: Mosser, "Chaucer's Scribe," Thaisen, "Trinity Gower D," and Mooney, "Locating Scribal Activity"; and in Tavormina, ed., *Sex, Aging, and Death*: Mooney, "Scribe," and Matheson, "Dialect."

13 See, for example, Wear, "Explorations," and Siraisi, "Changing Fortunes."

14 Johns, *Nature of the Book*, and Boffey, *Manuscript and Print*.

15 Cavallo and Storey, *Healthy Living*. Cavallo and Storey demonstrate how printers, rather than just authors, initially drove efforts to change the contents of medieval Italian healthy-living manuals in the early modern era to meet the needs of a new urban consumerist culture.

16 Griffin, "Reconsidering the Recipe."

17 Le Roy also printed the first illustrated book in France. Millar, "LeRoy," 286–7.

18 Atila, *Traictie tresutile*.

19 Gering was one of three Germans invited to establish a press at the Sorbonne in 1470 to produce Latin university texts. After 1472, he no longer worked at the Sorbonne, but continued to print until 1508. Renouard, *Répertoire*, 168–9.

20 "*kamiti epi[scopi] arusien[sis] civitatis: regni dacie, artis medicine exp[er]tissimi p[ro]fessoris*." Kamitus [Johannes Jacobi], *Regimen contra pestilentiam*.

21 Rand, "Elusive Canutus," 188. Rand provides a clear analysis of failed (and misguided) attempts to identify the fictitious "Kamiti/Kamitus" (later transcribed to "Canutus" at the British Library, which remains the name with which the tract is now identified). On the pre-modern "medical marketplace," see among others Cook, *Decline of the Old Medical Regime*, and Jenner and Wallis, eds., *Medicine and the Market*. Crisciani also speaks of the Paris Medical Faculty having "a corporate monopoly in the health/medical marketplace" ["*un maggior monopolio della corporazione sul mercato della salute*"] in "Città e medici," 18. On the medical marketplace of print, see Fissell, "Popular Medical Writing."

22 "*approuve par plusieurs docteurs en medecine*." Anonymous [Johannes Jacobi], *Remede tres utile*, A1.

23 Bisshop of Arusiens, *Here begynneth*, 1.

24 Despite the publication of numerous theories about this disease, it has not been unanimously identified.

25 Keiser, "Two Medieval Plague Treatises," 324, 319.

26 English manuscript copies include London, British Library (BL), Sloane MSS 1588 (ff. 275v–80v), 2270 (ff. 75r–7v), and 2276 (ff. 191r–9r); Oxford, Bodleian Library (Bodl.), Rawlinson MS A.393 (ff. 96r–9r); Cambridge,

Fitzwilliam Museum (Fitzwilliam), MS 261 (ff. 9v–19r); and Copenhagen, Det Kongelige Bibliotek, MS NKS 316c (ff. 1r–7v). The Latin version is found in Fitzwilliam MS 261 (ff. 1r–9r). Two other Latin copies were produced in Germany.

27 Paynel, *Moche Profitable Treatise*, A2.

28 Keiser has shown the textual similarities between a passage in Paynel's English tract and its counterpart in a French version printed by Antoine Caillaut in Paris c. 1489–91. Keiser, "Two Medieval Plague Treatises," 320.

29 Ibid., 319–20.

30 Warner, *Henry VIII's Divorce*, 83.

31 Greg, "Notes," 188.

32 Paynel, *De Morbo Gallico*, 1.

33 On early Tudor ideas about profitability, see Moore, "Gathering Fruit," and Wakelin, *Humanism*.

34 Moulton, *Myrour or Glasse of Helthe*. The spelling of Multon's name was changed to "Moulton" in the print versions. I follow that convention. Thus, my references to "Multon" are to the late fifteenth-century manuscript tract and references to "Moulton" are to the printed versions that appeared during and after the 1520s.

35 Greg, "Notes," 190.

36 Jones, "Medical Literacies," 32–3. More learned medical works, such as surgical and theoretical texts, appeared in Roman type, unreadable by those with only rudimentary reading skills. For an illustrated overview of the development of typographical styles and their use by printers in England and France, see Updike, *Printing Types*. On late medieval and early modern literacy levels and practices more generally, see Hackel "Rhetorics and Practices of Illiteracy"; Cressy, *Literacy*; and Houston, *Literacy*.

37 On the role and purpose of title pages, see among others Herman, "Excavating the Page," and McConchie, "Some Reflections." On the title pages of plague tracts specifically, see Ratia, "Investigating Genre."

38 Bisshop and Doctor of Physick of Denmarke, *Here after ensuith a litle treatise*.

39 Keiser, "Two Medieval Plague Treatises," 322.

40 *Conscriptum per me Raymundum Chalmelli magistrum in artibus et in medicina et medicum domini nostri pap*e." Leipzig, Universitätsbibliothek (UB Leipzig), MS 1178, cited in Sudhoff, "Pestshriften" (17), 37.

41 *Causa epydimie et preservatio ejusdem* and *Compendium breve contra epydimiam*, noted in Coville, "Écrits contemporains sur la peste," 363–7.

42 Chase, "Fevers, Poisons, and Apostemes," 154.

43 Ibid., 159–60.

44 Barkai, "Jewish Treatises," 12. At least twelve Jewish physicians practiced medicine in Avignon during fourteenth-century plague outbreaks. Jacob b. Solomon, physician to the pope's brother, also survived Avignon's outbreaks in 1361 and 1382 and wrote about his experiences, but not in a plague tract. On Jewish plague tracts more generally, see Einbinder, *After the Black Death.*

45 Copies survive in London, Society of Antiquaries of London (SAL), MS 101, f. 1v, and BL Additional MS 4897, ff. 262–5. For a discussion of these tracts in the context of health regimens, see Hardingham, "Regimen in Late Medieval England," 71–80.

46 On the latter, see Matheson, "John of Burgundy," 573–6.

47 Matheson, "Médecin sans Frontières?" 19. Several Latin copies of this shorter version also survive. For recent and more detailed discussions of John of Burgundy's tract, see Jones, "Itineraries and Transformations," and Jones and Honkapohja "From *Practica Phisicalia.*"

48 Singer, "Some Plague Tracts," 161. In terms of other popular medical texts in England, fewer than one hundred copies survive of either of the well-known Floridus Macer and *Agnus castus* herbals, in full or derivative versions. Keiser, "Vernacular Herbals," 300–1. In his consideration of what the extant number of a given manuscript means in terms of demand for it, Sargeant notes that even Chaucer's *Canterbury Tales*, Gower's *Confessio Amantis*, and Langland's *Piers Plowman* survive in less than one hundred copies each. "What Do the Numbers Mean?" 206. The high number of survivals of the John of Burgundy plague treatise is therefore quite impressive.

49 Malverne's tract survives in at least three copies: Sloane MS 59, ff. 186–9 and Bodl. Digby MSS 94, ff. 136–9v, and 147, ff. 53v–6r.

50 Sloane MS 3489, ff. 44r–51r. Keiser dates the treatise to c. 1475, but Kathleen L. Scott, who has studied the larger miscellany of which it once was a part, suggests that the "third quarter of the fifteenth century" is a better estimate. Scott, "Newly Discovered Booklets," 121.

51 BL Additional MS 25782, ff. 70r–7v.

52 For Blascus's tract, see Sloane MS 428; for Reguardati's tract, see Bodl. Ashmole MS 1475 (English) and Sloane MS 404 (Latin); the latter manuscript also contains a post-print (i.e., post-1485) scribal copy of the Bishop of Arusiens treatise. Jacobi's tract survives in SAL MS 101. The anonymous tracts appear in BL Egerton MS 2622 and Ashmole MSS 1435 and 1391.

53 Unattributed translation, adaptation, and copying were common practices across late medieval and early modern Europe, reflecting the "great store on the authority and authenticity [that was] bestowed on a text by the *auctor*." The longer a text had been circulating, and the higher the status of its author, the greater level of truth and authority it acquired. Pennycook, "Borrowing Others' Words," 205. For broader discussions of medieval authorship, see Partridge and Kwakkel, eds., *Author, Reader, Book,* and Minnis, *Medieval Theory of Authorship.*

54 Schurink, "Introduction," 2, considers translated, transformed texts to be originals in their own right.

55 The Oxford and Cambridge medical faculties were established in the early fourteenth century, some time after similar institutions were already operating on the Continent; medicine remained the smallest faculty in both universities until at least the fifteenth century.

56 Bartholomeus Anglicus and Gilbertus Anglicus, two of the most famous thirteenth-century encyclopaedic and medical writers from England, produced their works on the Continent (*De proprietatibus rerum*, c. 1240, and *Compendium Medicinae*, c. 1230–50, respectively). A century later, John of Gaddesden, author of the popular medical treatise *Rosa Medicinæ* (c. 1307), and John Ardene (1307–92), the famous surgeon, lived, worked, and wrote medical treatises in England, but neither wrote specifically about plague.

57 For medieval English medical students on the Continent, see Talbot and Hammond, *Medical Practitioners.* On foreign physicians and surgeons in English royal courts and noble households, see Rawcliffe, "Profits of Practice."

58 See, for example, excerpts in Horrox, *Black Death*, 111–15, and Sloane, *Black Death in London*, 22–4.

59 This belies the suggestion that all English plague treatises produced after 1500 "are original vernacular texts and not translations. The texts were written by English authors and they focus solely on the epidemics in England." Pahta and Ratia, "Treatises on Specific Topics," 98.

60 Fitzwilliam MS 261, f. 23r.

61 Voigts and Payne, "Medicine for a Great Household," 183–9.

62 Voigts, "Plague Saints," 103–7; and Voigts and Payne, "Medicine for a Great Household," 161–6.

63 Roger, "To Be Shut Up," 5–7.

64 Cooper, *Annals of Cambridge*, 1:275.

65 Voigts, "Plague Saints," 103.

66 The Scope manuscript is Berkeley Castle Muniments Select Book 89; it, and its relationship to Margaret, is discussed in detail in Voigts and Payne, "Medicine for a Great Household."

67 Fitzwilliam MS 261. For a description of the manuscript, see Wormold and Gilles, *Descriptive Catalogue*, 194–6.

68 Similarly, an anonymous *Regimen contra pestilenciam* written in Prague in 1371 was intended for Holy Roman Emperor Charles IV.

69 Paris, Bibliothèque nationale de France (BnF), NAF MS 4516 (c. 1371), ff. 97r–102v and Français MS 12323 (c. 1373), f. 135v–44r.

70 Boston, Countway Library of Medicine, Ballard MS 19.

71 BnF Latin MS 7138; and Bibliothèque nationale et universitaire de Strasbourg (BNU), MS 0.048.

72 Brussels, Koninklijke Bibliotheek van België/Bibliothèque royale de Belgique (KBR), MS II.1413, ff. 114r–16v; and Lille, Bibliothèque municipale, Médiathèque Jean Lévy, MS 863, ff. 132r–40v.

73 The Carcassonne translation is found in two fifteenth-century manuscripts: BnF Hébreu MSS 1191, ff. 141v–2v, and 1124, ff. 133v–40r. I am grateful to Susan Einbinder for her reading of these tracts; the translation is hers.

74 Trewythian's manuscript is Sloane MS 428. The tract also includes a few marginal sketches, which unfortunately have been lost; immediately preceding the plague treatise is a discussion of the causes and effects of a general pestilence in 1434.

75 Sloane MS 59, ff. 186–9; and BL Additional MS 5467, ff. 85–7.

76 Guild Book of the Barber-Surgeons of York: Egerton MS 2572, ff. 67–9; Southwell household: Cambridge, University Library (CUL), MS LL.1.18, ff. 3r–4v, 74r–5v; Chronicle and Cartulary of the Peterborough Abbey: BL Additional MS 39758, ff. 283–9. Medical compendium of St Mary's Priory, Coventry: BL Royal MS 12.G.IV, f. 158. Breviary of Muchelney Abbey, Somerset: BL Additional MS 43405, ff. 7v–9. Medical compendium of Durham Cathedral Priory: Durham, University Library, Cosin MS V.IV.I, ff. 2–4, 37–9. *Scotichronicon* of Inchcolm Abbey, Fife, Scotland: Cambridge, Corpus Christi College (CCC), MS 171, ff. 363v–4r. *Scotichronicon* of Paisley Abbey, Renfrewshire, Scotland: BL Royal MS 13.E.X, ff. 24v–5. Cartulary of St Mary's Abbey, Kelso, Roxburghshire, Scotland: Edinburgh, National Library of Scotland.

77 Norwich monk: CUL MS Ii.1.31, ff. 211r–v. Leicestershire parson: Rawlinson MS A.393, ff. 95r–6r. Yorkshire lord: Lincoln Cathedral MS A.5.2, ff. 300v–3r. London herald: BL Lansdowne MS 285, ff. 214r–v. London physician: London, Wellcome Collection (Wellcome) MS 550, ff. 108r–15r; London barber-surgeon: Sloane MS 706, ff. 267v–71v.

78 Honkapohja, *Alchemy*, 62–3.

79 Here, the commercial book trade was largely market-oriented; in its earliest days, the University of Paris, rather than guilds, controlled and oversaw much of the production of books concentrated around the colleges on the left bank of the Seine and in l'île de la Cité. During the fourteenth and fifteenth centuries, the University's monopolistic control weakened, and book production proliferated in areas outside traditional neighbourhoods.

80 For London, where manuscript book production converged by the early fifteenth century: Christianson, "Rise of London's Book-Trade" and "Evidence"; Gillespie and Wakelin, eds., *Production*; Raven, *Business of Books*; and Boffey, *Manuscript and Print*. For Paris, which was a major centre for commercial manuscript production in Northern Europe already in the thirteenth century: Fianu, "Métiers et espace," and Rouse and Rouse, *Manuscripts and Their Makers*. This is not to ignore production centres elsewhere, but to highlight the importance of these two cities in their respective kingdoms.

81 The large number of surviving practical, legal, scholarly, and literary manuscripts from the late medieval period, as compared to the earlier medieval centuries, is highly suggestive of growing literacy rates. This encompasses a wide spectrum from those who could read and write easily to those who were unable to read but could otherwise participate in activities that involved the use of written texts, so defining actual literacy levels is fraught with difficulty. The scholarly literature on this topic is quite large. For a good overview, see Jones, "Vernacular Literacy," especially 40–59; and Jones, "Discourse Communities."

82 Relying on sociolinguistic history (*l'histoire sociolinguistique*), Serge Lusignan argues that this region, which he calls the Picard nation (*la nation des Picards*), ran approximately from Abbeville in the west to Troyes in the south to the northern Low Countries in the east. *Essai d'histoire sociolinguistique*.

83 Bisshop of Arusiens, *Here begynneth*, 1.

84 BnF NAF MS 4516, f. 97r, and Français MS 12323, f. 135v.

85 Sloane MS 965.

86 Egerton MS 2572. On the guildbook, see Wragg, "Civic Relationship."

87 Honkapohja notes that six manuscripts associated with the Voigts-Sloane Group "display good craftsmanship" and some level of decoration, which "suggests that they were up-market items" produced by "professional scribes." Honkapohja, *Alchemy*, 5–15. See also Voigts, "Sloane Group."

88 Tokyo, Takamiya MS 33 (1475–99), f. 42v; and Cambridge, Gonville & Caius College, MS 336/72 (late 15th century), f. 144v

89 Fitzwilliam MS 261; and Wormold and Gilles, *Descriptive Catalogue*, 194–6.

90 Gonville & Caius MS 336/725 does contain marginal comments, suggesting that its owners made use of it at some point in time. I thank Alpo Honkapohja for his comments on this manuscript.

91 Unfortunately, in too many instances the original compendiums in which these tracts appeared were taken apart by later collectors and reassembled into new volumes to suit the collectors' interests. As part of this process, the margins were trimmed so that the new volume was uniform in size; this resulted sometimes in the loss of marginal notations. Such is the case for many of the manuscripts in the British Library's Sloane collection, for example.

92 Worcester MP: New Haven, Yale Center for British Art, Paul Mellon Collection, John Porter MS. Blystow rector: Bodl. Wood MS D.8. Incholm Abbey: CCC MS 171. Augustinian Monastery of St Marienwolde: BNU MS 0.048. Wharton: SAL MS 101. Thornton: Lincoln Cathedral MS 19. Charles Whyte, barber-surgeon: Sloane MS 776. German surgeon: BnF Latin MS 7138; Petrus de Oultre: KBR MS II.1413.

93 Dethick: Lansdowne MS 285. King: Sloane MS 1588.

94 Wellcome MS 674. For the revisions made to the plague tracts in this manuscript, see Jones, "Itineraries and Transformations" and Honkapohja, "Tracing."

95 Forman: Ashmole MSS 1403 and 1436. Collins: Sloane MS 1821. Boghurst: Sloane MS 349. Allaire: Wellcome MS 924. Boghurst's tract was transcribed and printed in 1894, while Allaire's is clearly laid out for print and includes a notice to readers.

96 Jacobi, *Regime de lepidimie*; Kamiti, *Regimen contra pestilentiam*; le Forestier, *Tractatus contre pestilentiam* and *Regime contre epidemie*. Le Forestier's work did not appear in print in England.

97 "*composé de plusieurs docteurs et autres grans clercs en medecine dedans avignon ou temps que la grant pestillence y regnoit et est approuvé. Avec aulcunes receptes tresprouffitables po[ur] la conservation des corps humains.*" Anonymous, *Souverain remede*, 1.

98 This text is quite different from the Jacobi/Kamiti tract, although Coste suggests that the two were the same tract. Whether the tract was translated from a Hebrew original has not yet been determined. Coste, *Représentations et comportements*, 119.

99 "*Pilules contre lepidimye et maulvais air composees et approuvees par maistre Jaques juif en avignon.*" Anonymous, *Souverain regime*, 5. A "maistre Jacque le Juyfz [d']Avignon" also appears in at least

one anonymous fifteenth-century manuscript treatise, now MS 419 in the Stadtbibliothek of Metz. I thank Susan Einbinder for discussing with me the possibilities of whom Havard's (and the earlier manuscript's) Jacques might have been. The name Isaac (Yitzhaq) often turns up in Romance languages as "Haqin," which could have been misconstrued as "Jacques." On Jewish physicians in Avignon and elsewhere, see Shatzmiller, *Jews*; Wickersheimer, *Dictionnaire*; and Pansier, "Les médecins juifs." On Jewish physicians in the medieval Islamic world and premodern Jewish medicine more generally, see Lev, *Jewish Medical Practitioners*, and Lehmhaus, ed., *Defining Jewish Medicine*, respectively.

100 Thayre, *Excellent and Best Approoved Treatise*, A2r, A6r.

101 Ibid., A6r, 36.

102 Ibid., A4r.

103 Phayer, *The Regiment of Life*. While the main text was also a translation (of the *Regimen Sanitatis Salerni*), the accompanying work on children's health was the first of its kind. Phayer's book appeared in at least nine editions until as late as 1722. The original work is de Houssemaine, *Régime singulier*.

104 Twyne, *New Counsell*; Drouet, *Consilium novum*; Hill, *Joyful Jewell*; and Fioravanti, *Del regimento*.

105 Lodge, *Treatise of the Plague*, 3–4.

106 Cuvelier, "Treatise of the Plague." The original tract is Valleriole, *Traicté de la peste*.

107 Parey, *Treatise of the Plague*; Van Diemerbroeck, *Several Choice* and *Treatise Concerning the Pestilence*; and Barbette, *Chirurgical and Anatomical Works*. See also Anonymous, *Succinct Account of the Plague*.

108 These include Gilbert Skeyne (1568), Thomas Brasbridge (1578), an anonymous "Learned Physician" (1592), Stephen Hobbes (1603), Thomas Thayre (1603), and Francis Herring (1603). John Caius penned an original treatise on the sweating sickness in 1552, following the genre's style.

109 Sloane MSS 786, 788, and 791. The works that Smith translated were by Andrés Laguna de Segovia (*Compendium curationis febris pestilentialis*, printed in 1542) and Leonhart Fuchs (*De medendis morbis*, book 4, chapter 12 [*de pestilentia*], printed in 1552).

110 Mead, *Short Discourse*. For the debates, see Jones, "Diseased Landscape," 108–9; Zuckerman, "Plague and Contagionism"; and Slack, *Impact of Plague*, 326–31, and "Perceptions of Plague."

111 Various, *Collection*; Browne, *Practical Treatise*; Bradley, *Plague at Marseilles*; and Anonymous, *Succinct Account*.

112 D'Andernach, *Instruction tresutile.*
113 Colin Jones counted two hundred individual authors, and forty anonymous ones, for 264 tracts printed in French or Latin between 1500 and 1770. "Plague and Its Metaphors," 102.
114 Among these authors are Nicolas de Houssemaine, dean of the Faculty of Medicine in Angers (1520); Jean Thibault, physician and astrologer to King François I (1531); Oger Ferrier, a royal physician and astrologer to Catherine de Medici (1548); Laurent Joubert, chancellor of the University of Montpellier (and later physician to Catherine de' Medici, Henri III, and Henri III of Navarre) (1564); Estienne Gourmelen, professor of medicine at the University of Paris (1581); Louis de Gardin, medical professor at the University of Douai (1617); royal physician J.S. de Saincte-Hillier (1623); Henry de Mello, professor of medicine at the University of Nantes (1625); François Ranchin, chancellor and professor in Montpellier's Faculty of Medicine (1640); and D.M. Pons, a physician in Montpellier's Faculty of Medicine (1720).
115 Here we find François Vallériole (1555), Sébastien Colin (1566), Guillaume Briet (1599), Pierre Drouet (1572), Nicolas de Nancel (1581); Jean Suau (1586), Jacques Moine and Pierre-Jean Fabre (1629), and Pierre Baux (1722), among many others.
116 B. Barralis, professor of medicine at the Paris Medical Faculty in the early seventeenth century, justified having translated a tract from Italian into French by noting that the Italian author's knowledge of plague was so well presented that nothing further could be added from local experience to improve it. "*ceste matier, l'ayant enrichie de si belles raisons, de si fortes authorités & d'experiences si sensibles, que j'estimay deslors qu'on ne pouuvoit rien adiouter à la perfection d'un tel ouurage.*" Barralis, trans., *Paradoxes de la peste*, A2. Royal councillors: Antoine Davin (1629) and Henry de Rochas d'Ayglun (1652); civic administrators and royal officials: Claude de Rubys (1577) and Pierre Rainssant (1668); health commissioner: Antoine Royet (1583); apothecaries: Nicolas Houël (1573) and Isaac Quatroux (1671); surgeons: Pierre André (1563), Ambroise Paré (1568), Jean Cassal (1589), Nicolas Habicot (1607), and Guillaume Potel (1629); Jesuits and other religious authors: Estienne Ydeley (1581), Jean Grillot (1629), and Abbé Martin Gaudereau (1721).
117 Coste, *Représentations et comportements*, 48–9. These are the tracts by the doctors from Basle (1519), Nicolas Houssemaine (1520), François Citoys (1623), Maurice de Toulon (1662), Paul Barbette (1675), and Francis Chicoyneau (1721).
118 Tonry, *Agency and Intention.*

119 Anonymous, *Treatise Concerning the Plague and the Pox*, D2.
120 Ibid., D2–3.
121 Ibid., 1.
122 Elizabeth Pickering, widow of Robert Redman, published an edition of Thomas Moulton's tract c. 1541.
123 On the former, see Slack, *Impact of Plague*, 62; on the latter, see Dobson, *Contours*, 403.
124 Tyrkkö, "Physical Dictionary (1657)," 175–6. On other women printers, see Driver, "By Me Elysabeth Pykeryng," and Bell, "Hannah Allen."
125 On "common good" as a key aspect of political thought, see Kempshall, *Common Good*.
126 Vadianus, *Ein kurtz und trüwlich underricht*. For Nourry's version, see Anonymous, *Regime contre la pestil[enc]e*. Nourry was a prolific printer, and among his many medical works were six editions of Arnaldus de Villanova's *Regimen sanitatus*. Although it misrepresents his medical production, see Lauvergnat-Gagnière, "Claude Nourry, imprimeur populaire?"
127 Anonymous, *Regime contro la pestilence*.
128 For a detailed study of that image and its role in plague tracts, see Jones, "Bubo Men?"
129 Coste, *Représentations et comportements*, 48–9.
130 Benedict, "French Cities," 8–9.
131 Pettegree, Walsby, and Wilkinson, eds., *French Vernacular Books*, 1:xiii.
132 Honkapohja, *Alchemy*, 23–4; Harris, "Patrons, Buyers and Owners," 216–17; Christianson "Rise of London's Book-Trade," 128–9.
133 Feather calls the failed local presses "the last heirs of the medieval tradition of localized book production for local use." *History of British Publishing*, 19. See also Raymond, ed., *Oxford History*; McKitterick, "University Printing"; and Barnard and Bell, "English Provinces."
134 Taavitsainen, et al., "Medical Texts," 12–13. Boffey discusses in some detail William Caxton's use of manuscript exemplars for his early books in *Manuscript and Print*.
135 Fissell has argued that a "real break with the late medieval manuscript tradition" occurred only in the 1650s. "Popular Medical Writing," 419. See also Slack, "Mirrors of Health," 238; and Bennett, *English Books*, vol. 1.
136 Some dates in figure 2.13 are approximate, as the *Short Title Catalogue* data do not always correlate with holding institutions' catalogues. The information in the catalogues likewise does not always match the books' colophons; where they exist, I have used the names and dates as they appear in the works themselves. The connections between the printers are well attested in the *British Book Trade Index*, accessed 1 April 2017,

http://bbti.bodleian.ox.ac.uk, and the *Oxford Dictionary of National Biography*, accessed 21 May 2017, http://www.oxforddnb.com.

137 Warner, *Henry VIII's Divorce*, 83–5. Redman apparently "drew liberally on blocks that belonged to other printers." Hodnett, *English Woodcuts*, 66. Although he does not discuss Redman directly, Johns's work on intellectual piracy and the battles for legitimacy between early modern printers is instructive here. Johns, *Nature of the Book* and *Piracy*.

138 Poultry Compter was a small prison run by the sheriff of London. It housed non-violent offenders, including those charged with religious dissent. The list of books these men are accused of having printed no longer survives, but since all were Protestant, one can assume that their banned books were reformist in nature. On the compter, see McGovern, "Compters."

139 Blayney, *Stationers' Company*, 401. The unnamed printer "for Rychard Jugge" has not been identified, but given that their tracts are identical, it may well have been Myddleton, Kele, or Toye.

140 Raven, *Business of Books*, 3.

141 Slack, *Impact of Plague*, 61.

142 The initial edition, published in 1656–57, was printed and sold by a printer (J.C.) and bookseller (Martha Harison) whose connection with the others is unknown.

143 Thomas Berthelet printed Thomas Paynel's new translation in 1534, and in 1536 Thomas Gybson printed the final edition.

144 Franssen and Simoni, "Jan van Doesborch."

145 On chapmen and women distributing books in England, see Newcomb, "Chapbooks," and Spufford, *Small Books*. For France, see Fontaine, *Histoire du colportage*.

146 "*Je donne ce Livre aux vivans, & à la posterité; S'il est censuré par les sçavans, & curieux, je souffriray patiemment leur jugement, & arresteray ma plume en m'escusant sur la priere de mes amis, qui ont desiré ceste premier piece de mes Opuscules: Que si on le juge passable, ie poursuiveray mon dessein, & donray bientost au jour la seconde Partie. Le premier Traicté de la Peste, n'est qu'un extraict, ou un abregé du grand que j'ay preparé en Latin.*" Ranchin, *Opuscules*, 2.

147 Slack, "Mirrors of Health," 247; and Coste, *Représentations et comportements*, 44. Unfortunately, many tracts acquired by English antiquarians and book collectors are bound into larger compendia (either contemporaneously by collectors or later by holding institutions) and trimmed to a standard size. At the Bibliothèque nationale de France, most printed tracts are kept as individual items, but are bound in cardboard. Little or no information is provided in either case about the

original state in which the tracts were acquired. This makes it difficult to determine whether treatises circulated as individual pamphlets or as part of small collections bound by booksellers.

148 There were no standard book sizes in this era, and the size noted here is a general approximation only. Instead, the term "quarto" commonly referred to a format in which each leaf or page represents one-quarter of the size of the original sheet of paper that was folded twice. Likewise, a page in a "folio" book represents one-half of the original sheet of paper, while a page in "octavo" represents one-eighth (the original sheet having been folded three times).

149 Slack, "Mirrors of Health," 246–7.

150 Pettegree, Walsby, and Wilkinson, eds., *French Vernacular Books*, x–xi; and Ratia and Suhr, "Medical Pamphlets." Keiser specifically refers to plague tracts as pamphlets in "Two Medieval Plague Treatises."

151 On this practice (in the English context), see Luborsky and Ingram, *Guide*, and Hodnett, *English Woodcuts*.

152 Boeckl, *Images of Plague*, and Marshall, "Manipulating the Sacred."

153 On representations of God as plague agent, see especially Marshall, "Manipulating the Sacred" and "God's Executioners."

154 Ydeley, *Des secrets souverains*, title page. On this image, see Jones, "Bubo Men?"

155 "*[parce] que [ce petit livre] est portatif, il est tresutile*, tant pour faire recouvrer la santé aux malades, que pour preserver ceux qui ne sont encore attaints de la maladie." Paré, *Traicte de la peste*, A3.

156 Johns, *Nature of the Book*, 34.

157 Cavallo and Storey, *Healthy Living*, especially chapter 2.

CHAPTER THREE

1 Kemp, *Brief Treatise*, 27.

2 Ibid., 2.

3 Ibid., 2, 45–6.

4 Foligno, "Short Casebook, 1348," in Aberth, *Black Death*, 48. The plague of Athens was described by Thucydides and mentioned by Galen, while Avenzoar discussed the pestilence of Crannon (making reference to Hippocrates) in the twelfth century.

5 Kemp, *Brief Treatise*, 9–10. Here, Kemp was referring to the works of the Italian, German, and Silesian physicians Ercole Sassonia (Hercules de Saxonia), Daniel Sennert, and Martin Weinrich, and the German scholar Johannes Heinrich Ursinus. Archaeological evidence of corpse desecration

reveals the long-standing belief in Eastern and Central Europe that the dead could rise to harm the living, and that plague could result from the *Nachtzehrer*'s chewing (the *Nachtzehrer* being a kind of vampire). Mortuary practices such as staking, decapitation, and covering corpses with stones were used to punish suspected plague carriers. See Barrowclough, "Time to Slay Vampire Burials?" Samuel Collins, personal physician to England's King Charles I, claimed in his unpublished manuscript that "Another cause assigned to the production of the plague (which rarely happens) are wichcrafts, as Historys relate … and which cannot be appeased till their bodys are dugg up & their heades cut of [sic], this cannot merite any credit were it not justified by the authority and testimony of most worthy and most celebrated Authour Hercules Saxonia." London, British Library (BL), Sloane MS 1821, f. 249r.

6 Kemp, *Brief Treatise*, 95–6.

7 Ibid., 39.

8 Ibid., 18, 14.

9 Ibid., 37–8.

10 Ibid., 43.

11 Ibid., 58–9.

12 Siraisi, *History, Medicine, and Traditions*, 65.

13 Kemp, *Brief Treatise*, 10.

14 Ibid., 42.

15 Ibid., 37–8.

16 See, among many others, Bull, *Thinking Medieval*; Guenée, *Comment on écrit l'histoire*; Woolf, "Memory and Historical Culture"; and Thompson, *Customs in Common*. For theories of memory as a historicization device, see Klein, *From History to Theory*; Kansteiner, "Finding Meaning in Memory"; Hutton, *History as an Art of Memory*; Connerton, *How Societies Remember*; and Hartog, *Regimes of Historicity*. On intentionally "un-remembered" histories, see Zemon Davis and Starn, "Introduction."

17 Carmichael, "Last Past Plague," and Wallis, "Dreadful Heritage."

18 Hecker, *Black Death*, i–ii. In fact, a few decades earlier, another German medical writer, Kurt Polycarp Joachim Sprengel, published a work entitled *Beiträge zur Geschichte der Medicin* (*Contributions to the History of Medicine*), which contained a long chapter about the origins, cause, and spread of the Black Death. I thank Nükhet Varlık for alerting me to this work. Hecker's work has been tremendously influential in framing all subsequent discussions of the Black Death, and indeed for creating the framework within which later historians have constructed the plague narrative. On this, see Getz, "Black Death," and more recently Varlık, "Why Is Black Death *Black*?"

19 Hecker, *Black Death*, ix.

20 "Report of the Paris Medical Faculty," in Horrox, *Black Death*, 158.

21 Foligno, "Short Casebook, 1348," in Aberth, *Black Death*, 48.

22 Ibn Khātimah quoted in Campbell, *Black Death*, 52n23. Emphasis added.

23 Petrarch, "Letters on Family Matters," in Aberth, *Black Death*, 72.

24 Arrizabalaga, "Facing the Black Death," 238–9.

25 Campbell, *Black Death*, 80. On this point, see also Chase, "Fevers, Poisons, and Apostemes"; Carmichael, "Universal and Particular," 34–8; and Jones, "Apostumes, Carbuncles, and Botches."

26 "*d'autres signes sont indiqués par les auteurs qui ne sont pas encore apparus chez nous, je n'en dis donc rien*." Paris, Bibliothèque nationale de France (BnF), Latin MS 11227, cited in Coville, "Écrits contemporains," 329.

27 "Astrological Causes of the Plague, Geoffrey de Meaux," in Horrox, *Black Death*, 167.

28 "Report of the Paris Medical Faculty," 161–2, 158. Emphasis added.

29 Córdoba, "Letter and Regimen," in Aberth, *Black Death*, 45–6. Emphasis added.

30 Much has been made of the fact that chroniclers writing at the time of the Black Death barely mentioned the pandemic at all, seemingly unaware that it was such a widespread and monumental event until they went on the Jubilee pilgrimage to Rome in 1350 and swapped stories. On this point, see Carmichael, "Universal and Particular," 19–20; and Michaud, "La peste, la peur et l'espoir." In his detailed survey of Italian, French, and German chronicles written as the epidemic unfolded, Gabriele Zanella found "that sustained consideration of the epidemic was quite rare in works written during 1348 or 1349 ... contemporary reports made in localities that were hit early were all situated within a larger context of crises – famines, war, earthquakes, and epidemic." Cited in Carmichael, "Universal and Particular," 19. However, reporting on mundane events, even if catastrophic, was not chroniclers' main goal. Intead, fourteenth-century chroniclers were more interested in men's – and especially their patron's – actions and behaviour than in other peripheral events. Even events like a calamitous epidemic that seem especially significant to us served only either "as an explanation that reveals the reasons for these [men's] actions and behavior" or as chronological reference points for other, seemingly more important, things. Zink and Lydon, "Time of the Plague," 272.

31 "Plague in France," in Horrox, *Black Death*, 55; for the Grey Friars: "*quadam inaudita pestilencia epidemia nominata infecti*," Gransden, "Fourteenth-Century Chronicle," 274; Fordun quoted in Jillings, *Scotland's Black Death*, 13.

32 Compare, for example, Thucydides's description of the Plague of Athens ("The bodies of dying men lay one upon another, and half-dead creatures reeled about the streets"), John of Ephesus's description of the First Plague Pandemic ("corpses which split open with no one to bury them ... [and] houses ... which suddenly became tombs for their inhabitants ...[and] highways which became deserted"), and Boccaccio's description of the Black Death ("As a result of this wholesale desertion of the sick by neighbours, relatives and friends ... many dropped dead in the open streets ... and the others who were dying all over the city, bodies were here, there and everywhere"). Thucydides, *History of the Peloponnesian War*; Witakowski, *Pseudo-Dionysius*, 74–5; and "Plague in Florence," in Horrox, *Black Death*, 30–2. This is not to suggest that medieval writers knew Thucycides's work well, as they did not; some translations of his work appeared in late fourteenth-century Aragon, and from there moved to Italy in the early fifteenth. Rather, the point here is to note the longterm continuity – or trope – of epidemic storytelling. Similar tropes filled biblical narratives of great disasters. On indirect knowledge of Thucydidean literary narrative, see Pade, "Renaissance." On the phenomenon of using Thucydidean trope in early modern plague narratives, see Anselment, "Thomas Sprat's *The Plague of Athens*." For other literary religious tropes in plague narratives, see Brockliss and Jones, *Medical World*, 67. Duffin argues that Thucydides's influence continues in today's descriptions of epidemic outbreaks in "Introduction," 4.

33 Carmichael, "Universal and Particular," 33.

34 Arrizabalaga, "Facing the Black Death," 238–9.

35 Rawcliffe, *Urban Bodies*, 361; Campbell, *The Great Transition*, 64. The decades between the Great Famine and the Black Death, by contrast, were considerably less healthy; these years also showed significant climate disruption. DeWitte's archaeological work on skeletal remains in London's East Smithfield plague pit shows a rather sickly lot, so much so that she saw the emergence of a healthier post-plague English population. DeWitte, "Survival"; DeWitte and Wood, "Selectivity"; and DeWitte and Kowaleski, "Black Death Bodies."

36 On animal epidemics, see Newfield, "Cattle Panzootic" and "Early Medieval Epizootics"; and Slavin, "Great Bovine Pestilence."

37 The Greek medical writer Rufus of Ephesus, writing centuries before the outbreak of the First Pandemic, recognized plague as a disease that existed even in his own day. Mulhall, "Plague before the Pandemics."

38 Procopius, *History of the Wars*, vol. 1, *Persian War*, book II, chapter 22, 453. On this, see Dinkova-Bruun, "Preface," vii, xi; and Forrai, "Procopius

Caesariensis," 211–36. I thank Monica Green for bringing these secondary sources to my attention.

39 In Istanbul, however, Byzantine historians who received patronage from the Ottomans continued that tradition of scholarship.

40 The early ninth-century Byzantine chronicle of Theophanes Confessor drew from sixth-century sources and was known in the West through Anastasius Bibliothecarius's late ninth-century Latin translation. It spoke of the pandemic only in passing. I thank Anthony Kaldellis for his suggestions about possible transmission routes of First Pandemic writing into the Western chronicle tradition. Email correspondence, 25 March 2016. Re-engagement with Syriac sources took even longer.

41 Memory of the First Plague Pandemic was preserved and passed on for centuries through a wide variety of Islamicate writing: poetry, hadith commentaries, chronicles, Qur'an commentaries, medical texts, and theological and spiritual writings. References to the earlier outbreaks were then incorporated into plague tracts in the fourteenth century. See Conrad, "Arabic Plague Chronologies and Treatises." Fancy elaborates on this tradition, demonstrating that Arabic commentaries on ancient medical texts, medical encyclopedias, and specialist tracts alike discussed plague in some detail between the ninth and mid-fourteenth centuries. Consequently, when plague arrived (again) in Muslim-ruled western Eurasia and North Africa in the late 1340s, authors were able to turn to vivid descriptions of the disease in standard medical works to understand its causes, symptoms, and possible treatments. Fancy, "Knowing the Signs of Disease." I am not aware of any similar practice in the Jewish tradition. There is no notion of a first pandemic in Jewish literature; if anything, the biblical plagues, of which there are a number (included from the Prophets), were looked to as the first. Both the Bible and the Talmud include multiple discussions of plague, but these include disease, natural disasters, famines, and miraculous events that were oftentimes conflated. Jewish legal/rabbinic discussions of plagues throughout the centuries invariably referred to the biblical and Talmudic passages and not to any secular disease event. Indeed, while the borrowing of prayer and poetic themes from previous pandemics was common, there is little reference in Jewish literature to the history of pandemics outside of the Jewish experience. I thank Susan Einbinder and Eddie Reichman for discussing this point with me. On the custom of reciting the *Pittum haketoret*, which traces back to one of the first plagues mentioned in the Bible, see Einbinder, *Writing Plague*.

42 Of sixth-century knowledge, Little notes that "Greek and Roman medical writers, who commented on and anthologized the works of Hippocrates,

apparently knew of plague … not as a disease experienced or observed, but as one heard about from the far side of the Mediterranean." "Life and Afterlife," 9.

43 Phillips attributes this to the fall of the Roman Empire in the West and the narrowing of political horizons. Phillips, *Medieval Expansion*, 6.

44 Email correspondence with Alessandra Foscati, 23 March 2016. See also Foscati, *Ignis sacer*, xii.

45 "*inaudita … et nulla fuit talis.*" Chauliac, *Inventarium*, 1:118.

46 "*Antiqui siquidem in causis talium morborum diminute et superficialiter transiverunt … vel quia causas illorum vel modos actionis causarum ignoraverunt quia morbus est incognitus suis non cognitis causis vel modus actionis eorum … Postquam itaque vidi dicta antiquorum super morbis epidimicis tractancium, aspexi etiam tractatus diversos doctorum modernorum.*" Leipzig, Universitätsbibliothek (UB Leipzig), MS 1178, cited in Sudhoff, "Pestshriften" (17), 37–8.

47 "Treatise of John of Burgundy," in Horrox, *Black Death*, 192.

48 Goldstein and Pingree, "Levi ben Gerson's Prognostication," 7.

49 Carmichael notes the difficulties that some Black Death-era tract writers had reconciling astrological explanations with the epidemic. Carmichael, "Universal and Particular," 23. Jacquart compares some Italian and French discussions about astrological explanations of plague in the early fifteenth century. Jacquart, "Theories." See also Chase, "Fevers, Poisons, and Apostemes."

50 "*grans guerres mutacions de royaumes et de sects et … de paup[er]acions de richesce de m[ou]lt et … destruccion de sectes de sarrasins.*" BnF NAF MS 4516, f. 100v. A fifteenth-century English translation notes "this pestilence come by … [the] co[n]iu[n]ccion þat was made byfore s. anno 45to, for his trases and effects enduren yit … but þit coruptyng of the aire is not alone cause of moreyne but also habonndance of humors corupt in hem þ[a]t dien." Sloane MS 3449, f. 10v–11r, 5v. In other words, plague resulted from the combination of the ongoing effects of the malicious conjunction and people's humoral susceptibility to infection.

51 "*Et pour ce q[ue] eu ceste instans epidemie, ainsi que de nouvel reco[m] menciee.*" BnF NAF MS 4516, f. 98r.

52 The major outbreaks were in 1360–62, 1367–69, 1373–75, 1381–83, 1389–93 (England only), and 1399–1402. Numerous smaller localized outbreaks also occurred before 1400. The list of French outbreaks comes from Chase, "Fevers, Poisons, and Apostemes," 156, and Biraben, *Les hommes et la peste*, 1:377–8. The list of English outbreaks comes from Bolton, "Looking for *Yersina pestis*," 33, and Rawcliffe, *Urban Bodies*, 361–4.

53 "*Eodem anno mortalitas generalis oppressit populum que dicebatur Pestis Secunda*." Martin, *Knighton's Chronicle*, 184.

54 For example: "*Mesme celle ane fuist la secunde pestilence parmy Engleterre*"; "*Lan mille CCCLXIX fuist la tierc pestilence parmy Engleterre et en plusours autres terres*"; and "*Mesme celle an mille CCCLXIII [sic for CCCLXXIII] comensast le quart pestilence en plusours villes en Engleterre*." Galbraith, *Anonimalle Chronicle*, 50, 58, 77.

55 "*tamen pestilencia fuit multo minor quam precedens anno* 13mo." Gransden, "Fourteenth-Century Chronicle," 275; "*Eodam anno [1379], tempore aestivali tanta pestis exorta est in partibus Borealibus ex iniquo sidere, quanta nunquam antea visa fuit*" and "*Eo tempore [1391] mortalitas tanta succrevit in Northfolchia et multis aliis Comitatibus, ut non impar magnis pestilentiis censeretur*." Riley, *Thomas Walsingham*, 1:409 and 2:203, respectively. The Westminster monk John of Reading commented "there was at this time [1361] death without sorrow – just as there was in 1349." "The Second Pestilence," in Horrox, *Black Death*, 87.

56 "*L'an de la major mortaudat*," "*grant mortalitat*," "*an pestilencial de mortalitat*," "*mortalitat granda*," and so on. Dumas, *Santé et société*, 304–5. A similar trend appeared in Italian chronicles; Matteo Villani, for example, wrote "the wondrous mortality of *anguinaia* began anew this year [1363], similar to that which had its beginning in the years 1348 to 1350." Carmichael, *Plague and the Poor*, 11.

57 "*Et hoc manifeste vidimus in illa ingenti et inaudita mortalitate que apparuit nobis in Avinione anno domini millesimo* ccc^{o} xlviii^{o} *… Post vero, anno 60° … revenit ad nos mortalitas*." Chauliac, *Inventarium*, 1:117–19.

58 "*est mortalitas nunc de anno presenti 1382 … unius magne comete, que apparuit de anno … lapso 1381 de mense novembris fere per totum mensem*." UB Leipzig MS 1178, cited in Sudhoff, "Pestshriften" (17), 39.

59 "*Volo aliqua de pestilencia scribere que nos frequencius invadit quam fecerit antiquos*." Quoted in Chase, "Fevers, Poisons, and Apostemes," 163n3.

60 "Report of the Paris Medical Faculty," 161.

61 "*Et pour ce q[ue] eu ceste instans epidemie, ainsi que de nouvel reco[m] menciee et par succession de temps encore & encore retournera car nest mie maintenant la fin*." BnF NAF MS 4516, f. 98r.

62 "*Et non displiceat quia propter ipsius mirabilitatem et providenciam si iterum accideret narrabo eam*." Chauliac, *Inventarium*, 1:117–19.

63 "*Cum morbi pestilenciales qui hactenus fuerunt, sunt et erunt, prout praesumitur in diversis regionibus*." Erfurt, Universitätsbibliothek (UB Erfurt), Amplonian MS Q.194, cited in Sudhoff, "Pestschriften" (5), 48.

64 Astrological theories of history often spoke to recurrent or long-term impacts of nefarious astrological combinations, and writers who spoke most openly about plague's recurrence also emphasized the conjunction's role in causing it.

65 "*Item fis un autre traictie de la distinccion des maladies pestilencieuses des autres maladies qui se [com]mence cu[m] nimiru[m] p[ro]pt[er] instans tempus epidemiale, &c. ... e par experience longue de xx. ans et plus en m[ou]lt de lieux ou epidemie a regne.*" BnF NAF MS 4516, f. 98r, 101v. In Horrox's translation of a later Latin copy, John claimed to have "more than twenty-four years of experience." "Treatise of John of Burgundy," 192. Since the treatise was ostensibly written in 1365, twenty-four years (and even twenty years, as some copies say) of experience is clearly an exaggeration if he is talking specifically about plague. However, it makes more sense if the French version, produced in 1371, is in fact the earliest version, or if John was simply referring to his experience with epidemics in general.

66 Johannes Jacobi: "*il eut jadis une pestilence à Montpellier et je n'ai pu éviter la communauté parce que j'allais de maison en maison pour soigner les malades ... et ainsi j'ai survécu à une telle pestilence. Mes collègues étaient incrédules que j'aie gardé la vie.*" Quoted in Dumas, *Santé et société*, 314–15.

67 Carmichael's "Universal and Particular" shows that 78 per cent of Latin tracts written between the late 1350s and 1400 did so. I thank her for sharing her raw data with me.

68 "*apostematibus et antracibus in exterioribus, potissime in subasellis et inguinibus ... revenit ad nos mortalitas ... cum febribus, bochiis, carbunculis, et antracibus.*" Chauliac, *Inventarium*, 1:117–19.

69 Carmichael, "Universal and Particular," 37. Emphasis added.

70 Oxford, Bodleian Library (Bodl.), Rawlinson MS A.429, f. 85v.

71 Jacquart, "Theory," 142–3, 147.

72 "*Mais plus souvent en peult venir lapostume qui tellement en prent plusieurs qui fait venir de ce siecle tres durement plusieurs.*" Atila, *Traictie tresutile contre la peste*, 5.

73 Hartog, *Regimes of Historicity*, 17.

74 Brockliss and Jones, *Medical World*, 19. Large regional or national outbreaks are noted in England for the years 1407, 1413, 1417–21, 1426–27, 1433–34, 1439–40, 1450, 1457–59, 1463–64, 1467, 1471, 1473, 1478–80, 1487, and 1499–1500. Numerous localized outbreaks are interspersed, and a similarly long list of outbreaks followed in the sixteenth century. Rawcliffe, *Urban Bodies*, 364–71; and Keiser, "Two Medieval Plague

Treatises," 302. For France, Biraben's list (admittedly unreliable) suggests that in only three years during the entire fifteenth century (1403, 1419, and 1447) were there no reports of multiple/widespread plague outbreaks. Biraben, *Les hommes et la peste*, 1:378–81.

75 McCormick notes that a similar process marked writing about the First Pandemic, in that documentary records of outbreaks grew increasingly scarce after c.600. McCormick, "Gregory of Tours," 48.

76 Martin, *Knighton's Chronicle*. See also Woolf, "Historical Writing in Britain," 473–96.

77 Hedeman, *The Royal Image*, 181.

78 Nichols, *Chronicle of the Grey Friars of London*, 16, 22, 24, 26; and McLaren, *The London Chronicles*, 40, 236.

79 "*la mortalité si tres cruelle … on ne avoit oncques veu ne ouy parler de mortalité qui fust si desvée*." Tuetey, *Journal d'un Bourgeois de Paris*, 115.

80 Aston, "Death," 204. Carmichael also suggests that lower mortality may have led chroniclers to see repeated outbreaks "as though they were more a nuisance than a serious threat … [as such, the epidemics] became peripheral to [more] important events." Carmichael, *Plague and the Poor*, 62. On the decline of chronicle writing, see Gransden, *Historical Writing*, 342, and Bellaguet, *Chronique du religieux de Saint-Denys.*

81 Quoted in Ormrod, "Politics of Pestilence," 176.

82 "*Et ergo audiendi non sunt medici pitagorici jubentes tempore pestilentiali fieri usum ceparum et aliarum rerum excessive calidarum*." Amplonian Q.194, cited in Sudhoff, "Pestschriften" (5), 50; "*Tempore pestilentiali vitentur loca et infirmi et non exea tur de mane stomacho jejuno*." Heidelberg, Universitätsbibliothek MS Palatinus Germanicus 558, cited in Ibid., (5), 54.

83 An examination of German tracts transcribed by Karl Sudhoff in the early twentieth century, by contrast, shows that some of them seem to have continued referring to the Black Death well into the fifteenth century.

84 Rawlinson MS A.429, f. 85v.

85 Sloane MS 3489, f. 44r. Emphasis added.

86 Moulton, *This is the Myrour or Glasse of Helthe*, (<1530), 2. Emphasis added.

87 Moulton, *This is the Myrour or Glasse of Helthe*, (c. 1566), 7; Moulton, *Compleat Bone-Setter*, B1.

88 Matheson, "Médecin sans Frontières?," 27. The tracts are in Sloane MS 3285 (c. 1406–07) and Cambridge, Cambridge University Library (CUL), MS LL.1.18 (late 15th century).

89 "*la peste: qui lors ou peu au paravant regnoit bien forte en Lorraine … Et pour ce que je veoy à l'oeil que le temps present tend à la mesme disposition.*" D'Andernach, *Instruction tresutile*, 3–4.

90 Bysshop and Doctor of Physick of Denmarke, *Here after ensuith a litle treatise*, 2.

91 Phayer, *The Regiment of Life*, 3v.

92 "*co[n]gnoistre comme[n]t elles vienne[n]t & comment elles doibue[n]t retourner.*" Thibault, *Le thresor du remede*, A1.

93 Paynel, *Moche Profitable Treatise*, 1.

94 Jones, "Information and Science," 100.

95 Carmichael, "Last Past Plague," 158.

96 "*ce lieu de Sedan estant pour la seconde fois rudement assailli de peste.*" Courcelles, *Traite de la peste*, 2.

97 "*Et a ce propos recite Dalescus de tarenta que en lan mil trois ce[nt]s iiii xx et vii. Il regna a monpellier ung tel catarre et reume pestilentiel q[ue] a grand peine il eschapa la dixiesme partie du peuple sans les enfa[n]s … Sembablement en lan mil quatre cens quatre vingts et cinq. En la cite de londres et pays denviron Il commencea … une telle fiebvre pestilentielle et si furieuse que plusieurs mouroient soudainement.*" Le Forestier, *Le regime contre epidimie*, 2. According to Geneviève Dumas (personal correspondence, 17 December 2016), Montpellier's urban chronicle makes no reference to an epidemic for the year 1387. However, there is a mortality episode noted in 1397, and city officials consulted with doctors to determine if it was plague. The scribe, tract author, or printer may have mistaken that year for 1387.

98 Guerin, *Traicte tresexcellent*.

99 "*les lieux maritimes, ou exposez au Midi … c'est la seule raison … qu'il y a des lieux … qui sont plus sujets que les autres.*" Courcelles, *Traite de la peste*, 34.

100 For similar observations about Italian plague tracts, see Carmichael, "Last Past Plague," and Cohn, *Cultures of Plague*. Cohn's study features narrative plague histories with local interest anecdotes, while Carmichael points to physician (or health official) testimonials.

101 Carmichael, "Last Past Plague," 133.

102 Wrightson, *Earthly Necessities*, 3.

103 William Wotton, *Reflections*, quoted in Houston and Pincus, "Introduction," 3. See also Withington, *Society in Early Modern England*.

104 Duris, *Quelle révolution scientifique?*

105 This somewhat oversimplifies the argument in Subrahmanyam, "On World Historians," as non-Europeans also engaged in this type of history writing,

at around the same time. In addition to their geographic scope, universal and global histories also differ in their aesthetic criteria and their sense of symmetry.

106 Quoted in Siraisi, "Anatomizing the Past," 1.

107 Siraisi, *History, Medicine, Traditions*, 65. See also Siraisi, "Anatomizing the Past." In his tract on the sweating sickness, John Caius likewise included a long historical discussion of that disease and others. Caius, *Boke, or Counseill*. See also Nutton, "John Caius, Historian," and Goulding, "Histories of Science." I also thank Craig Martin for sharing his unpublished work with me, as it explores some of these same themes.

108 Carmichael, "Last Past Plague," 158. See also Pomata, "*Praxis Historialis,*" and Siraisi, *History, Medicine, Traditions*.

109 "*la contagion de peste qui a esté ceste presente annee en la ville de Lyon*." Rubys, *Discours sur la contagion*, title page.

110 "*la peste survenue à Bourdeaux, cest an 1599*." Briet, *Discours sur les causes de la peste*, title page.

111 "*ce qui s'est passé de plus mémorable en cette ville, depuis the mois d'août de l'an 1628 jusques au mois d'octobre de l'an 1629*." Grillot, *Lyon affligé de contagion*, title page.

112 Woolf calls this "the medium-term past" in "Memory and Historical Culture," 296.

113 "*je me souviens que en l'an 1555. estant lors jeune escolier à Padouë, je vis pe[n]dre & estrangler un medecin Espaignol, & quelques uns … [parce qu'ils] infectoient ledittes maisons avec certains emplastres*." Rubys, *Discours sur la contagion de peste*, 9.

114 Joubert, *Traitté de la peste*, 11.

115 "*La peste … est comme une mauvaise beste, qui en tue plusieurs … Ce qui a esté veu depuis quinze ou seize ans ença, d'une noble & fameuse ville, limitrophe, appelee Trente*." Nancel, *Discours tresample*, 13–14.

116 Brasbridge, *Poore Man's Jewell*, 3.

117 "*depuis l'an cinq cens quatre vingt seize, jusque à present sans aucune recompense, chose estrange veu qu'il ny a ville en vostre Royaume où les chirurgiens ne soient gag[n]ez annuellement & perpetuellement pour ce sujet, excepté votre ville de Paris*." Potel, *Traicté de la peste*, 4.

118 "*cette Ville, apres avoir possedé une parfaite santé pour le regard de la maladie contagieuse, l'espace de quarante années ou environ; ayant oublié l'affliction receuë depuis les années 1581. jusques en l'année 1587*." Chevalier, *L'ordre public*, 1.

119 Under the Ancien Régime, the *parlement* was a provincial appellate court of the Kingdom of France. It was not only the court of final appeal of the

judicial system: laws and edicts issued by the crown only became official in their respective jurisdictions when the parlements accepted them. While both the modern French term *parlement* (legislature) and the English word parliament derive from this older French term, the Ancien Régime parlements were not legislative bodies and cannot be equated with today's governmental structures.

120 Holt, "King in Parlement," 516.

121 Aubert, *Traite contenant les causes*, 5; Houël, *Traité de la peste*, 4; and Briet, *Discours sur les causes de la peste*, 10.

122 "*depuis cinq ou six ans, la France au cœur de laquelle … la ville de Paris, peult rendre, fidel tesmoignage, de l'inconvenient & perte, quelle a souffert, par sa cruelle contagion … les hommes y sont demeurez plongez de plus en plus.*" Le Lievre, *Epydimyomachie*, A6.

123 "*plusieurs excelents personnages, curieulx, du repos, & tranquilité, de l'esconomye humaine, ce soient employes pour arracher, & effaßer, du cœur des hommes, ce facheux caractere, de discorde, & mauvaise plante de guerre, publiant par tous aux oreilles de chacun, la douceur, benefice, & vilité, de la paix.*" Ibid.

124 Kemp, *Brief Treatise*, A2.

125 Clarke, *Historian's Guide*.

126 Wither, *Britain's Remembrancer*, title page.

127 Ibid.

128 Rawcliffe, *Urban Bodies*, 68. For a contemporary reading of the bills of mortality from London, Westminster, and Norwich in 1603, see Chettle, *A True Bill*.

129 Jenner, "Plague on a Page," 226. See also Harding, "Reading Plague."

130 Jenner, "Plague on a Page," 266.

131 The City of London's weekly bills of mortality were publicly available from the early 1560s; by the late 1620s, annual summaries also appeared. For an overview of the genre, see Ratia, "Bills of Mortality." Systematic reporting of causes of death by locality began in Europe as a result of the recurrent plague epidemics: Florence's civic burial registers and Milan's civic death registers were among the earliest, commencing in the late fourteenth and mid-fifteenth centuries, respectively. Alter and Carmichael, "Classifying the Dead." See also Carmichael, "Registering Death" and "Legal Foundations."

132 Graunt, *Reflections*, 1–2.

133 Graunt, *London's Dreadful Visitation*, A2.

134 Anonymous, *Weekly Bill of Mortality*; and Bell, *London's Remembrancer*. See also Graunt, *Natural and Political Observations*.

135 Thayre, *Excellent and Best Approoved Treatise*, 3.
136 Anonymous, *Especiall Observations*, 2. Emphasis added.
137 Boghurst, *Loimographia*, 3.
138 Revel, "Autour d'une épidémie ancienne," 979. See also Panel, *Trois Opuscules*.
139 Slauter, "Write Up Your Dead," 6. On later developments in these kinds of bills in both England and France, see Rusnock, *Vital Accounts*, especially chapter 6.
140 Belmas, "Pouvoir politique et catastrophe sanitaire."
141 Details of the debate between Jouyse and Lamperiere are found in Coste, *Représentations et comportements*, 603–7. See also Jouyse, *Examen du livre de Lamperiere*, and Lamperiere, *Traité de la peste* and *L'Ombre de Nécrophore*.
142 "*Ce que l'on estimoit avoir esté fait par les Aethiopiens, à la terrible Peste des Athenie[n]s, que recite Thucydide.*" Ferrier, *Remedes*, 9.
143 Ibid., 7–13.
144 Siraisi, *History, Medicine, and Traditions*, 15; and Wear, *Knowledge & Practice*, 35.
145 Coste, *Représentations et comportements*, 15.
146 Runciman, *Fall of Constantinople*, xi; Pade, "Renaissance," 26; Forrai, "Procopius Caesariensis," 212–13; and Soll, "Uses of Historical Evidence," 153. For a good, albeit brief, discussion of the differences in the development of English and French historical thought and practice, see Woolf, "Erudition."
147 Brasbridge, *Poore Man's Jewell*, 3.
148 There were a few exceptions: Guy de Chauliac's works remained especially popular, and other early tract authors such as Johannes Jacobi, Gentile da Foligno, and Raymond Chalin de Vinario saw their treatises printed in the fifteenth and sixteenth centuries. In 1623, Guillaume Potel relied on and repeated Guy de Chauliac's explanations of the disease, since he "talked about the great pestilence of his time" ("*où il parle de ceste grande pestillence qui fur de son temps*"). Potel, *Traicté de la peste*, 27. Aside from Chauliac, however, references to medieval medical writers are largely absent from the early modern plague tracts.
149 Dinkova-Bruun, "Preface," xi–xii; Soll, "Uses of Historical Evidence," 156; Carmichael, "Last Past Plague," 149; Pade, "Thucydides' Renaissance Readers"; and Schlatter, "Thomas Hobbes and Thucydides," 350. See Hobbes, *Eight Bookes*, and Sprat, *Plague of Athens*.
150 Anselment, "Thomas Sprat's *The Plague of Athens*," 11. The Plague of Athens was not the disease that we now call plague, and Thucydides did

not describe buboes; however, other physical symptoms that he noted – fever, dry mouth, convulsions, and headaches – resonated with early modern readers. Thucydides's descriptions of the epidemic's social impacts were also profoundly familiar.

151 Siraisi, *History, Medicine, and Traditions*, 94, and "Anatomizing the Past," 10. See also Siraisi, "Cardano," 346, 353–4.

152 Siraisi, "Anatomizing the Past," 6.

153 "*Mathieu Villani historien Flore[n]tin escript que ceste grande peste qui advint de son temps en Italie, qui fut lez annees 1346.47.48.& 49. pendant laquelle Jean boccace escrivit son Decameron.*" Rubys, *Discours sur la contagion*, 8.

154 "*la peste est quelque fois universelle, comme celle qui est descrite par Gui de Cauliac, laquelle fust en l'an 1348. apres avoir commencé premierement en Orient & en apres environné & circui presque tout le monde.*" Joubert, *Traitté de la peste*, 11.

155 Siraisi, *History, Medicine, and Traditions*, 102–5. See also Palmer, "Girolamo Mercuriale," and Nutton, "With Benefit of Hindsight."

156 Mercuriale, *De peste*, in Siraisi, *History, Medicine, and Traditions*, 104.

157 College des Maistres Chirurgiens jurez de Paris, *Traicté de la peste*, 7, 11. The first outbreak is the Antonine Plague of 165–80 CE, the second is the First Plague Pandemic outbreak in Rome in 590.

158 "*Jacob. de partib. recite que ceste maladie commençant l'an 1385. & continuant par cinq années, emporta plus de la moitié du monde.*" Sainct-Hillier, *Loimologie*, 13–14.

159 Vigier, "Traitté de la Peste," 315–16.

160 Chettle, *True Bill*, 1.

161 Gadbury, *London's Deliverance Predicted*, 6.

162 Anonymous, *Shutting Up*, 6.

163 Graunt, *Reflections*, 25, 28, 30.

164 Anonymous, *Weekly Bill of Mortality*, n.p.

165 Bradley, *Plague at Marseilles Consider'd*, A7r.

166 Ibid., title page.

167 Ibid., 12. See also Anonymous, *Late Dreadful Plague*.

168 Bradley, *Plague at Marseilles Consider'd*, A3.

169 Ibid., 12–13.

170 Brookes, *History*, 5–6.

171 Ibid., 6.

172 Ibid., 7.

173 Ibid., 12. Brookes is off here by one year, as the sweating sickness was noted first in 1485.

174 Ibid., 17. Noteworthy here is the fact that in the margins of the account is the finding aid "Pestilence with Inflammation of the Lungs, 1348." Brookes also provides a lengthy description of pneumonic symptoms, and suggests that this form of plague spread first, followed by the bubonic version.

175 Ibid., 18.

176 Quincy, *Essay*, 25.

177 Browne, *Practical Treatise*, 4. It is not clear if Browne was referring to Andrewes Burrell, who wrote a treatise on afflictions among seamen in the English navy in 1649, but was not a physician.

178 Ibid., 38.

179 Ibid., 55.

180 Mead, *Short Discourse*, A3.

181 Mead, *Discourse*, 23.

182 Ingram, *Historical Account*, 5.

183 Ibid., iv.

184 Ibid., 44–9.

185 "*La Peste qui ravage la Ville de Marseille, est un Contagion que tout le monde doit assez connoître par ses tristes effects.*" Boyer, *Dissertation abregée*, 3.

186 "*on peut conclure de-là, que la Peste est un genre, & non pas une espece de maladie. Les symptomes particuliers qui l'ont caracterisée autrefois, seront les especes de ce genre … elle fut nommée Coqueluche … Enfin, l'inguinaire ou la Peste à Bubons, qu'on prétend n'avoir commencé qu'au sixième siècle.*" Baux, *Traité de la peste*, 5–7. Baux also misdates the initial sweating sickness outbreak of 1485.

187 Manget, *Traité de la peste*, 39–42.

188 "*Ouvrage necessaire a tous jeunes Medecins & Chirurgiens destinez au secours des Pestiferez.*" Pestalozzi, *Avis de precaution*, title page.

189 For example: "*Il semble que des Auteurs Medecins & Historiens se soient fait un deffi, a qui donneroit l'idée la plus outrée de la Contagion de la Peste, en racontant des Histoires*" (Joubert, *Reflexions*, 1), and "*Les Histoires nous fournissent sur cela tant d'exemples si extraordinaire qu'on auroit de la peine à les croire*" (Goiffon, *Relations et dissertation*, 56–7).

190 "*nous pouvons dire, qu'il n'en a jamais donné l'exemple si terrible que celui que nous venons de voir dans la peste a desolé la ville de Marseille en 1720 … on ose assurer, que de toutes celles que les Historiens raportent, que les Auteurs de Médecine décrivent, & que nos Négociants & nos gens de mer ont vu dans les différentes Contrées du Levant; aucune n'a été si rapide dans ses progrès, ni si violente dans ses effets que celle-ci.*"

Bertrand, *Relation historique*, 8, 483. See also Gordon, "Confrontations with the Plague," 18.

191 "*Les troubles & les désordres de la contagion, des désolations extrêmes, une mortalité générale, des évenemens singuliers étoient un sujet bien digne d'un Historien.*" Bertrand, *Relation historique*, 370.

192 Hecker, *Black Death*, xi–xii.

193 Ibid., ix–x.

194 Ibid., 130–5.

195 Carmichael, "Last Past Plague," 134.

196 A key exception is Clarke and Rawcliffe, eds., *The Fifteenth Century*.

CHAPTER FOUR

1 "*On ne marque presque jamais, ni le progrès ni la durée de la Peste dans un Estat; on ne dit mot de plusieurs Lieux qui ont été affligez; ce qui fait croire que plusieurs Pestes dont on a parlé, pouvoient être la même qui avoit passé d'une Ville ou d'un Royaume à l'autre, ou qui s'étoit renouvellée, parce qu'elle n'avoit pas été suffisamment éteinte.*" Baux, *Traité de la peste*, 16.

2 "*Nous n'avons pas crû devoir nous étendre davantage sur ce qui regard l'origine de la Peste: cette recherche n'est pas d'une grande utilité; il est assez indifferent pour le soulagement des malades.*" Ibid., 17. Baux wrote his comments in July 1721, but the tract was published the following year.

3 *Biographie universelle*, 581.

4 The *Grand Saint Antoine* has loomed large in scholarship about the Plague of Provence, buttressed by the fact that accounts blaming the ship, its crew, and its cargo for importing plague into the city from the Levant can be found in archives throughout the Atlantic world. However, these accounts simply repeated the story coming out of Marseille itself, which in turn was based largely on French diplomatic and economic interests. Even in that city not everyone agreed with the "it arrived via ship" narrative. Further, there are almost no records of outbreaks in the eastern Mediterranean at this time: just one in Greece in July 1719 and one in Damascus in November 1719. The next recorded outbreaks are *after* the outbreak in Marseille. This does not mean that there might not have been outbreaks when the ship passed through Levantine ports, but there is no evidence that there were. Ancient DNA evidence also does not support a Levantine origin for the outbreak. See Varlık, "Rethinking the History of Plague," 287–9.

5 Around 500 BCE, Alcmaeôn of Crotôn explicitly suggested that disease is "sometimes affected by external causes, such as certain waters or a particular site." Quoted in Freeman, *Ancilla*, 40–1. The Hippocratic treatises *Airs, Waters, and Places* and *On the Nature of Man* elaborated that specific topographical and climatic features defined local people's health, and that epidemics were caused by infected air. Galen added to this the idea of "miasma."

6 On medieval medical writers who examined the relationship between local environments and disease, see Aberth, *Environmental History*, 13–18. For early modern applications, see Wear, "Place, Health, and Disease." For such ideas in health regimens and plague tracts, see Cavallo and Storey, eds., *Conserving Health* and Jones, "Diseased Landscape," respectively.

7 On medieval and early modern "otherness," see Benveniste and Costas, "Heterodoxies."

8 "*Il est donc certain, que si Marseille avoit été le foyer de l'infection, la mortalité auroit dû y être plus grande ou qu'elle auroit dû n'être pas confiderable dans les Lieux qui en sont éloignez.*" Baux, *Traité de la peste*, 10.

9 "*ces Villes où la mort fait sa moisson.*" Ibid., 8.

10 "*Nous voyons entrer la Peste en France; nous la voyons passer de Ville en Ville, de Province en Province.*" Ibid., 13.

11 But see note 4, this chapter.

12 Baux, *Traité de la peste*, 2–3, 15–17.

13 Signoli, et al., "Paleodemography and Historical Demography."

14 Brockliss and Jones, *Medical World*, 350–3.

15 The scholarship here is large and growing. On theories of space and place, see among others Lefebvre, *Production de l'espace*; Foucault, "Questions on Geography"; Lussault, *L'Homme spatial*; Stock and Vöhringer, *Spatial Practices*; Lévy and Lussault, "*Espace*"; and de Certeau, *Practice*. On specific uses or practices of space/place, see Lévy, *L'espace légitime;* Kümin, *Political Space*; Hanawalt and Kobialka, *Medieval Practices of Space*; *Construction de l'espace au Moyen Âge*; Buttimer and Seamon, *Human Experience*; Foucault, *Folie et Déraison;* and Gilchrist, "Medieval Bodies."

16 Lefebvre, *Writings on Cities*; Rawcliffe, *Urban Bodies*; Rawcliffe and Weeda, eds., *Policing the Urban Environment*; Fay, *Health and the City*; Porter, *Health, Civilization, and the State*; Granshaw and Porter, *The Hospital in History*; Barnes, *The Great Stink*; Corbin, *The Foul and the Fragrant*; Fitzpatrick and LaGory, *Unhealthy Places*; Anderson, *Colonial Pathologies*; McFarlane, "Governing the Contaminated City"; Geltner, "Healthscaping"; Touati, *Maladie et société*; and Dobson, *Contours of Death*.

17 Gregory likely followed the typical "rogation days" pattern around the city that was used for all kinds of catastrophes. In the Christian tradition, rogation days are days of prayers and fasting, observed by the litany of the saints and processions. The major rogation is held on 25 April, while minor rogations are held on Monday through Wednesday preceding Ascension Thursday. Plague processions were largely grafted onto earlier penitence processions, but they followed a clear geographic route. On earlier processions against the threat of plague, see Stoclet, "Consilia humana." See also Horden, "Ritual and Public Health," for a good discussion of the spatial aspects of early anti-plague rituals. For later re-enactments of these processions and their adaptation to public health requirements, see Chiu, "Singing on the Street."

18 Crawshaw, *Plague Hospitals*, 86. Rawcliffe shows that, like people whose uncivil behaviours were believed to bring pollution and disease into the civic body, diseased bodies were best removed to a place outside the town's boundaries. Rawcliffe, *Urban Bodies*.

19 Koch, *Disease Maps*, 55.

20 Anonymous, *Shutting Up*, 5.

21 Córdoba, "Letter and Regimen," in Aberth, *Black Death*, 46.

22 "Report of the Paris Medical Faculty," in Horrox, *Black Death*, 162.

23 Anticipating plague's arrival in the Iberian Peninsula months earlier, Jacme d'Agramont had justified writing his tract on people's fears of the "epidemics or pestilence and mortality of people [that] reign and have reigned in some parts and regions neighbouring ours." Duran-Reynals and Winslow, "Jacme d'Agramont," 57.

24 "Astrological Causes of the Plague, Geoffrey de Meaux," in Horrox, *Black Death*, 167.

25 "*pestilenciam epydimialem que nunc grassatur in mundo*." Lille, Bibliothèque municipale, Médiathèque Jean Lévy, MS 863, f. 151.

26 "Importance of Prayer," in Horrox, *Black Death*, 114.

27 "Intercessionary Processions (1)" in Ibid., 111.

28 Petrarch, "Letters on Family Matters," 72.

29 "Plague Seen from Tournai," in Horrox, *Black Death*, 46, 49.

30 Procopius, *History of the Wars*, vol. I, book II, chapter 22, 453.

31 Ibid., vol. VI, chapter 23, 275.

32 Ibid., vol. I, book II, chapter 22, 453; Ibid., vol. VI, chapter 23, 275; Witakowski, *Pseudo-Dionysius*, 74–7.

33 Croke, *Chronicle of Marcellinus*, 50. Adomnán, the late seventh-century abbot of Iona, devoted a chapter of his *Vita Columbae* to "the plague, which in our own time twice visited the greater part of the world ...

including Italy, the Roman States, and the Cisalpine provinces of Gaul, with the States of Spain also, which lie beyond the Pyrenees, these islands of the sea, Scotia (Ireland) and Britain." Reeves, *Life of Saint Columba.* While popular in the Scottish and Irish hagiographical tradition, the *Vita Columbae* was not widely known.

34 McCormick, "Gregory of Tours," 38.

35 Pope Gregory I also acknowledged that the pestilence he faced "was ravaging Italy, Africa, and the East." Stathakopoulos, *Famine and Pestilence*, 332–3.

36 Sharp, "Isidore of Seville," 57. As noted in chapter 1, other medical writing about the First Plague Pandemic appears to have been completely unknown in the West; although John of Alexandria, Stephanus of Athens, and Paul of Aegina all described the symptoms of bubonic plague they too did not place their clinical accounts into any wide geographical context. Mulhall, "Confronting Pandemic."

37 See chapter 3 for the absence of the First Plague Pandemic from the fourteenth-century collective memory.

38 Carmichael, "Universal and Particular," 19.

39 Greengrass, *Christendom Destroyed*, xxvi–xxvii.

40 "Plague in France according to Jean de Venette," in Horrox, *Black Death*, 55; Luce, *Chroniques de J. Froissart*, 4:100; Martin, *Knighton's Chronicle*, 94; and "Plague according to Thomas Walsingham," in Horrox, *Black Death*, 66.

41 Carmichael, "Universal and Particular," 29–30.

42 "*Et nomino eam ingentem quia totum mundum vel quasi occupavit … ille non occupaverunt nisi unam regionem, ista totum mundum.*" Chauliac, *Inventarium*, I:118.

43 On the shedding of long-standing epistemological paradigms for others, see Foucault, *The Order of Things*.

44 Jacme d'Agramont, for example, distinguished the causes of a universal pestilence that affects "a whole region or … several" from those of "a pestilence particular and appropriate to one city only." Duran-Reynals and Winslow, "Jacme d'Agramont," 63, 68.

45 "Astrological Causes of the Plague," 170.

46 London, British Library (BL), Additional MS 27582, f. 70r.

47 "*sudore continuo interficiebat cuius febris adventus incepit sua vexilla extendere in anglia in civitate londonia decimanona die mensis septembris anno domini 1485.*" Le Forestier, *Tractatus contra pestilentiam*, A2r.

48 One exception was Raymond Chalin de Vinario, who reported that the 1381–82 epidemic simultaneously affected the eastern, western, and

northern parts of the world: "*Nam fuit eodem anno et est adhuc in tota Syria, Grecia, in Ytalia, in Alemania, in Anglia, in Scotia, in Francia, in Yspania et Naverra, quamuis plus in una regione quam in alia et in uno loco quam in alio secundum exigenciam agencium et secundum disposicionem.*" Leipzig, Universitätsbibliothek (UB Leipzig), MS 1178, cited in Sudhoff, "Pestshriften" (17), 39. Some Italian and German writers made similar observations, but they were far fewer in the French treatises.

49 "*Et hoc manifeste vidimus in illa ingenti et inaudita mortalitate que apparuit nobis in Avinione.*" Chauliac, *Inventarium*, 1:117.

50 "*Post vero, anno 60°, pontificatus domini Innocencii sexti anno octo … revenit ad nos mortalitas.*" Ibid., 1:119.

51 I discuss these locations, and their váriants, in more detail in "Itineraries and Transformations."

52 Paris, Bibliothèque nationale de France (BnF), NAF MS 4516, ff. 97r, 98r.

53 "*Vidi tamen quod quidam nobilis curatus fuit, quern tenuiin cura in Montepessulano, qui habuit apostema pestilentiale in leo inguine et fleubotomatus fuit de vena pedis.*" Erfurt, Universitätsbibliothek (UB Erfurt), Amplonian MS Q.194, cited in Sudhoff, "Pestschriften" (5), 53.

54 "*ad utilitatem tocius comitatus insignis ville Montispessuli.*" Munich, Staatsbibliothek MS Latin 372, cited in Ibid., (17), 53.

55 Cambridge, Trinity College (TCC), MS R.14.52, f. 153v.

56 Rawcliffe, *Urban Bodies*, 364–71; and Stathakopoulus, *Famine and Pestilence*, 120.

57 Oxford, Bodleian Library (Bodl.), Rawlinson MS A.429, f. 85v.

58 Kurath, *Middle English Dictionary*, 573–5.

59 On how local dialects anchored medical texts to specific places, see Taavitsainen, "Scriptorial 'House-styles,'" 211.

60 Matheson, "Médecin sans Frontières?," 27.

61 BL Sloane MS 3489, ff. 44r–51r.

62 Moulton, *Myrour or Glass of Helthe*, B1–2.

63 Phayer, *Goodly Bryefe Treatise*, L3.

64 Anonymous, *Present Remedies*, A3.

65 Kellwaye, *Defensative Against the Plague*, A4v.

66 Skene, *Ane breve descriptioun of the pest*, A1.

67 Brasbridge, *Poore Mans Jewell*, A2.

68 Ibid., A3.

69 Skene, *Ane breve descriptioun of the pest*, A1. Jillings points out however, that Skene did not actually experience plague in Aberdeen, so his recourse to observation was more rhetorical device than fact. Jillings, "Medical Advice?" 313.

70 Twyne, *New Counsell*, A2.

71 Griffiths and Jenner, eds., *Londinopolis,* 2. The population increased from about 50,000 to 200,000–250,000 between 1500 and 1600, while the city's proportion of England's total population increased from about 2 per cent to more than 5 per cent. See also Boulton, "London 1540–1700," and Slack, "Great and Good Towns."

72 Merritt, "Perceptions and Portrayals," 1–3.

73 Stow, *Survey of London*, 1.

74 Platter, *Travels*, cited in Boulton, "London 1540–1700," 315.

75 Merritt, "Perceptions and Portrayals," 1–3, 22.

76 Clapham, *Epistle*, A3.

77 Recent mapping of the rise and spread of plague in London strongly suggests that the disease was endemic in the city during the sixteenth and seventeenth centuries. Cummins, Kelly, and Ó Gráda, "Living Standards."

78 Bradwell, *Watch-Man*, 1; and I.D., *Salomon's Pest-house*, 1.

79 Taylor, *Fearefull summer*. See also Dekker, *Wonderfull yeare*.

80 Herring, *Certaine Rules*, 3.

81 Thayre, *Excellent and Best Approoved Treatise*, 1, A2.

82 Anonymous, *Especiall Observations*, B1; and Bradwell, *Watch-Man*, 1.

83 Kemp, *Brief Treatise*, 14.

84 Hodges, *Loimologia,* 2.

85 De Garencières, *Mite*; J.V., *Golgotha*; and Quarles, *Londons Disease*.

86 Boffey's recent work on book production in London also emphasizes the city's depiction in literary and other works. *Manuscript and Print*.

87 For Newcastle-upon-Tyne, see Wrightson, *Ralph Tailor's Summer*; for East Stoke and Newark, see Jennings, "Anatomy of a Civil War Plague" and "Stinking, Miserable, Infected Town." See also Slack, *Impact of Plague,* and Dobson, *Contours of Death*, 383–449.

88 Anonymous, *Especiall Observations*, B1.

89 The scholarship on early modern plague literature is vast. See, among others, Totaro and Gilman, ed., *Representing Plague*; Gilman, *Plague Writing*; Healy, *Fictions of Disease*; and Achinstein, "Plagues and Publication."

90 Gatford, *Logos alexipharmakos*, 1–2.

91 Vincent, *Gods Terrible Voice*. Two anonymous tracts printed in Oxford by Leonard Lichfield in 1644 were generic in their discussion of geography: *Concerning the Constitution* and *Physicall Directions*.

92 Physician in York, *Treatise of the Plague*, title page, 6.

93 On the non-linear link between book production and marketing, see Ornato, *La face cachée*.

94 While Paris's population by 1600 was more than three times the size of Rouen and more than five times the size of Lyon or Marseille, London's was at least *fifteen* times the size of the next largest English city, Norwich. Boulton, "London 1540–1700," 316; and *Atlas Historique de Paris*, accessed 25 August 2017.

95 "*Pour vous advertir en considera[n]t que au pays Da[n]jou & autre part la peste a este et est de si grande violence.*" De Houssemaine, *Ung regime singulier*, 59.

96 Phayer, *Regiment of Life*.

97 In *Cultures of Plague*, Cohn also notes that tract writers from the 1570s onwards shifted their discussion from a regional/global narrative to a story of plague in the particular place where they lived and had some claim to eyewitness experience. In some ways, the shift from remote to local allowed them to avoid deciding what were the ultimate causes of plague. The questions became instead, how did it get *here*, and why did it become so devastating?

98 Mizauld, *Singuliers et secours contre la peste*.

99 André, *Traite de la peste*, 6. His experience was apparently gained in Paris, Toulouse, Montpellier, and Lyons, as well as on the battlefields in Scotland, Boulogne, Metz, and in Germany.

100 Rubys, *Discours sur la contagion*.

101 "*qui ne souffre quelque delay, on n'a pas tousiours le loisir ni la commodité, se servir en son temps, de Medecins. Mais toutesfois, vous vous pouvés servir de moy.*" Gardin, *La Chasse-peste*, 2.

102 "*la maladie Pestilente de ceste ville de Paris.*" Rochas, *Discours tresutile*, 5; for Toulouse, see Rochas d'Ayglun, *Examen ou raisonnment*.

103 "*La seconde [sorte de contagion est] le co[m]merce ou transport des matiers qui facilement s'imbibent du venin de la peste comme il arriva il y a trois ans a Paris par des marchas de Roüan.*" Robin, *Advis sur la peste*, 13.

104 "*toute peste qui a este aux Villes & aux villages est seulement venuë par communication des personnes qui ont porté la mal co[m]me il c'est remarque … a Dijon dans dans une seule maiso[n] jusques a present appportée de Beaune par un homme que l'on dit qui servoit aux pestes audit Beaune.*" Ibid.

105 For contemporary concerns about changes in early modern France, see Benedict, "French Cities," and Davis, *Society and Culture*.

106 "*Tout le monde s'effraye & tremble, pour ainsi dire, au seul nom de peste: à peine ce mal commence t-il à se manifester quelque part dans une ville que les plus proches prennent d'abord l'allarme et qu'ils se croïent perdus sans ressource.*" Bouillet, *Avis et remèdes*, 1.

107 Anonymous, *Some Customs Consider'd.*

108 See Wear, *Knowledge & Practice*, 305–7. Theories that linked disease outbreaks with earthquakes and volcano eruptions were not new, of course, having existed during Antiquity. They came into vogue again in this era, linked to chemical and mechanical theories and their new perception of natural disasters. See Gordon, "Confrontations with the Plague."

109 "*Certes maintena[n]t que nous voyons le peril emine[n]t nous talloner de si prés, que ia la contagio[n] a fait bresche, par sa malignité occulte, en plusiers endroits de vostre ville (Messieurs de Tours) & petit à petit s'advance, pour endommager de plus en plus tant ceux de la ville, comme des faulx-bourgs & villages.*" Nancel, *Discours tresample*, 3.

110 "*Voila ce que nous en attendions, il est advenu, nous le voyons à l'oeil.*" Ibid., 4.

111 "*je sçay d'asseurance, que la contagion nous est venuë de Paris: laquelle nous ont apportée … aucuns povres religieux Jacobites, fuiants, & porta[n]ts leur mort en leur sein.*" Ibid., 115. The term "Jacobite" was synonymous with Jacobin or member of the mendicant Dominican Order, suggesting that Nancel linked these religious men with the spread of both disease and religious dissension during France's Wars of Religion. The Dominicans were deeply engaged in spreading the principles of the Counter-Reformation, and had preached and incited violence against local Protestant populations throughout the kingdom. Their arrival in Tours presaged more death and destruction.

112 "*[ils] nous ont fraternellement communiqués … & aucuns merciers & contreporteurs, lesquels pensants gaigner quelque arge[n]t, ont hazardé leur vie.*" Ibid., 115.

113 "*comme j'ay dit, [la peste] nous a[v]ait esté importee non des ve[n]ts, mais par forains & peregrins venants de Paris.*" Ibid., 116.

114 Collas, *Histoire d'un quartier de Tours.*

115 Nancel, *Discours tresample*, 5.

116 Knecht, *French Wars of Religion*; Nicholls, "Protestants, Catholics and Magistrates"; and Heller, *Conquest of Poverty*, 134.

117 "*le chef & coeur de la France.*" Nancel, *Discours tresample*, 4.

118 "*Au reste, je n'ay encore leu, ni entendu par aucun rescrit de Messieurs les Medecins de Paris, d'où la peste a pris en ce lieu là, sa première origine.*" Ibid., 115.

119 "From all such procedures great infection of the air occurs, in Paris, in Avignon and in Lerida." Duran-Reynals and Winslow, "Jacme d'Agramont," 69.

120 "Report of the Paris Medical Faculty," 161. Emphasis added. The assumption that southerly winds were unhealthy was integral to *Airs, Waters, and Places*: "southern" climates were considered invariably hot and humid, which threatened the health of "northerners" more accustomed to changing seasons. Fear of hot places continued well into the early modern era among colonizers and colonists. See Wear, "Place, Health, and Disease"; Kupperman, "Fear of Hot Climates"; and Linte, "'Hot Climates' and Disease."

121 Arrizabalaga, "Facing the Black Death," 275. On the directionality of window openings, see Dumas, "La fenêtre en temps d'épidémie," 157–65.

122 The terrestrial causes of plague were emphasized most strongly in Iberian, Italian, and German tracts.

123 Rawcliffe, *Urban Bodies;* Fay, *Health and the City*; Geltner, "Healthscaping"; Leguay, *La pollution au Moyen Age*; and Jones, "Diseased Landscape."

124 Pullan, "Plague and Perceptions," and Palmer, "Ad una sancta perfettione." Cohn and Henderson also point to perceptions that a link existed between plague and the poor in Italian texts but delay its inception to the mid- to later sixteenth century. Cohn, *Cultures of Plague*, and Henderson, "Charity and Welfare."

125 I thank Aleksandra Pfau for reminding me to include lepers in this discussion. Medieval lepers were included among those suspected of causing plague; while they were rarely if ever mentioned directly in the plague tracts (and so are not treated at length here), they *were* targeted by public health measures that aimed to cleanse the air in most urban areas. Some French civic and royal ordinances from the late fourteenth century explicitly mentioned lepers as a danger to public health. The movement especially of non-local lepers, like those of "foreign" paupers and vagabonds, were controlled (or at least attempts were made to control them) as part of the effort to control the spread of diseases like plague. Pfau, "Lepers in the Streets." Similar measures were implemented in England; see Rawcliffe, *Leprosy*, 274–84.

126 Smaller charitable lay almshouses did survive, providing shelter to the "impotent, but self-caring, poor who were ... unable to earn their living due to age, disease, or disability ... The residents were usually elderly, infirm, and relatively poor, but could look after themselves when they joined the almshouse." Lennard-Brown, "Almshouses," 16–17. Chapters 2 and 7 of Lennard–Brown's dissertation provide extended discussions of the link between poverty and population and of urban poverty, respectively. I am grateful to her for sharing her dissertation with me.

127 On comparative early modern poverty, see Jütte, *Poverty and Deviance*, and Beier, *The Problem of the Poor*.

128 Categories of poor included working versus non-working; urban versus rural; and deserving (moral or respectable and thus worthy of harity) versus undeserving (immoral or criminal and thus not worthy of charity). Siena mentions religion only in passing as a factor that caused attitudes to harden against the poor, pointing instead to the deepening and expanding reach of poverty that caused opinions to toughen. *Rotten Bodies*, 12.

129 Roger, "To Be Shut Up," 3.

130 Siena's recent work highlights the tendency of the early modern British to blame their epidemics on the poor. His book focuses primarily on class dynamics (and the embodiment of social rank) in the eighteenth century, but his observations are (as he notes) equally applicable to the seventeenth century and, I would argue, even the sixteenth. One of Siena's key questions that speaks well to this book is why, despite the intellectual gulf that separated writers of different centuries, the language they used to blame the poor for plague (and later epidemic typhus and cholera) remained essentially unchanged. The answer, he finds, lay in an ongoing fear of epidemic disease, plague having cast a long shadow, combined with the use of "history as a medical tool," wherein lessons from the past demonstrated that plague epidemics tended to begin among the poor. *Rotten Bodies*, 1–2.

131 College of Physicians, *Certain Necessary Directions*, A4r. For a longer discussion of this, see Slack, *Poverty and Policy* and *Impact of Plague*; and Wear, *Knowledge & Practice*, 281–6.

132 Slack, "Books of Orders," 8.

133 Slack, *Impact of Plague*, 151–64; and Cummins, Kelly, and Ó Gráda, "Living Standards and Plague," 2–18. The location of Black Death-era and later plague pits (emergency cemeteries) beyond London's walls – the East and West Smithfield and Clerkenwell pits, for example, lie just beyond the eastern and northern edges of the city – and the lack of documentary evidence about whose remains are interred there or where they had resided does not tell us much about which parishes were hit first or hardest in the early decades and centuries of the Second Pandemic. The parish-by-parish collation of causes of deaths, which ultimately generated the bills of mortality, commenced only in the sixteenth century.

134 In "Overlapping Circles," Griffiths points to tensions evident in the late sixteenth century as the boundaries between so-called moral citizens and the criminal underworld – and the geographical neighbourhoods that housed each – became increasingly blurred. As Siena notes in *Rotten Bodies*, the increasing numbers of vagrants, criminals, alehouses, and

crowded slums across the urban landscape, in addition to institutions for the poor (hospitals, orphanages, and, later, workhouses), also visually reinforced the idea that poorer neighbourhoods were both a blight and a threat to public health and safety. Pelling emphasizes what she calls the "skirting" nature of urban living among the upper- and middle-classes in the seventeenth century: town-dwellers (here Pelling looks specifically at the membership of the London College of Physicians) who studiously avoided the very urban environments that made city living potentially dangerous through "vigilant seasonal and 'semi-detached' patterns of living." Outbreaks of plague and smallpox intensified this "'skirting' mentality," increasing its socially divisive effects. Pelling, "Skirting the City?," 156.

135 Jenner, "Plague on a Page," 265. On the mental images inspired by the broadsheets, see also Monteyne, *Printed Image*, 73–112.

136 Slauter, "Write Up Your Dead." See also Greenberg, "Plague, the Printing Press"; Rawcliffe, *Urban Bodies*, 68; and Slack, *Impact of Plague*, 128–9, 239.

137 Wrightson, *Ralph Tailor's Summer*, 33.

138 Sullivan, "Physical and Spiritual Illness," 81.

139 As I discuss in chapter 5, by the eighteenth century, writers like Richard Mead were able to recast the poor as those who lived in crowded, filthy, foreign cities, enabling a suspicious finger to be pointed at the Ottoman Empire.

140 As Siena rightly notes, "medical treatises [like plague tracts] provided an effective [and scientifically legitimate] medium for advancing claims about class that were unlikely to be challenged on finicky details" about to whom exactly the phrase "the poor" referred. *Rotten Bodies*, 8.

141 Herring, *Certaine Rules*, C1.

142 Ibid., C1.

143 Wear, *Knowledge & Practice*, 284.

144 Elyot, *Castel of Helth*, 12.

145 Brasbridge, *Poore Man's Jewell*, A8.

146 Lodge, *Treatise of the Plague*, A3.

147 Bullein, *Dialogue*, 28.

148 Bradwell, *Watch-man*, 46.

149 Hodges, *Loimologia*, 15.

150 Kemp, *Brief Treatise*, 14.

151 Mead, *Short Discourse*, 38.

152 As Siena notes, for tract writers like Mead, it was well understood and accepted that "the poor represented a uniquely contagious threat, and ... their liberty was more expendable than that of the more affluent readers of his learned treatise." *Rotten Bodies*, 57.

153 Davis, *Society and Culture;* Mouysset, "La peste de 1628 en Rouergue"; Audouin-Rouzeau, *Les chemins de la peste*; Davis, "Poverty and Poor Relief" and "Poor Relief, Humanism and Heresy"; and Béroujon, *Peuple et pauvres.* Unfortunately, much of the detailed French historiography on the poor says little about plague, and vice versa. A study of population movements, however, reveals that in the city of Dijon, poor recent immigrants without local ties died in a proportionately greater number during the plague outbreak of 1400 than did those who had lived in the city for a longer period of time. Galanaud et al., "Mortality and Demographic Recovery."

154 Murphy, "Plague Ordinances."

155 In her work on early modern Seville, *Plague and Public Health,* Bowers also points to the sometimes creative movement of merchants in and out of plagued cities, often flouting ordinances that were meant to prohibit such travel.

156 "*manger mechantes viandes ... grains pourris, & autres vilenies.*" Ferrier, *Remedes Preservatifs*, 7. On popular errors, see Coste, *La littérature des « Erreurs populaires ».*

157 "*les exhalations putrides qui s'eslevent coustumierent es lieux ou il y-a affluence de povres gens.*" Courcelles, *Traite de la peste*, 34. "*le menu peuple ... qui habitent en lieux fort sales et ords, & qui en tout temps vivent salement.*" Joubert, *Traitté de la peste*, 61.

158 The language of plague did enter French discourse about the poor: Jones notes that the broad movement to institutionalize the poor was predicated, in part, on an assumption that they were "as contagious as a plague victim." "Languages of Plague," 48.

159 Croissainte, *Brief Journal*, 6–10, cited in Siena, *Rotten Bodies*, 58.

160 Plenty of Protestant writing about plague in England evoked a strong sense of anti-Catholicism, divine chastisement, and providential expectations, yet this practice rarely spilled over into the medically oriented plague tracts. For a recent discussion of the religious links made between plague, war, and Catholic enemies in the early seventeenth century, see Rolfe, "Fatal and Memorable."

161 The wars are typically divided into a number of different phases, although their respective dates are the subject of continued historical debate. For works on the Wars of Religion, see among many others Le Roux, *Guerres de Religion*; Knecht, *French Wars of Religion*; Gould, *Catholic Activism*; Holt, *French Wars of Religion*; and Constant, *Les Français.*

162 Davis, "The Sacred and the Body Social," 41, 42.

163 This pattern was not replicated in England, since Jews had been expelled from the entire kingdom in the 1290s and had not yet re-established themselves in any great numbers. There is a small but important scholarship on this. See among others, Einbinder, *After the Black Death*; Colet et al., "Black Death and Its Consequences"; Raspe, "The Black Death in Jewish Sources"; Cohn, "The Black Death and the Burning of Jews"; and Winkler, "Approach of the Black Death" and "Clamor of the People." For contemporary accounts of the atrocities from the perpetrators' perspective, see Horrox, *Black Death*, 207–26.

164 Naphy, *Plagues, Poisons, and Potions.*

165 Protestant scapegoats were also blamed for causing outbreaks in Padua, Ljubljana, Graz, and elsewhere. Fabbri, "Continuity and Change," 191. See also Bercé, "*Rumeurs et épidémies*," and Coste, *Représentations et comportements*, 655–63.

166 "*mettres des gibets par tous les carrefours, avec escripteaux par lesquels lesdits engraisseurs estoyent asseurez que si tost qu'ils seroyent prins, ilz seroyent aussi tost attachez & penduz ausdits gibetez, sans autre forme ny figure de proces*"; "*Les seulz heretiques deceuz par la predestination de Calvin … moururent à tas.*" Rubys, *Discours sur la contagion*, 19, 32. For an assessment of Rubys's work in the context of ritualized religious violence, see Semmens, "Plague, Propaganda and Prophetic Violence." See also Leonardo, "Cut Off This Rotten Member," and Brenot, "La Peste soit des Huguenots," for the integration of disease into the Catholic rhetoric against Protestants more generally.

167 "*estimant par là accueillir ce non moins saige que fidelle & affectionneé serviteur du Roy & de la couronne de France, le seigneur de la Mante, gouverneur & Cappitaine de laditte citadelle, ou du moins l'estonner tellement par la mort de ses soldatz, qu'ilz le contraindroient d'abondonner la place.*" Rubys, *Discours sur la contagion*, 35.

168 The tract was not Rubys's only work that linked Protestants to plague and to the fate of the Catholic community. In his 1604 history of the city of Lyon, he once again accused the local Protestant population of having deliberately spread plague in 1564 and 1576. Rubys, *Histoire veritable*, 401–2, 428. For a discussion of Rubys's larger role in the battles between Catholics and Protestants in Lyon, see Hartley, "War and Tolerance."

169 The "greasing" conspiracies appear to have been limited to Lyon, perhaps because of its close commercial ties with cities in Switzerland and Germany where such conspiracies were particularly popular. Naphy, *Plagues, Poisons, and Potions.*

170 "*meschans & cruelz ho[m]mes … qui, ou par vengeance, ou espoir de quelque malheureux … assemblent beaucoup d'ordures, & infections, pour les semer en plusieurs lieux.*" Ferrier, *Remedes Preservatifs et curatifs*, 8–9. Plague *engraisseurs* had also been accused and executed in Toulouse in 1530.

171 "*Dieu veut imprimer ceste creance aux hommes, que les rebellions contre l'Eglise … sont tousiours suivies de chastimens rigoureux.*" Grillot, *Lyon affligé de contagion*, 6.

172 Ibid., 40. Suspected *engraisseurs* were also hanged in Rouen in 1629.

173 Hodges, *Loimologia*, 36.

174 Ibid., 64.

175 Ibid., 142.

176 "*Les causes des Fièvres malignes & des maladies populaires sont originaires du pays ou elles produisent leurs effets, & ne passent aucunement dans d'autres ni voisins ni éloignés: Celle de la Peste est étrangère.*" Goiffon, *Relations*, 48.

177 "*il paroit que les Maladies épidémiques contagieuses, & les épidémiques non contagieuses différent par la nature de leurs causes dont l'une n'a qu'une modique & petite origine, & l'autre une source abondante, étendue & générale.*" Ibid., 41.

178 "*Ces sortes de maladies ont toujours une source vaste & dépendent d'une grande quantité de matière gâtée & corrompuë … & nullement qu'elle y ait été transférée.*" Ibid., 43.

179 "*je pense qu'on n'ôsera pas douter que la cause ne soit trés-limitée.*" Ibid., 42.

180 Carmichael, "Plague Persistence," 162–8; Murphy, "Plague Ordinances," 152; and Tomić and Blažina, *Expelling the Plague.*

181 On new evidence about the earliest such quarantine measures in England, see Roger, "To Be Shut Up." Other measures were in place throughout the kingdom to forestall plague epidemics; see Rawcliffe, *Urban Bodies.*

182 College of Physicians, *Certain Necessary Directions*, B3v.

183 Slack, *Impact of Plague*, 245. Also useful here is Raymond, "Newspaper."

184 Anonymous, *Brief Relation of the Plague at Naples.*

185 "*mon opinion sur ce que dessus, est, qu'on voit ordinairement, que la peste se met aux Villes grandes & fort peuplées: comme au grand Caire, à Constantinople, à Paris, à Tholouse, à Lyon, (à quoy la nature du lieu fait quelque chose).*" Davin, *Tres singulier traité*, 45.

186 Physician in York, *Treatise of the Plague*, 13.

187 Thomson, *Loimotomia,* 20.

188 "*Pendant les dix-huits années que j'ai fait la Mission dans la Turquie, l'Armenie, la Perse, l'Arabie & l'Inde, je me suis trouvé une infinité de fois dans des Villes affligées de Peste.*" Gaudereau, *Relation*, 13.

189 Rose, *Theorico-practical*, v.
190 Mead, *Short Discourse*, A2.
191 Bradley, *Plague of Marseilles*, 1.
192 Mead, *Short Discourse*, 20.
193 Rose, *Theorico-practical*, 9.
194 "*la peste … qui alarme tant toute l'Europe.*" Manget, *Traité de la peste*, 1.
195 "*L'air de Marseille est exempt de toutes ces infections.*" Bertrand, *Relation historique*, 18.
196 "Report of the Paris Medical Faculty," 162.
197 They also echo the "from the east" trajectories established during the First Plague Pandemic. Writers in the sixth century pointed to the southeast Mediterranean, with Egypt and Ethiopia being the most commonly named origins of plague. The first *recorded* outbreak was in Pelusium, on the eastern Nile Delta, but that was simply when it was noticed among human populations and, importantly, written about. See Green and Jones, "Evolution and Spread," 44–6.
198 Mussis, "Arrival of the Plague," 16–21. "Tartar" was a blanket term used by Western Europeans to describe someone from northern and Central Asia beyond the Caspian Sea (the region itself was called Tartary). The term "Tatar" generally referred to the same group of people; both words were associated variously with the Mongols and the Turkic inhabitants of Central Asia. The word "Saracen" primarily referred to Arab Muslims, but was also applied to other Muslims such as Turks or Persians.
199 Boccaccio, *Decameron*, 4.
200 "Arrival of the Plague," 16, 18.
201 Villani, "Chronicle," in Aberth, *Black Death*, 19–20.
202 Bartsocas, "Two Fourteenth-Century Greek Descriptions," 395.
203 Dols, "Ibn al-Wardī," 448–51.
204 Green, "Climate and Disease," 12–19; Green, "Four Black Deaths"; and Green and Fancy, "Plague and the Fall of Baghdad."
205 Carmichael, "Universal and Particular," 27. The historiography that has blindly accepted Mussis's account at face value, often framing the Caffa siege as an early example of biological warfare, is long and need not be repeated here.
206 Barker, "Laying the Corpses to Rest," 100.
207 Barker's work is especially useful here, as she dissects the meanings of the Byzantine chroniclers' narrative geography of plague's early movement. Ibid., 102.
208 Barker also notes that Mussis conflated events of multiple sieges into one: catapults had been used in an earlier siege at Caffa (albeit not to throw

corpses over the walls) but not during the most recent one he associated with plague. Ibid., 101–2.

209 On Mongol-European relations, see Jackson, *Mongols and the West*; Di Cosmo, "Black Sea Emporia"; Abu-Lughod, *Before European Hegemony*; Campbell, *The Great Transition*, 126–30; and most recently, with significant new details, Barker, "Laying the Corpses to Rest."

210 "Plague according to Thomas Walsingham," in Horrox, *Black Death*, 66.

211 Similar problems arise with terms such as "India," since there was a multiplicity of "Indies" in the medieval vocabulary, each referring to a different geographical space. Accounts of plague's origin in, or passage through, India are therefore not as straightforward as they might seem. Phillips, *Medieval Expansion*, 192.

212 Al-Wardī, "Essay on the Report of the Pestilence," in Aberth, *Black Death*, 17.

213 Cited in Campbell, *Black Death*, 51–2n23.

214 Córdoba, "Letter and Regimen," 49.

215 "*Ista pestilencia invalescit, ad nostra loca propinqua se extendit, ut patet in multis locis, unde Remis et in locis vicinis.*" BnF Latin MS 11227, cited in Coville, "Écrits contemporains," 328.

216 See the special 2018 issue of *Afriques* and Guérin, "Exchange of Sacrifices."

217 Phillips, *Medieval Expansion*, 239; and Campbell, *The Great Transition*, 386.

218 Khanmohamadi, *Light*, 3. See also see also O'Doherty, *Indies*, and Allen, ed., *Eastward Bound*.

219 Dalché criticizes scholars who see these medieval sources as "*de pures abstractions livresques sans rapport avec l'espace réel, répétées sans critiques et sans recours à ce que nous considèrerons comme relevant de l'expérience.*" Dalché, "Représentations géographiques savantes," 13. See also Bouloux, "L'espace habité"; Lilley, ed., *Mapping Medieval Geographies*; Tomasch and Gilles, eds., *Text and Territory*; and Edson, *World Map*.

220 Phillips, *Medieval Expansion*, 191.

221 Higgins, *Writing East*, 2–3. See also Campbell, *Witness*.

222 Higgins, *Writing East*, 5. I take the term "medieval Orientalism" from Higgins.

223 The phrases come from Lilley, *Mapping Medieval Geographies*, 4.

224 Abu-Lughod describes eight interconnected thirteenth-century trading zones that stretched from England in the West to China and and South-East Asia in the East. The Venetians and Genoans' commercial enterprises

in the eastern Mediterranean connected them to trading zones that stretched much further east. Abu-Lughod, *Before European Hegemony.*

225 "*retrogradando de Alamania et de partibus septentrionalibus, revenit ad nos mortalitas.*" Chauliac, *Inventarium*, 1:119.

226 Phillips, *Medieval Expansion*, 205. Compare to McCleery, "From the Edge of Europe," which speaks to the circulation and construction of new knowledge about disease more generally.

227 *Orders Thought Meet*, A3.

228 Rubys, *Discours sur la contagion*, 33–4.

229 "*Ce mal est transporté d'ailleurs, & non nay avec nous ... veint un estra[n] gier, dit on, venant d'Espagne.*" Briet, *Discours sur les causes*, 9, 13.

230 "*La Ville de Rouën estoit parfaictement purgée de la maladie contagieuse il y avoit beaucoup d'anées ... [et] elle avoit deja presque oublié toutes les douleurs que cette fascheuse maladie luy avait causé par le passé.*" Anonymous, *Estat general*, 16.

231 Kinzelbach, "Infection, Contagion, and Public Health"; Arrizabalaga, "Facing the Black Death," 259–60; and Slack, *Impact of Plague*, 197–310.

232 Koch, *Disease Maps.*

233 Ibid., 31.

234 Ibid., back cover, 36. Emphasis added. For an interesting discussion of things purposely not shown on early modern maps, see Harley, *New Nature of Maps*, especially chapter 3, "Silences and Secrecy: The Hidden Agenda of Cartography in Early Modern Europe."

235 Cohn, *Cultures of Plague*, 95.

236 Quincy, *Essay*, 25–6.

237 Even through the mid-sixteenth century, though, the Continental translation, production, and wide dissemination of Claudius Ptolemy's *Geography* and its world maps were not replicated in England. Roland, "After poyetes and astronomyers," 127–51. Nevertheless, although Lavezzo has suggested that England's geographic marginalism was cultivated as a form of cultural exceptionalism that continued into the early modern era (*Angels on the Edge*), Roland argues (129–30) that "Looking beyond the evidence of map production, it becomes apparent that English readers and printers did participate in the changing geographic culture of Europe: missing from assessments of an isolated or indifferent English geographical imagination is the international context of the English book trade and the role of literary and popular texts in the development of a narrative English geographical imagination." The lack of English-produced world maps clearly did not equate with a lack of knowledge about or interest in the broader world.

238 Headley, "Geography and Empire," 1121–2.

239 Ibid., 1124.

CHAPTER FIVE

1 Mead, *Short Discourse*, 18.

2 Ibid., 2–3.

3 Kinglake, *Eothen*, 7.

4 Brownrigg, *Considerations*, 25. Seeking to "throw further light on the Medical History of the Plague," the physician Patrick Russell wrote an entire account of the Aleppan outbreaks of 1760–62. *Treatise of the Plague.*

5 Clot, *De la peste*, 6.

6 On the International Sanitary Conferences, see Harrison, "Disease, Diplomacy and International Commerce" and Carvalho and Zacher, "International Health Regulations." The examples noted here are discussed in more detail in Varlık, "Oriental Plague."

7 In the *Punch* magazine, see, for example, John Leech's "A Consultation about the State of Turkey" of 17 September 1853; the unattributed cartoon "The Two Sick Men" of 18 August 1860; and Bernard Partridge "The Reversion" of 7 April 1915.

8 Varlık, "Oriental Plague," 61.

9 Varlık, *Plague and Empire*, 186. Varlık notes that Constantinople ultimately became an infamous "plague hub."

10 "*Car entre autre choses elle est propre contre la peste, & toutes defluxions.*" Belon du Mans, *Observations*, 51. Emphasis added.

11 Mead, *Short Discourse*, 5.

12 Mead, *Discourse on the Plague*, 71.

13 Mead, *Short Discourse*, 6–7.

14 Ibid., 9.

15 Ibid., 27–8.

16 Ibid., 10.

17 Ibid., 18.

18 Varlık, "Oriental Plague," 76. There is a large literature on Europe and its cultural and geographical Others, both historical and modern. On the theory of Otherness in identity-building, see Gifford, "Defining Others." Despite criticisms, the classic work on Orientalism as Other remains Said, *Orientalism*. On the medieval construction of the east as Other, see Tolan, *Saracens*. On early modern travellers to the east, see among many options Brentjes, *Travellers from Europe*; Borromeo, *Voyageurs occidentaux*; MacLean, *Rise of Oriental Travel*; Bisaha, *Creating East and West*;

Çırakman, *From the "Terror of the World"*; and Yérasimos, *Voyageurs*. On discontinuities in European perceptions of the Islamic Other, see Wintle, "Islam." Stephanie Leitch has analyzed how early sixteenth-century German prints of the native inhabitants of the newly discovered Americas, Africa, and Asia were first "release[d] … from the shackles of a visual tradition of exotica that had grouped them together with marvelous beings, monstrous races, wild men, and barbaric Others, and considered them instead as fully human" until European colonial projects later in the century reconfigured them as infidels and savages. Leitch, *Mapping Ethnography*, 2. I thank Ann Carmichael for noticing this reference. On European Othering in the New World, see also Greenblatt, *Marvelous Possessions*. It is not difficult to stretch Leitch's visual analysis to a more text-based one that reconfigured the Turk from a potentially barbaric but otherwise useful Other into one that was diseased and decrepit.

19 See the discussion in chapter 4, note 4 that outlines the problematic nature of this account of plague's arrival in Marseille.

20 Hodges, *Loimologia*, 30. Hodges wrote his tract in 1672; this translated version appeared in 1721.

21 College of Physicians, *Certain Necessary Directions*, 2.

22 England was quite late in applying quarantines and shipping restrictions on goods and vessels coming from suspected plague ports. Such measures had been used in the medieval Byzantine Empire and were instituted by trading city-states on, or connected to, the Mediterranean during fourteenth-century post-Black Death outbreaks. Tomić and Blažina, *Expelling the Plague*, and Varlık, "Beyond Eurocentric Histories."

23 Kemp, *Brief Treatise*, 15.

24 Gadbury, *London's Deliverance*, 10.

25 Anonymous, *Shutting Up*, 6.

26 Hodges, *Loimologia*, 29, 46.

27 Cummins, Kelly, and Ó Gráda, "Living Standards," 17.

28 Ibid., 1, 30. According to the Bills of Mortality, the first recorded deaths from plague in this outbreak (between December 1664 and May 1665) were actually in St Giles in the Fields. The first deaths in Westminster are noted only after mid-June 1665.

29 Varlık, *Plague and Empire*, 73. Varlık demonstrates clearly the falsity of De Busbeq's claims. On the problem of using European sources for Ottoman history, see Faroqhi, *Approaching Ottoman History*, especially 110–43. See also Brentjes, *Travellers from Europe*.

30 Parker, *Books*; and Faroqhi, *Approaching Ottoman History*, 111, 113.

31 Çırakman (*From the "Terror of the World"*) and Pippidi (*Visions*) emphasize the wide variety of perspectives that European writers offered about the Ottoman Empire. Çırakman suggests, for example, that French writers tended towards more positive portrayals than Germanic writers because of the latter's proximity to the western borders of the Ottoman Empire. French attitudes towards the Ottomans also remained positive longer than did the English ones. *From the "Terror of the World,"* 35–6.

32 Grelot, *Late Voyage*, 188. See also Nicolay, *Les quatre premiers livres.*

33 Grelot, *Late Voyage*, 192–4.

34 "*Les Turcs vivent long-temps, & sont peu sujets aux maladies, & nous en avons beaucoup de dangereuses qu'ils ne connaissent point … Je croy que cette grande santé leur vient en partie à cause des bains dont ils usent si souvent.*" Thévenot, *Relation d'un voyage*, 70.

35 "*D'ailleurs il ne se passe guere d'années que cette ville ne soit ataquée de la peste, qui toutefois n'y est pas si fort qu'en Chrétienté.*" Tavernier, *Les six voyages*, 78. See also Pippidi, *Visions*, 53–4. This is not to suggest that these writers did not also have some very negative things to say about the Ottoman Empire. Nicolay, for example, described the Turks as the most barbarous, avaricious, and cruel people in the world. It is clear in some of the travel accounts that the purpose of highlighting the positive aspects of the Ottoman Empire was simply to shame Christian readers into being more charitable. On this point, see Malcolm, "Positive Views of Islam," 199.

36 Mundy, *Travels*, quoted in MacLean, *Rise of Oriental Travel*, 229n8.

37 Moryson, *Itinerary*, 2:100–1.

38 Robson, *Newes from Aleppo*, 11.

39 Ibid., 13–4.

40 Ricaut, *History of the Present State*, 319. Stray dogs and cats were likewise blamed for plague in Europe. Gratien's work on nineteenth- and twentieth-century Ottoman Cilicia, including Alexandretta/Iskenderun, shows that negative images of the region's unhealthiness continued almost to the present day. Gratien, "Ottoman Quagmire." I am grateful to him for sharing with me both his embargoed dissertation and a chapter of his forthcoming book. See also Varlık, *Plague and Empire*, 78–9.

41 Varlık, *Plague and Empire*; and McCleery, "From the Edge," 68–9. Urban environmental amelioration projects in England, both medieval and early modern, are addressed in detail in Rawcliffe, *Urban Bodies*; Fay, *Health and the City*; and Skelton, *Sanitation in Urban Britain.* Similar works exist for other European sites, including France, pointing to an ongoing Europe-wide effort to healthscape urban centres from at least the later medieval era onward.

42 Lambarde and Camden are quoted in Wear, "Place, Health, and Disease," 447. See also Wear, "Making Sense"; Jones, "Diseased Landscape"; and Varlık, "Oriental Plague." For contemporary interest in the topographical and geographical dichotomy between healthy and unhealthy places, and a modern analysis of the reality of differential disease patterns by geography in England, see Dobson, *Contours of Death*. For the slightly later French interest in landscapes of disease, see Peter, "Disease and the Sick."

43 Wear, "Place, Health, and Disease," 451.

44 Cited in Ibid.," 458. On the Carolinas, see McCandless, *Slavery*. See also McNeill, *Mosquito Empires*; Merrens and Terry, "Dying in Paradise"; and Earle, "Environment, Disease and Mortality." Cagle provides an interesting case study of how late fifteenth- and early sixteenth-century Portuguese explorers initially relied on *Airs, Waters, and Places* traditions to deem the West African coast on the south side of the Senegal River as especially healthy and suitable for settlement; a few decades of personal encounters with new diseases and unfamiliar conditions convinced them otherwise. Cagle, "Beyond the Senegal."

45 Cited in Brazeau, *Writing a New France*, 5. On the difficulties of winter, see especially chapter 1.

46 Van Linschoten, *Voyage*, 1:240, cited in Pearson, "Thin End of the Wedge," 153; see also 153–6 for European accounts of other diseases.

47 Kochhar, "The Truth Behind the Legend," 259. See also Wang, "Imperial Landscape."

48 Scholarly literature on fear of diseased colonial spaces and bodies largely focuses on later centuries: Anderson, *Colonial Pathologies*; Arnold, *Colonizing the Body*; McFarlane, "Governing the Contaminated City"; Peckham, ed., *Empires of Panic*; and Swanson, "The Sanitation Syndrome."

49 Shakow, "Marks of Contagion," xii.

50 Isom-Verhaaren, *Allies with the Infidel*, 114–40. On earlier European-Ottoman relations, see Housley, *Crusading*.

51 Brotton, *This Orient Isle*, 8.

52 For a recent re-examination of the impact of the battle of Lepanto, see Brummet, "Lepanto Paradigm Revisited."

53 Anonymous, *Weekly Bill of Mortality*, 1.

54 Thomson, *Loimotomia*, 20.

55 Rose, *Theorico-practical*, 19.

56 Bradley, *Plague of Marseilles Cons'd*, 11–12.

57 Quincy, *Essay*, 255.

58 Mead, *Discourse*, 24.

59 Browne, *Practical Treatise*, 14.

60 Gordon's work on the Enlightenment points to the increasing idealization of the city, especially among French writers, as one impetus behind the large upswing in plague writing during and following the outbreak in Marseille: "The more the city became an imaginary scene of productive and aesthetic exchange," he writes, "the more it became important to banish death from view." Gordon, "The City and the Plague," 69–70. French authors' attempts to portray their cities as clean, healthy places in contrast to the filthy cities of the Orient were a key part of this process.

61 "*les contrées du Levant [qui] sont souvent désolées par la peste.*" Bertrand, *Relation historique*, 25.

62 "*On trouve en Asie une infinité de lieux qui en sont infectez.*" Gaudereau, *Relation des differentes especes de peste*, 18. As Varlık notes, by the eighteenth century "a considerable number of European medical writers [were going to] the Orient, [observing] the plague, and [writing] about it. In this manner, these medical writers joined other travelers who created the discursive map of the Orient as an infected landscape." "Oriental Plague," 78.

63 "*Mais nous observons seulement que nôtre Europe a souffert peu de Pestes qu'elle ne doive aux levains qui lui en ont été aportés des pays Orientaux, où elle régne ordinairement (particuliérement chés les Turcs, tantôt dans un lieu, tantôt dans un autre).*" Manget, *Traité de la peste*, 17.

64 Varlık, "Oriental Plague," 58; and Jones "Diseased Landscape."

65 "*Nous voyons entrer la Peste en France; nous la voyons passer de Ville en Ville, de Province en Province; & nous trouvons d'ailleurs dans les Auteurs l'Histoire de tant Pestes, qui ont été portées en Europe, & qui se sont communiquées d'un Royaume à l'autre, que nous pourrions croire avec quelque apparence de raison, que cette Maladie est étrangere.*" Baux, *Traité de la peste*, 13.

66 "*Nous trouverions en foüillant dans les Historiens, un grand nombre de ces Pestes qui sont venuës de quelque partie de l'Affrique ... On trouveroit sans doute dans les Auteurs un grand nombre d'autres Pestes venuës du Levant.*" Ibid., 14–15.

67 "*Cette Maladie est ordinaire en Egypte; mais ... elle n'y est pas fort dangereuse ... de sorte qu'y ayant un continuel commerce d'Egypte à Constantinople, & la predestination à laquelle les Turcs s'arrêtent, les empêchant d'y établir aucun ordre, le mal se communique par toute la Turquie, où' il fait bien d'autres ravages qu'en Egypte. Le commerce qu'on a en presque de tout temps dans le Levant, a dû souvent fournir l'occasion aux Negocians de porter la Peste par toute l'Europe.*" Ibid., 14–15.

68 "*de Levant où ce mal avoit longument regné.*" Rubys, *Discours sur la contagion*, 8.

69 "*Or la peste est quelque fois universelle, comme celle qui est descrite par Gui de C[h]auliac, laquelle fust en l'an 1348 apres avoir commencé premierement en Orient & en apres environné & circui presque tout le monde.*" Joubert, *Traitté de la peste*, 11.
70 Graunt, *Reflections*, D1–2.
71 Anonymous, *Weekly Bill of Mortality*, n.p.
72 For a useful discussion of the changes in meaning of "the East" and of "Asia" over a longer period of time than is addressed here, see Lewis and Wigen, *Myth of Continents*, 47–103. I thank Nükhet Varlık for this reference.
73 Browne, *Practical Treatise*, 14. Browne's thoughts about a Mongolian role in the spread of plague are interesting, given current research pointing in the same direction. See Green, "Four Black Deaths," and Fancy and Green, "Plague and the Fall of Baghdad."
74 Mead, *Short Discourse*, 2.
75 Mead, *Discourse*, 26, 22.
76 "*Il est vrai que dès les premiers tems ce Royaume étoit regardé comme la source des maladies pestilentielles.*" Gaudereau, *Relation*, 21.
77 Knolles, *Generall Historie*, A6, A1, 1. For mention of "plagues," see pages 20, 67, 91, 99, 102, 119, and 184, among others.
78 One estimate suggests that about 3,500 titles on the Turks were published in Europe between 1501 and 1600 alone. Heywood, "Sir Paul Rycaut," 34.
79 McJannet, "History Written by the Enemy," 399.
80 Ricaut, *History*, 151.
81 "*La peste qui est un fleau ordinaire dans les terres du Turc.*" Mézeray, *Histoire générale*, 156.
82 "*La peste nous vient de l'Asie, & depuis deux mille ans toutes les pestes qui ont paru en Europe y ont été transmises par la communication des Sarrasins, des Arabes, des Maures, ou des Turcs avec nous, & toutes les pestes n'ont pas eu chez nous d'autre source.*" Jaucourt, "Peste," in *Encyclopédie*, 12:452.
83 Brownrigg, *Considerations*, 2. As recent research shows, plague movement in that period was actually in the opposite direction, from west to east, into rather than out of the Ottoman Empire. Varlık, *Plague and Empire*, 131–59.
84 Justus Hecker used the term *morgenländische Pest* – which is translated in the English version as "oriental plague." Hecker, *Black Death*, 4–6. For a thorough discussion of the impact of Hecker's terminology on plague historiography, see Varlık, "Oriental Plague."
85 Clot, *De la peste*, 4.

CONCLUSION

1 Defoe, *Journal*, 20.
2 The phrase comes from Carmichael, "Last Past Plague."
3 Healy, "Defoe's Journal," 26.
4 Defoe, *Journal*, 95, 72.
5 Ibid., 17.
6 Ibid., 23. Siena discusses in some detail Defoe's earlier *Due Preparations for the Plague*, which advocated emptying the city of its poor to prevent the eruption of disease. Siena, *Rotten Bodies*, 63–9.
7 Defoe, *Journal*, 246.
8 Phayer's reissued and Bradley's new tracts, for example, appeared in the "Advertisements and Notices" section of *Post Boy* for the week of 24–27 February 1722, while Defoe's *Journal* appeared during the week of 15–17 March.
9 Mayer, "The Reception of *A Journal of the Plague Year*," 531–2.
10 The exemplar used here for John of Burgundy is translated from the French version.
11 "*les maistres du temps present usent plus es choses dessus dittes de experience que ceuls qui nous ont passes. Et ainsi quil est dit … experience fait lart.*" Paris, Bibliothèque nationale de France (BnF), NAF MS 4516, f. 102r.
12 "*a suyvi la descriptio[n] des Arabes, com[m]e il fait partout, broüillant infinis mots Arabiques, & pervertissant en plusieurs endroits l'inte[n]tion des bons autheurs Grecs: lesquels il n'a ni leu, ni suyvi, ni entendu.*" Nancel, *Discours tresample*, 164.
13 Mead, *Short Discourse*, A2–3.
14 The first editions of Mead's book omit treatments, but they are added to later versions. See Mead, *Discourse on the Plague*, 151–64.
15 "*dont it advient q[ue] par le influence des corps s[u]r celesteaux causeeme[n]t & de fait, li-airs soit de piece a corrumpus & effect pestilentcieux apparus … causa le Infeccion de pluseurs.*" BnF NAF MS 4516, 97r.
16 "*Cestoit bien raison, puis que Paris, le chef & cœur de la France, patissoit; que tous les autres membres & dependa[n]ces souffrissent … qu'estant comme le centre, il envoyast par toute la circonference, & distribuast de son malheur; comme jadis florissant, il departissoit de ses bie[n]s, dons & faveurs, tant pour le bon reglement de justice, comme de toutes bonnes ars, sciences, & disciplines; comme aussi de ses marcha[n]dises & traffique.*" Nancel, *Discours tresample*, 4.

17 As noted earlier, religious writers from the time of the Black Death had drawn on biblical analogies, but the spread of humanist approaches and access to newly available historical texts allowed authors to discuss current outbreaks in the context of recorded epidemics of the past.

18 Mead, *Short Discourse*, 18.

19 Jones, "Languages of Plague," 46.

20 On the influence of plague experience on the development of English prose satire, for example, see Kerwin, "Writing the Plague."

21 Goldberg has cautioned that "If the plague was 'universally understood' as divine punishment for sin in society, it may be that the perspective of the legislators, drawn primarily from the landed elite, and the chroniclers, an educated and predominantly clerical cadre whose sympathies lay with the ruling order of society, represents only one interpretation of that sin … [in the case of England, that of a] conservative, London-minded view." This points to the critical importance of knowing who the writers were: not simply a generic cadre of writers, but individuals with political and religious sympathies that were played out through their treatises. Goldberg, "Introduction," 10–11.

22 "Residual orality" refers to verbal expressions of thought and knowledge that are not necessarily replicated in print, even in cultures in which writing and print are widely used. Ong, *Orality and Literacy*, 41.

23 Carmichael, "Last Past Plague," 142.

24 "*A celle cause jay voulu escripre ce petit regime pour aider, secourir, et subvenir a ung chascun qui sera ou pourroit estre prins et touche de epidimie et pestilence. Et quiconqꝫ se voudra lyre et entendre sa[n]s soy ennuyer plus que jay fait a lordonner il luy proufitera plus que romans ne croniques ou bien souvent plusiers passent le te[m]ps. Et par tant je metꝫ fin a ce present regime fait et compose par maistre Thomas le forestier docteur en medecine.*" Le Forestier, *Regime contre epidimie*, F8.

Bibliography

MANUSCRIPT AND ARCHIVAL SOURCES

Boston

Francis A. Countway Library of Medicine, Center for the History of Medicine

Brussels

Koninklijke Bibliotheek van België/ Bibliothèque royale de Belgique

Cambridge

Cambridge University Library
Corpus Christi College
Fitzwilliam Museum
Gonville & Caius College
Trinity College

Copenhagen

Det Kongelige Bibliotek

Durham

Durham University Library

Edinburgh

National Library of Scotland

Lille

Bibliothèque municipale, Médiathèque Jean Lévy

Lincoln

Lincoln Cathedral

London

British Library: Additional, Cotton, Egerton, Lansdowne, Royal, and Sloane Collections
Society of Antiquaries
Wellcome Collection

New Haven

Yale Center for British Art, Paul Mellon Collection

Oxford

Bodleian Library: Ashmole, Digby, Rawlinson, and Wood Collections

Paris

Bibliothèque nationale de France: French, Hebrew, and Latin Collections

Strasbourg

Bibliothèque nationale et universitaire de Strasbourg

Tokyo

Takamiya Collection

PUBLISHED SOURCES

Aberth, John. *The Black Death: The Great Mortality of 1348–1350: A Brief History with Documents*. Boston, MA: Bedford/St Martins, 2005.
– *Doctoring the Black Death: Europe's Late Medieval Medical Response to Epidemic Disease*. Lexington, KY: Rowman and Littlefield, 2021.
– *An Environmental History of the Middle Ages: The Crucible of Nature*. London: Routledge, 2013.
Abu-Lughod, Janet L. *Before European Hegemony: The World System A.D. 1250–1350*. Oxford: Oxford University Press, 1989.
Achinstein, Sharon. "Plagues and Publication: Ballads and the Representation of Disease in the English Renaissance." *Criticism* 34, no. 1 (1992): 27–49.
Adams, Thomas R., and Nicolas Barker. "A New Model for the Study of the Book." In *A Potencie of Life: Books in Society: The Clark Lectures 1986–1987*, edited by Nicolas Barker, 5–39. London: British Library, 2001.
Agramont, Jacme d'. "Regiment de Preservacio a Epidimia o Pestilencia e Mortaldats." Translated by M.L. Duran-Reynals and C.E.A Winslow. *Bulletin of the History of Medicine* 23 (1949): 57–89.
Afriques. Special Issue "Sillages de la peste noire en Afrique subsaharienne: une exploration critique du silence." No. 9 (2018).
Agrimi, Jole, and Chiara Crisciani. *Les consilia médicaux*. Translated by Caroline Viola. Turnhout, BE: Brepols, 1994.
Alexander, John T. *Bubonic Plague in Early Modern Russia: Public Health and Urban Disaster*. Baltimore, MD: The Johns Hopkins University Press, 1980.
Allen, Rosamund, ed. *Eastward Bound: Travel and Travellers, 1050–1550*. Manchester, UK: Manchester University Press, 2004.
Alter, George C., and Ann G. Carmichael. "Classifying the Dead: Toward a History of the Registration of Causes of Death." *Journal of the History of Medicine and Allied Sciences* 54, no. 2 (1999): 114–32.
Andernach, Jehan Guinter d'. *Instruction tresutile, par laquelle un chacun se pourra maintenir en santé tant au temps de peste comme en autre temps*. Argentine, FR: au Pelican, 1547.
Anderson, Warwick. *Colonial Pathologies: American Tropical Medicine, Race, and Hygiene in the Philippines*. Durham, SC: Duke University Press, 2006.
André, Pierre. *Traité de la peste et de cure d'icelle*. Poitiers, FR: N. Logeroys, 1563.

Anonymous. *A Brief Relation of the Plague at Naples, in the Year M.DC. LVI*. London: J. Grismond, 1665.
– *Concerning the Constitution of an Aire Infected and How to Know Plague-sores and Carbuncles.* Oxford: Leonard Lichfield, 1644.
– *Especiall Observations and Aprroved Physicall Rules.* London: B. Alsop and T. Fawcet, 1625.
– *Estat general de ceux qui sont morts de peste au lieu de santé et dans la ville de Rouen.* Rouen, FR: Laürens Machuël, 1668.
– *The Late Dreadful Plague at Marseilles Compared with that Terrible Plague in London in the Year 1665.* London: H. Parker, 1721.
– *Physicall Directions in Time of Plague.* Oxford: Leonard Lichfield, 1644.
– *Present Remedies Against the Plague: Shewing Sundrye Preservatives for the Same.* London: John Danter, 1592.
– *Regime contre la pestil[enc]e ce faict et compose par messieurs les medecins de la cite de Basle en allemaigne.* Lyon, FR: Claude Nourry, c. 1514.
– *Regime contro la pestilence per les medecins de Basle.* Venice, IT: n.p., c. 1519.
– [Johannes Jacobi]. *Remede tres utile contra fievre pestilencieuse.* Paris: Ulrich Gering, c. 1480.
– *The Shutting Up Infected Houses as It is Practised in England Soberly Debated.* London: n.p., 1665.
– *Some Customs Consider'd Whether Prejudicial to the Health of This City.* London: for Eman. Matthews, 1721.
– *Souverain remede co[n]tre Lepidimye bosse et maulvais aer.* Lyon, FR: Martin Havard, c. 1501.
– *A Succinct Account of the Plague at Marseilles … Translated from the French by a Physician.* London: for S. Buckley, 1721.
– *A Treatise Concerning the Plague and the Pox.* London: Gertrude Dawson, 1652.
– *The Weekly Bill of Mortality: With a Lamentable Relation of Many Visitations by the Plague in Times Past.* London: Tho. Milbourn, 1665.
Anselment, Raymond A. "Thomas Sprat's *The Plague of Athens*: Thucydides, Lucretius, and the 'Pindaric Way.'" *Bulletin of the John Rylands Library* 78, no. 1 (1996): 3–20.
Arnold, David. *Colonizing the Body: State Medicine and Epidemic Disease in Nineteenth-Century India.* Berkeley: University of California Press, 1993.
Arrizabalaga, Jon. "Facing the Black Death: Perceptions and Reactions of University Medical Practitioners." In *Practical Medicine from Salerno*

to the Black Death, edited by Luis García-Ballester, Roger French, Jon Arrizabalaga, and Andrew Cunningham, 237–88. Cambridge, Cambridge University Press, 1994.

– "*Pestis Manufacta*: Plague, Poisons and Fear in Mid-Fourteenth-Century Europe." In *"It All Depends on the Dose": Poisons and Medicines in European History,* edited by Ole Peter Grell, Andrew Cunningham, and Jon Arrizabalaga, 62–80. London and New York: Routledge, 2018.

Aston, Margaret. "Death." In *Fifteenth-Century Attitudes: Perceptions of Society in Late Medieval England*, edited by Rosemary Horrox, 202–28. Cambridge: Cambridge University Press, 1994.

Atila. *Traictie tresutile contre la peste.* Paris: Gaspard Philippe, c. 1505.

Atlas Historique de Paris. http://paris-atlas-historique.fr/4.html

Aubert, Jacques. *Traite contenant les causes, la curation, & preservation de la peste.* Lausanne, FR: Jean le Preux, 1571.

Audouin-Rouzeau, Frédérique. *Les chemins de la peste: le rat, la puce, et l'homme.* Rennes, FR: Presses Universitaires de Rennes, 2003.

Barbette, Paul. *The Chirurgical and Anatomical Works of Paul Barbette … Together with a Treatise of the Plague.* London: J. Darby, 1672.

Barkai, Ron. "Jewish Treatises on the Black Death (1348–1500): A Preliminary Study." In *Medicine from the Black Death to the French Disease,* edited by Roger French, Jon Arrizabalaga, Andrew Cunningham, and Luis García-Ballester, 6–25. Aldershot, UK: Ashgate, 1998.

Barker, Hannah. "Laying the Corpses to Rest: Grain, Embargoes, and *Yersinia pestis* in the Black Sea, 1346–48." *Speculum* 96 no. 1 (2021): 97–126.

Barker, S.K., and Brenda M. Hosington, eds. *Renaissance Cultural Crossroads: Translation, Print and Culture in Britain, 1473–1640.* Leiden, NL: Brill, 2013.

Barnard, John, and Maureen Bell. "The English Provinces." In *The Cambridge History of the Book in Britain*, volume IV, edited by John Barnard and D.F. McKenzie, 665–86. Cambridge: Cambridge University Press, 2002.

Barnes, David S. *The Great Stink of Paris and the Nineteenth-Century Struggle against Filth and Germs.* Baltimore, MD: Johns Hopkins University Press, 2006.

Barralis, B., trans. *Paradoxes de la peste.* Paris: Fleury Bourriquant, 1620.

Barroso, Efrén de la Peña. "Un *Regimen sanitatis* contra la peste: El Tratado del licenciado Vázquez." *Asclepio* 44, no. 2 (2012): 397–416.

Barrowclough, David. "Time to Slay Vampire Burials? The Archaeological and Historical Evidence for Vampires in Europe." Discussion Paper. Cambridge: Red Dagger Press, 2014. http://www.academia.edu/8854480/Time_to_Slay_Vampire_Burials_The_Archaeological_and_Historical_Evidence_for_Vampires_in_Europe.

Barry, Jonathan. "'Compleat Physician' and Experimentation in Medicines: Everard Maynwaring (c. 1629–1713) and the Restoration Debate on Medical Practice in London." *Medical History* 62, no. 2 (2018): 155–76.

Bartsocas, Christos S. "Two Fourteenth-Century Greek Descriptions of the Black Death." *Journal of the History of Medicine and Allied Sciences* 21, no. 4 (1966): 394–400.

Baux, Pierre. *Traité de la peste.* Toulouse, FR: Jean Guillemette, 1722.

Beier, Alan L. *The Problem of the Poor in Tudor and Early Stuart England.* New York: Routledge, 2003.

Bell, John. *London's Remembrancer: Or a True Accompt of Every Particular Weeks Christnings and Mortality in All the Years of Pestilence within the Cognizance of the Bills of Mortality.* London: E. Cates, 1665.

Bell, Maureen. "Hannah Allen and the Development of a Puritan Publishing Business, 1646–51." *Publishing History* 26 (1989): 5–66.

Bellaguet, M.L., trans. *Chronique du religieux de Saint-Denys, contenant le règne de Charles VI de 1380 à 1422.* Paris: Editions du Comité des travaux historiques et scientifiques, 1994.

Belmas, Élisabeth. "Pouvoir politique et catastrophe sanitaire: la « publication » des épidémies de peste dans la france moderne." *Parlement[s], Revue d'histoire politique* 25 (2017): 31–54.

Belon du Mans, Pierre. *Les observations de plusieurs singularités et choses memorables.* Paris: Hierosme de Marnef et Guillaume Cauellat, 1588.

Benedict, Philip. "French Cities from the Sixteenth Century to the Revolution: An Overview." In *Cities and Social Change in Early Modern France*, edited by Philip Benedict, 7–68. London: Routledge, 1992.

Bennett, H.S. *English Books & Readers.* Volume 1: *1475 to 1557: Being a Study in the History of the Book Trade from Caxton to the Incorporation of the Stationers' Company.* Cambridge: Cambridge University Press, 1969.

Benveniste, Henriette-Rika, and Costas Gaganakis. "Heterodoxies: Construction of Identities and Otherness in Medieval and Early Modern Europe." *Historein* 2 (2000): 7–12.

Bercé, Yves-Marie. "*Rumeurs et épidémies: les semeurs de peste.*" In *La vie, la mort, la foi, le temps: mélanges offerts à Pierre Chaunu*, edited by Jean-Pierre Bardet and Madeleine Foisil, 85–94. Paris: Presses universitaires de France, 1993.

Béroujon, Anne. *Peuple et pauvres des villes dans la France moderne: De la Renaissance à la Révolution*. Paris: Armand Colin, 2014.

Bertrand, Jean-Baptiste. *Relation historique de tout ce qui s'est passé à Marseille pendant la dernière peste*. Cologne: Pierre Marteau, 1723.

Bertrand, Michel Jean-Baptiste. *Observations faites sur la peste qui règne à présente à Marseille et dans la Provence*. Lyon, FR: A. Laurens, 1721.

Biographie universelle, ancienne et moderne. Tome troisième. Paris: Michaud Frères, 1811.

Biraben, Jean-Noël. *Les hommes et la peste en France et dans les pays européens et méditerranéens*. 2 volumes. Paris: Mouton, 1975–6.

Bisaha, Nancy. *Creating East and West: Renaissance Humanists and the Ottoman Turks*. Philadelphia: University of Pennsylvania Press, 2004.

Bisshop of Arusiens. *Here begynneth a litill boke necessarye & behouefull agenst the Pestilence*. London: William Machlinia, 1485.

Bisshop and Doctor of Physick of Denmarke. *Here after ensuith a litle treatise*. London: Thomas Gybson, 1536.

Blayney, Peter W.M. *The Stationers' Company and the Printers of London, 1501–1557*. Cambridge: Cambridge University Press, 2013.

Boccaccio, Giovanni. *Decameron*. Translated by G.H. McWilliam. 2nd edition. Harmondsworth, UK: Penguin Classics, 2003.

Boeckl, Christine M. *Images of Plague and Pestilence: Iconography and Iconology*. Kirksville, MO: Truman State University Press, 2000.

Boecler, Johann. *Recueil des observations qui ont étées faites sur la maladie de Marseille*. Strasbourg, FR: Jean Regnauld Doulssecker, 1721.

Boffey, Julia. *Manuscript and Print in London c. 1475–1530*. London: The British Library, 2012.

Boghurst, William. *Loimographia: An Account of the Great Plague of London in the Year 1665*, edited by Joseph Frank Payne. London: Shaw and Sons for the Epidemiological Society of London, 1894.

Bolton, J.L. "Looking for *Yersina Pestis*: Scientists, Historians and the Black Death." In *The Fifteenth Century XII: Society in an Age of Plague*, edited by Linda Clark and Carole Rawcliffe, 15–38. Woodbridge, UK: Boydell, 2013.

Borromeo, Elisabetta. *Voyageurs occidentaux dans l'Empire ottoman (1600–1644)*. 2 volumes. Paris: Maissoneuve & Larose, 2007.

Bos, Gerrit. "The Black Death in Hebrew Literature: Ha-Ma'amar be-Qaddahot ha-Dever (Treatise on Pestilential Fever)." *European Journal of Jewish Studies* 5, no. 1 (2011): 1–52.

– *Maimonides, On the Elucidation of Some Symptoms and the Response to Them (Formerly Known as On the Causes of Symptoms). A New Parallel Arabic-English Translation.* Leiden, NL: Koninklijke Brill, 2019.

– *Maimonides, On the Regimen of Health. A New Parallel Arabic-English Translation.* Leiden, NL: Koninklijke Brill, 2019.

Bos, Gerrit, and Guido Mensching. "The Black Death in Hebrew Literature: Abraham Ben Solomon Hen's *Tractatulus de pestilentia.*" *Jewish Studies Quarterly* 18, no.1 (2011): 32–63.

Bos, Kristin I., Alexander Herbig, Jason Sahl, Nicholas Waglechner, Mathieu Fourment, Stephen A. Forrest, Jennifer Klunk, et al. "Eighteenth Century *Yersinia pestis* Genomes Reveal the Long-Term Persistence of an Historical Plague Focus." *eLife* 5 (2016): e12994.

Bouillet, Jean. *Avis et remèdes contre la peste.* Béziers, FR: E. Barbut, 1721.

Bouloux, N. "L'espace habité." In *La Terre: connaissance, représentations, mesure au Moyen Âge*, edited by Patrick Gautier Dalché, 259–441. Turnhout, BE: Brepols, 2013.

Boulton, Jeremy. "London 1540–1700." In *The Cambridge Urban History of Britain, Volume 2: 1540–1840*, edited by Peter Clark, 315–46. Cambridge: Cambridge University Press, 2000.

Bowers, Kristy Wilson. *Plague and Public Health in Early Modern Seville.* Rochester, NY: University of Rochester Press, 2013.

Boyer, Jean-Baptiste-Nicolas. *Dissertation abregée sur la maladie de Marseille.* Toulon, FR: Louis Mallard, 1720.

Bradley, Richard. *The Plague at Marseilles Consider'd.* London: for W. Mears, 1721.

Bradwell, Stephen. *Physick for the Sicknesse, Commonly Called the Plague.* London: for Benjamin Fisher, 1636.

– *A Watch-Man for the Pest.* London: John Dawson, 1625.

Brasbridge, Thomas. *The Poore Mans Jewell.* London: George Bishop, 1592.

Brazeau, Brian. *Writing a New France, 1604–1632: Empire and Early Modern French Identity.* London: Routledge, 2009.

Brenot, Anne-Marie. "La Peste soit des Huguenots: Étude d'une logique d'exécration au XVIe siècle." *Histoire, économie et société* 11, no. 4 (1992): 553–70.

Brentjes, Sonja. *Travellers from Europe in the Ottoman and Safavid Empires, 16th–17th Centuries: Seeking, Transforming, Discarding Knowledge.* New York: Routledge, 2010.

Briet, Guillaume. *Discours sur les causes de la peste survenue a Bourdeaux, cest an 1599 auec la preservation & curation d'icelle.* Bordeaux, FR: Millanges, 1599.

British Book Trade Index. http://bbti.bodleian.ox.ac.uk.

Brockliss, Laurence, and Colin Jones. *The Medical World of Early Modern France.* Oxford: Clarendon Press, 1997.

Brooke, John. "Thinking Big about the Plague." *Inference* 4, no. 2 (2018). https://inference-review.com/letter/thinking-big-about-the-plague.

Brookes, Richard. *A History of the Most Remarkable Pestilential Distempers that have Appeared in Europe for Three Hundred Years Last Past.* London: A. Corbett, 1721.

Brotton, Jeremy. *This Orient Isle: Elizabethan England and the Islamic World.* London: Allen Lane, 2016.

Brough, William. *A Preservative Against the Plague of Schisme.* London: for I. Clarke, 1650.

Browne, Joseph. *A Practical Treatise of the Plague and All Pestilential Infections that have Happen'd in this Island for the Last Century.* 2nd edition. London: for J. Wilcox, 1720.

Brownrigg, William. *Considerations on the Means of Preventing the Communication of Pestilential Contagion, and of Eradicating It in Infected Places.* London: for Lockyer Davis, 1771.

Brummet, Palmira. "The Lepanto Paradigm Revisited: Knowing the Ottomans in the Sixteenth Century." In *The Renaissance and the Ottoman World*, edited by Anna Contadini and Claire Norton, 63–93. Aldershot, UK: Ashgate, 2013.

Bull, Marcus Graham. *Thinking Medieval: An Introduction to the Study of the Middle Ages.* New York: Palgrave Macmillan, 2005.

Bullein, William. *A Dialogue Bothe Pleasant and Pitifull, Wherein is a Godlie Regimente Against the Feuer Pestile[n]ce.* London: Ihon Kyngston, 1578.

Buttimer, Anne, and David Seamon, eds. *The Human Experience of Space and Place.* London: Croom Helm, 1980.

Bysshop and Doctor of Physick of Denmarke. *Here after ensuith a litle treatise.* London: Thomas Gybson, 1536.

Cagle, Hugh. "Beyond the Senegal: Inventing the Tropics in the Late Middle Ages." *Journal of Medieval Iberian Studies* 7, no. 2 (2015): 197–217.

Caius, John. *A Boke, or Counseill Against the Disease Commonly Called the Sweate.* London: Richard Grafton, 1552.

Calamy, Edmund. *Englands Antidote, Against the Plague of Civill Warre.* London: by I.L. for Christopher Meredith, 1645.
Campbell, Anna Montgomery. *The Black Death and Men of Learning.* New York: Columbia University Press, 1931. Reprint, New York: AMS Press, 1966.
Campbell, Bruce M.S. *The Great Transition: Climate, Disease, and Society in the Late-Medieval World.* The 2013 Ellen McArthur Lectures. Cambridge: Cambridge University Press, 2016.
Campbell, Mary B. *The Witness and the Other World: Exotic European Writing, 400–1600.* Ithaca, NY: Cornell University Press, 1988.
Carmichael, Ann G. "The Last Past Plague: The Uses of Memory in Renaissance Epidemics." *Journal of the History of Medicine and Allied Sciences* 53, no. 2 (1998), 132–60.
– "The Legal Foundations of Post-Mortem Diagnosis in Later Medieval Milan." In *Death and Disease in the Medieval and Early Modern World: Perspectives from Across the Mediterranean and Beyond*, edited by Lori Jones and Nükhet Varlık. York, UK: York Medieval Press, 2022 (forthcoming).
– *Plague and the Poor in Renaissance Florence.* Cambridge: Cambridge University Press, 1986.
– "Plague Persistence in Western Europe: A Hypothesis." *The Medieval Globe* 1, no. 1 (2014): 157–92.
– "Registering Death and Causes of Death in Late Medieval Milan." In *Death in Medieval Europe: Death Scripted and Death Choreographed*, edited by Joëlle Rollo-Koster, 209–36. London: Routledge, 2017.
– "Universal and Particular: The Language of Plague, 1348–1500." In *Pestilential Complexities: Understanding Medieval Plague*, edited by Vivian Nutton, 17–52. London: Wellcome Trust Centre for the History of Medicine, 2008.
Carvalho, Simon, and Mark Zacher. "The International Health Regulations in Historical Perspective." In *Plagues and Politics: Infectious Disease and International Policy*, edited by Andrew T. Price-Smith, 235–61. London: Palgrave Macmillan, 2001.
Carvallo, Sarah. "The Empirical Turn of Medicine in England, 1660–1690." *Archives Internationales d'Histoire des Sciences* 67, no. 178 (2017): 75–112.
Cavallo, Sandra, and Tessa Storey, eds. *Conserving Health in Early Modern Culture: Bodies and Environments in Italy and England.* Manchester, UK: Manchester University Press, 2017.

– *Healthy Living in Late Renaissance Italy.* Oxford: Oxford University Press, 2013.

Certeau, Michel de. *The Practice of Everyday Life.* Translated by Steven Rendall. Berkeley: University of California Press, 1984.

Chartier, Roger. *The Order of Books: Readers, Authors, and Libraries in Europe between the Fourteenth and Eighteenth Centuries.* Translated by Lydia G. Cochrane. Stanford, CA: Stanford University Press, 1994.

Chase, Melissa P. "Fevers, Poisons, and Apostemes: Authority and Experience in Montpellier Plague Treatises." *Annals of the New York Academy of Sciences* 441, no. 1 (1985): 153–70.

Chauliac, Guy de. *La grande chirurgie de M. Gui de Chauliac ... restituée nouvellement à sa dignité par M. Laurens Joubert.* Lyon, FR: Estienne Michel, 1579.

– *Inventarium sive chirurgia magna*, edited by Michael McVaugh. 2 volumes. Leiden, NL: Brill, 1997.

Chettle, Henry. *A True Bill of the Whole Number that Hath Died in the Cittie of London.* London: I. Roberts for John Trundle, 1603.

Chevalier, Guillaume. *L'ordre public pour la ville de Lyon, pendant maladie contagieuse.* Lyon, FR: Antoine Valançol, 1670.

Chicoyneau, François. *Relation exacte et fidèle de ce qui s'est passé de plus remarquable à Marseille.* Nancy, FR: s.p., 1721.

Chicoyneau, François, François Verny, et Jean Soulier. *Observations et reflexions.* Toulouse, FR: Claude-Gilles Lecamus, 1720.

Chiu, Remi. "Singing on the Street and in the Home in Times of Pestilence: Lessons from the 1576–78 Plague of Milan." In *Domestic Devotions in Early Modern Italy*, edited by Maya Corry, Marco Faini, and Alessia Meneghin, 27–44. Leiden, NL: Brill, 2018.

Christianson, C. Paul. "The Rise of London's Book-Trade." In *The Cambridge History of the Book in Britain*, volume III, edited by Lotte Hellinga and J.B. Trapp, 128–47. Cambridge: Cambridge University Press, 1999.

– "Evidence for the Study of London's Late Medieval Manuscript-Book Trade." In *Book Production and Publishing in Britain 1375–1475*, edited by Jeremy Griffiths and Derek Pearsall, 87–108. Cambridge: Cambridge University Press, 1989.

Çırakman, Asli. *From the "Terror of the World" to the "Sick Man of Europe": European Images of Ottoman Empire and Society from the Sixteenth Century to the Nineteenth.* New York: Peter Lang, 2002.

Clapham, Henoch. *An Epistle Discoursing upon the Present Pestilence.* London: T.C., 1603.

Clarke, Linda, and Carole Rawcliffe, eds. *The Fifteenth Century XII: Society in an Age of Plague*. Woodbridge, UK: Boydell Press, 2013.

Clarke, Samuel. *The Historian's Guide, or, Britain's Remembrancer*. London: W. Crook, 1690.

Clot, A.B. *De la peste observée en Égypte. Recherches et considérations sur cette maladie*. Paris: Fortin, Masson, 1840.

Cohn, Samuel K., Jr. "The Black Death and the Burning of Jews." *Past & Present* 196, no. 1 (2007): 3–36.

– *Cultures of Plague: Medical Thinking at the End of the Renaissance*. Oxford: Oxford University Press, 2010.

Colet, Anna, Josep Xavier Muntané i Santiveri, Jordi Ruíz Ventura, Oriol Saula, M. Eulàlia Subirà de Galdàcano, and Clara Jáuregui. "The Black Death and Its Consequences for the Jewish Community in Tàrrega: Lessons from History and Archeology." *The Medieval Globe* 1 (2014): 63–96.

Colin, Sébastien. *Traicté de la Peste et de sa guerison*. Poitiers, FR: Enguilbert de Marneuf, 1566.

Collas, Rolande. *Histoire d'un quartier de Tours: Le Sanitas des origines à nos jours*. Paris: Office d'édition et de diffusion du livre d'histoire, 1994.

College des Maistres Chirurgiens jurez de Paris. *Traicté de la peste*. Paris: Nicolas Buon, 1606.

College of Physicians. *Certain Necessary Directions, as well for the Cure of the Plague, as for Preventing the Infection*. London: Robert Barker, 1636.

Connerton, Paul. *How Societies Remember*. Cambridge: Cambridge University Press, 1989.

Connolly, Margaret, and Linne R. Mooney, eds. *Design and Distribution of Late Medieval Manuscripts in England*. York, UK: York Medieval Press, 2008.

Conrad, Lawrence I. "Arabic Plague Chronologies and Treatises: Social and Historical Factors in the Formation of a Literary Genre." *Studia Islamica* 54 (1981): 51–93.

Constant, Jean-Marie. *Les Français pendant les guerres de religion*. Paris: Hachette Littératures, 2002.

Constructions de l'espace au Moyen Age: pratiques et représentations. XXXVIIe Congrès de la Société des historiens médiévistes de l'enseignement supérieur public. Paris: Publications de la Sorbonne, 2007.

Cook, Harold J. *The Decline of the Old Medical Regime in Stuart London*. Ithaca, NY: Cornell University Press, 1986.

Cooper, Charles Henry. *Annals of Cambridge*. Volume 1. Cambridge: Warwick and Co., 1842.

Corbin, Alain. *The Foul and the Fragrant: Odor and the French Social Imagination*. Cambridge, MA: Harvard University Press, 1986.

Coste, Joël. *La littérature des « Erreurs populaires », Une ethnographie médicale à l'époque moderne*. Paris: Champion, 2002.

– *Représentations et comportements en temps d'épidémie dans la littérature imprimée de peste (1490–1725): Contribution à l'histoire culturelle de la peste en France à l'époque moderne*. Paris: Honoré Champion Éditeur, 2007.

Courcelles, François de. *Traite de la peste clair et tres-utile*. Sedan, FR: Abel Riuery, 1595.

Coville, Alfred. "Écrits contemporains sur la peste de 1348 à 1350." In *Histoire littéraire de la France* 37, 325–90. Paris: Imprimerie National, 1938.

Crawshaw, Jane L. Stevens. *Plague Hospitals: Public Health for the City in Early Modern Venice*. Burlington, VT: Ashgate, 2012.

Crespo, Fabian. "Leprosy in Medieval Europe: An Immunological and Syndemic Approach." In *Death and Disease in the Medieval and Early Modern World: Perspectives from Across the Mediterranean and Beyond*, edited by Lori Jones and Nükhet Varlık. York, UK: York Medieval Press, 2022 (forthcoming).

Cressford, Craig, Christiana L. Scheib, Meriam Guellil, Marcel Keller, Craig Alexander, Sarah A. Inskip, and John E. Robb. "Beyond Plague Pits: Using Genetics to Identify Responses to Plague in Medieval Cambridgeshire." *European Journal of Archaeology*. Published online 17 June 2021. https://doi.org/10.1017/eaa.2021.19.

Cressy, David. *Literacy and the Social Order*. Cambridge: Cambridge University Press, 1980.

Crisciani, Chiara. "Città e medici di fronte alla peste." *Rivista per le Medical Humanities* 29, no. 8 (2014): 11–23.

Croke, Brian, trans. *The Chronicle of Marcellinus. Byzantina Australiensia* series, volume 7. Sydney: Australian Association for Byzantine Studies, 1995.

Cui, Yujun, Chang Yu, Yanfeng Yan, Dongfang Li, Yanjun Li, Thibaut Jombart, Lucy A. Weinert, et al. "Historical Variations in Mutation Rate in an Epidemic Pathogen, *Yersinia pestis*." PNAS 110, no. 2 (2013): 577–82.

Cummins, Neil, Morgan Kelly, and Cormac Ó Gráda. "Living Standards and Plague in London, 1560–1665." *Economic History Review*, 69, no. 1 (2016): 3–34.

Cunningham, Andrew. "Transforming Plague: The Laboratory and the Identity of Infectious Disease." In *The Laboratory Revolution in*

Medicine, edited by Andrew Cunningham and Perry Williams, 209–44. Cambridge: Cambridge University Press, 1992.

Cuvelier, Eliane. "'A Treatise of the Plague' de Thomas Lodge (1603): Traduction d'un ouvrage médical français." *Études Anglaises* 21, no. 4 (1968): 395–403.

Dalché, Patrick Gautier. "Représentations géographiques savantes, constructions et pratiques de l'espace." In *Construction de l'espace au Moyen Âge : pratiques et représentations*. XXXVIIe Congrès de la SHMESP (Mulhouse, 2–4 juin 2006), 13–38. Paris: Publications de la Sorbonne, 2007.

Davin, Antoine. *Tres singulier traité de la generale et particuliere preservation, & de la vraye & asseurée curation de la Peste*. Grenoble, FR: Richard Cocson, 1629.

Davis, Barbara Beckerman. "Poverty and Poor Relief in Sixteenth-Century Toulouse." *Historical Reflections/Réflexions Historiques* 17, no. 3 (1991): 267–96.

Davis, Natalie Zemon. "Poor Relief, Humanism and Heresy: The Case of Lyon." *Studies in Medieval and Renaissance History* 5 (1968): 215–75.

– "The Sacred and the Body Social in Sixteenth-Century Lyon." *Past & Present* 90 (1981): 40–70.

– *Society and Culture in Early Modern France: Eight Essays*. Stanford, CA: Stanford University Press, 1975.

Davis, Natalie Zemon, and Randolph Starn. "Introduction." *Representations* 26, special issue: Memory and Counter-Memory (1989): 1–6.

Debus, A.G. *The French Paracelsians: The Chemical Challenge to Medical and Scientific Tradition in Early Modern France*. Cambridge: Cambridge University Press, 1991.

Defoe, Daniel. *A Journal of the Plague Year: Being Observations or Memorials of the Most Remarkable Occurrences, as well Public as Private, which Happened in London During the Last Great Visitation in 1665*. London: for E. Nutt, J. Roberts, A. Dodd, and J. Graves, 1722.

Dekker, Thomas. *The Wonderfull Yeare 1603; Wherein is Shewed the Picture of London, Lying Sicke of the Plague*. London: Thomas Creede, 1603.

DeLacy, Margaret. *The Germ of an Idea: Contagionism, Religion, and Society in Britain, 1660–1730*. New York: Palgrave Macmillan, 2016.

DeWitte, Sharon N. "Survival in the Context of Urbanization and Environmental Change in Medieval and Early Modern London, England." In *Disease and the Environment in the Medieval and Early Modern Worlds*, edited by Lori Jones. London: Routledge, 2022 (forthcoming).

DeWitte, Sharon N., and Maryanne Kowaleski. "Black Death Bodies." *Fragments* 6 (2017): 1–37.

DeWitte, Sharon N., and James W. Wood. "Selectivity of Black Death Mortality with Respect to Preexisting Health." *PNAS* 105, no 5 (2008): 1436–41.

Di Cosmo, Nicola. "Black Sea Emporia and the Mongol Empire: A Reassessment of the Pax Mongolica." *Journal of the Economic and Social History of the Orient* 53 (2010): 83–108.

Dinkova-Bruun, Greti. "Preface." In *Catalogus Translationum et Commentariorum: Mediaeval and Renaissance Latin Translations and Commentaries, Annotated Lists and Guides*, volume 11, edited by Greti Dinkova-Bruun, Julia Haig Gaisser, and James Hankins, vii–xvi. Toronto: Pontifical Institute of Mediaeval Studies, 2016.

Dobson, Mary J. *Contours of Death and Disease in Early Modern England*. Cambridge: Cambridge University Press, 1997.

Dols, Michael. "Al-Manbijī's 'Report of the Plague': A Treatise on the Plague of 764–65/1363–64 in the Middle East." In *The Black Death: The Impact of the Fourteenth-Century Plague*, edited by Daniel Williman, 65–76. Binghamton, NY: Center for Medieval and Early Renaissance Studies, 1982.

– "Ibn al-Wardi's *Risalah al-Naba''An al-Waba'*: A Translation of a Major Source for the History of the Black Death in the Middle East." In *Near Eastern Numismatics, Iconography, Epigraphy and History: Studies in Honor of George C. Miles*, edited by George C. Miles and Dickran A. Kouymjian, 443–55. Beirut, LB: American University of Beirut, 1974.

Driver, Martha. "'By Me Elysabeth Pykeryng': Women and Book Production in the Early Tudor Period." In *Manuscripts and Printed Books in Europe 1350–1550: Packaging, Presentation and Consumption*, edited by Emma Cayley and Susan Powell, 115–19. Liverpool, UK: Liverpool University Press, 2013.

Drouet, Pierre. *Consilium novum de pestilentia*. Paris: Andream Wechelum, 1572.

Duffin, Jacalyn. "Introduction: Lessons and Disappointments." In *SARS in Context: Memory, History, Policy*, edited by Jacalyn Duffin and and Arthur Sweetman, 1–17. Montreal and Kingston: McGill-Queen's University Press, 2006.

Dumas, Geneviève. "La fenêtre en temps d'épidémie : air et miasmes à Montpellier aux XIVe et XVe siècles." In *Par la fenêtre : études de littérature et de civilisations médiévales*, actes du colloque du CUERMA, 157–65. Aix-en-Provence, FR: Presses universitaires de Provence, 2003.

– *Santé et société à Montpellier à la fin du Moyen Âge. The Medieval Mediterranean: Peoples, Economies and Cultures, 400–1500* series, volume 102. Leiden, NL: Brill, 2015.

Duris, Pascal. *Quelle révolution scientifique? Les sciences de la vie dans la querelle des Anciens et des Modernes (XVIe–XVIIIe siècles)*, Paris: Hermann, collection "Les collections de la République des Lettres," 2016.

Earle, Carville. "Environment, Disease and Mortality in Early Virginia." *Journal of Historical Geography* 5, no. 4 (1979): 365–90.

Echenberg, Myron J. *Plague Ports: The Global Urban Impact of Bubonic Plague, 1894–1901*. New York: New York University Press, 2007.

Edson, Evelyn. *The World Map, 1300–1492: The Persistence of Tradition and Transformation*. Baltimore, MD: Johns Hopkins University Press, 2007.

Eggert, Katherine. *Disknowledge: Literature, Alchemy, and the End of Humanism in Renaissance England*. Philadelphia: University of Pennsylvania Press, 2015.

Einbinder, Susan. *After the Black Death: Plague, Trauma and Commemoration among Iberian Jews*. Philadelphia: University of Pennsylvania Press, 2018.

– *Writing Plague: Jewish Writing, Memory, and the Great Italian Plague (1630–31)*. Philadelphia: University of Pennsylvania Press, 2022 (forthcoming).

Eisenberg, Merle, and Lee Mordechai. "The Justinianic Plague: An Interdisciplinary Review." *Byzantine and Modern Greek Studies* 43, no. 2 (2019): 156–80.

Elyot, Thomas. *The Castel of Helth Gathered and Made by Syr Thomas Elyot Knyghte, Out of the Chiefe Authors of Physyke*. London: Thomas Bertheleti, 1539.

Eroshenko, Galina A., Nikolay V. Popov, Zhanna V. Al'khova, Lyubov M. Kukleva, Alina N. Balykova, Nadezhda S. Chervyakova, Ekaterina A. Naryshkina, and Vladimir V. Kutyrev. "Evolution and Circulation of *Yersinia pestis* in the Northern Caspian and Northern Aral Sea Regions in the 20th-21st Centuries." *PLOS One* 16, no. 2 (2021): e0244615.

Fabbri, Christiane Nockels. "Continuity and Change in Late Medieval Plague Medicine: A Survey of 152 Plague Tracts from 1348 to 1599." PhD dissertation, Yale University, 2006.

– "Treating Medieval Plague: The Wonderful Virtues of Theriac." *Early Science and Medicine* 12, no. 3 (2007): 247–83.

Fabre, Pierre-Jean. *Traicté de la Peste selon la doctrine des Medicins Spagyriques*. Toulouse, FR: Raimond Colombiez, 1629.

Fancy, Nahyan. "Knowing the Signs of Disease: Plague in the Arabic Medical Commentaries Between the First and Second Pandemics." In *Death and Disease in the Medieval and Early Modern World: Perspectives from Across the Mediterranean and Beyond*, edited by Lori Jones and Nükhet Varlık. York, UK: York Medieval Press, 2022 (forthcoming).

Fancy, Nahyan, and Monica H. Green. "Plague and the Fall of Baghdad (1258)." *Medical History* 65, no. 2 (2021): 157–77.

Faroqhi, Suraiya. *Approaching Ottoman History: An Introduction to the Sources*. Cambridge: Cambridge University Press, 1999.

Fay, Isla. *Health and the City: Disease, Environment and Government in Norwich, 1200–1575*. Woodbridge, UK: Boydell Press, 2015.

Feather, John. *A History of British Publishing*. 2nd edition. London: Routledge, 2006.

Ferrier, Oger. *Remedes Preservatifs et curatifs de peste*. Lyon, FR: Jean de Tournes, 1548.

Fianu, Kouky. "Métiers et espace: topographie de la fabrication et du commerce du livre à Paris (XIIIe–XVe siècles)." In *Patrons, Authors and Workshops: Books and Book Production in Paris around 1400*, edited by Godfried Croenen and Peter F. Ainsworth, 21–46. Louvain, FR: Peeters, 2006.

Fioravanti, Leonardo. *Del regimento della peste*. Venice, IT: Andrea Revenoldo, 1565.

Fissell, Mary E. "Making Meaning from the Margins: The New Cultural History of Medicine." In *Locating Medical History: The Stories and Their Meanings*, edited by Frank Huisman and John Harley Warner, 364–89. Baltimore MD: The Johns Hopkins University Press, 2006.

– "Popular Medical Writing." In *Oxford History of Popular Print Culture*, volume 1, *Cheap Print in Britain and Ireland to 1660*, edited by Joad Raymond, 418–31. Oxford: Oxford University Press, 2011.

Fitzpatrick, Kevin, and Mark LaGory. *Unhealthy Places: The Ecology of Risk in the Urban Landscape*. New York: Routledge, 2000.

Fontaine, Laurence. *Histoire du colportage en Europe:(XVe–XIXe siècle)*. Paris: Editions Albin Michel, 1993.

Forrai, Réka. "Procopius Caesariensis." In *Catalogus Translationum et Commentariorum: Mediaeval and Renaissance Latin Translations and Commentaries, Annotated Lists and Guides*, volume 11, edited by Greti Dinkova-Bruun, Julia Haig Gaisser, and James Hankins, 211–36. Toronto: Pontifical Institute of Mediaeval Studies, 2016.

Foscati, Alessandra. *Ignis sacer: Una storia culturale del 'fuoco sacro' dall'antichità al Settecento*. Micrologus Library 51. Firenze, IT: Sismel Edizioni del Galluzzo, 2013.

Foucault, Michel. *Folie et Déraison: Histoire de la folie à l'âge classique*. Paris: Libraire Plon, 1961.

– *The Order of Things: An Archaeology of the Human Sciences*. New York: Routledge, 2005.

– "Questions on Geography." In *Power/Knowledge: Selected Interviews and Other Writings 1972–1977*, edited by Colin Gordon, translated by Colin Gordon, Leo Marshall, John Mepham, and Kate Soper, 63–77. New York: Pantheon Books, 1980.

Franssen, P.J.A., and A.E.C. Simoni. "Jan van Doesborch (?–1536), Printer of English Texts." *Quaerendo* 16, no. 4 (1986): 259–80.

Freeman, Kathleen. *Ancilla to the Pre-Socratic Philosophers*. Cambridge, MA: Harvard University Press, 1948.

Furholt, Martin. "Massive Migrations? The Impact of Recent aDNA Studies on Our View of Third Millennium Europe." *European Journal of Archaeology* 21 (2018): 159–91.

Gadbury, John. *London's Deliverance Predicted: In a Short Discourse Showing Causes of Plague in General*. London: J.C. for E. Calvert, 1665.

Gage, Kenneth L., and Michael Y. Kosoy. "Natural History of Plague: Perspectives from More than a Century of Research." *Annual Review of Entomology* 50 (2005): 505–28.

Galanaud, Pierre, Anne Galanaud, Patrick Giraudoux, and Henri Labesse. "Mortality and Demographic Recovery in Early Post-Black Death Epidemics: Role of Recent Emigrants in Medieval Dijon." *PLOS ONE* 15, no. 1 (2020): e0226420.

Galbraith, V.H., ed. *The Anonimalle Chronicle, 1333 to 1381: From a MS. Written at St Mary's Abbey, York*. Manchester, UK: Manchester University Press, 1970. Originally published in 1927.

García-Ballester, Luis, Lola Ferre, and Eduard Feliu. "Jewish Appreciation of Fourteenth-Century Scholastic Medicine." *Osiris* 6 (1990): 85–117.

Gardin, Louis du. *La Chasse-peste, ou les remedes singuliers et familiers dont chascun se poura servir pour se preserver en temps pestiferé*. Douay, FR: Pierre Auroy, 1617.

Garencières, Theophilus de. *A Mite Cast into the Treasury of the Famous City of London, Being a Brief and Methodical Discourse of the Nature, Causes, Symptomes, Remedies and Preservation from the Plague, in this Calamitous Year, 1665, Digested into Aphorismes*. London: Thomas Ratcliffe, 1665.

Gatford, Lionel. *Logos alexipharmakos, Or, Hyperphysicall Directions in Time of Plague*. Oxford: Henry Hall, 1644.

Gaudereau, Martin. *Relation des differentes especes de peste que reconnoissent les Orientaux*. Paris: Jacques Quillau, 1721.

Geltner, Guy. "Healthscaping a Medieval City: Lucca's Curia viarum and the Future of Public Health History." *Urban History* 40, no. 3 (2013): 395–415.

Getz, Faye Marie. "Black Death and the Silver Lining: Meaning, Continuity, and Revolutionary Change in Histories of Medieval Plague." *Journal of the History of Biology* 24, no. 2 (1991): 265–89.

Giffin, Karen, Aditya Kumar Lankapalli, Susanna Sabin, Maria A. Spyrou, Cosimo Posth, Justina Kozakaitė, Ronny Friedrich, et al. "A Treponemal Genome from an Historic Plague Victim Supports a Recent Emergence of Yaws and Its Presence in 15th Century Europe." *Scientific Reports*, 10, no. 9499 (2020). https://doi.org/10.1038/s41598-020-66012-x.

Gifford, Paul. "Defining Others: How Interperceptions Shape Identities." In *Europe and its Others: Essays on Interperception and Identity*, edited by Paul Gifford and Tessa Hauswedell, 13–38. Oxford: Peter Lang, 2010.

Gil-Sotres, Pedro. "Derivation and Revulsion: The Theory and Practice of Medieval Phlebotomy." In *Practical Medicine from Salerno to the Black Death*, edited by Luis Garcia-Ballester, Roger French, Jon Arrizabalaga, and Andrew Cunningham, 110–55. Cambridge: Cambridge University Press, 1994.

Gilchrist, Roberta. "Medieval Bodies in the Material World: Gender, Stigma, and the Body." In *Framing Medieval Bodies*, edited by Sarah Kay and Miri Rubin, 43–61. Manchester, UK: Manchester University Press, 1994.

Gillespie, Alexandra, and Daniel Wakelin, eds. *The Production of Books in England 1350–1500*. Cambridge: Cambridge University Press, 2011.

Gilman, Ernest B. *Plague Writing in Early Modern England*. Chicago, IL: University of Chicago Press, 2009.

Goiffon, Jean-Baptiste. *Relations et dissertation sur la peste du Gévaudan*. Lyon, FR: P. Valfray, 1722.

Goldberg, P.J.P. "Introduction." In *The Black Death in England*, edited by W.M. Ormrod and P.G. Lindley, 1–16. Stamford, UK: Paul Watkins, 1996.

Goldstein, Bernard R., and David Pingree. "Levi ben Gerson's Prognostication for the Conjunction of 1345." *Transactions of the American Philosophical Association* 80, no. 6 (1990): 1–60.

Gordon, Daniel. "The City and the Plague in the Age of Enlightenment." *Yale French Studies* 92 (1997): 67-87.

– "Confrontations with the Plague in Eighteenth-Century France." In *Dreadful Visitations: Confronting Natural Catastrophe in the Age of Enlightenment*, edited by Alessa Johns, 3–29. New York: Routledge, 1999.
Gould, Kevin. *Catholic Activism in South-West France, 1540–1570.* Aldershot, UK: Ashgate, 2006.
Goulding, Robert. "Histories of Science in Early Modern Europe: Introduction." *Journal of the History of Ideas* 67, no. 1 (2006): 33–40.
Gransden, Antonia. "A Fourteenth-Century Chronicle from the Grey Friars at Lynn." *English Historical Review* 72, no. 283 (1957): 270–8.
– *Historical Writing in England.* 2 volumes. London: Routledge and Kegan Paul, 1974–82.
Granshaw, Lindsay, and Roy Porter, eds. *The Hospital in History.* London: Routledge, 1989.
Grant, Edward. *A Source Book in Medieval Science.* Volume 1. Boston, MA: Harvard University Press, 1974.
Gratien, Chris. "The Ottoman Quagmire: Malaria, Swamps, and Settlement in the Late Ottoman Mediterranean." *International Journal of Middle East Studies* 49, no. 4 (2017): 583–604.
Graunt, John. *London's Dreadful Visitation: Or, A Collection of all the Bills of Mortality for the Present Year …* London: E. Cotes, 1665.
– *Natural and Political Observations, Mentioned in a Following Index, Upon the Bills of Mortality.* London: Thomas Roycroft, 1662.
– *Reflections on the Weekly Bills of Mortality for the cities of London and Westminster.* London: Samuel Speed, 1665.
Green, Monica H. "Climate and Disease in Medieval Eurasia." In *Oxford Research Encyclopedia of Asian History.* Oxford: Oxford University Press, 2018.
– "Editor's Introduction to Pandemic Disease in the Medieval World: Rethinking the Black Death." *The Medieval Globe* 1 (2014): 9–26.
– "The Four Black Deaths." *The American Historical Review* 125, no. 5 (2020): 1601–31.
– "The Historian, the Archaeologist, and the Geneticist: Pandemic Thinking." Presentation at the Society for Medieval Archaeology Annual Conference, *The Long Black Death: New Perspectives.* York, UK, 5 July 2019.
– "Putting Africa on the Black Death Map: Narratives from Genetics and History." *Afriques* 9 (2018). http://journals.openedition.org/afriques.
– "Taking 'Pandemic' Seriously: Making the Black Death Global." *The Medieval Globe* 1 (2014): 27–62.

Green, Monica H., and Lori Jones. "The Evolution and Spread of Major Human Diseases in the Indian Ocean World." In *Disease Dispersion and Impact in the Indian Ocean World*, edited by Gwyn Campbell and Eva-Maria Knoll, 25–57. London: Palgrave, 2020.

Greenberg, Stephen. "Plague, the Printing Press, and Public Health in Seventeenth-Century London." *Huntington Library Quarterly* 67, no. 4 (2004): 508–27.

Greenblatt, Stephen. *Marvelous Possessions: The Wonder of the New World*. Chicago, IL: University of Chicago Press, 1991.

Greengrass, Mark. *Christendom Destroyed: Europe 1517–1648*. London: Allen Lane, 2014.

Greg, W.W. "Notes on the Types, Borders, ETC., Used by Thomas Berthelet." *The Library* TBS-8, no. 1 (1906): 187–220.

Grelot, Guillaume-Joseph. *A Late Voyage to Constantinople*. Translated by J. Phillips. London: John Playford, 1683.

Griffin, Carrie. "Reconsidering the Recipe: Materiality, Narrative and Text in Later Medieval Instructional Manuscripts and Collections." In *Manuscripts and Printed Books in Europe 1350–1550: Packaging, Presentation and Consumption*, edited by Emma Cayley and Susan Powell, 135–49. Liverpool, UK: Liverpool University Press, 2013.

Griffiths, Paul. "Overlapping Circles: Imagining Criminal Communities in London, 1545–1645." In *Communities in Early Modern England: Networks, Place, Rhetoric*, edited by Alexandra Shepard and Phil Withington, 115–133. Manchester, UK: Manchester University Press, 2000.

Griffiths, Paul, and Mark S.R. Jenner, eds. *Londinopolis, c. 1500–c. 1750: Essays in the Cultural and Social History of Early Modern London*. Manchester, UK: Manchester University Press, 2000.

Grillot, P. Jean. *Lyon affligé de contagion, ou narré de ce qui s'est passé de plus memorable en ceste Ville, depuis le mois d'Aoust de l'an 1628 jusques au mois d'Octobre de l'an 1629*. Lyon, FR: François de la Bottiere, 1629.

Gruber, Henry. "Indirect Evidence for the Social Impact of the Justinianic Pandemic: Episcopal Burial and Conciliar Legislation in Visigothic Hispania." *Journal of Late Antiquity* 11, no. 1 (2018): 193–215.

Guenée, Bernard. *Comment on écrit l'histoire au XIIIe siècle: Primat et le Roman des roys*. Paris: CNRS Editions, 2016.

Guerin, Jacques. *Traicte tresexcellent contenant la vraye maniere d'estre preservé de peste en temps dangereux*. Anvers, FR: Christophle Plantin, 1567.

Guérin, Sarah M. "Exchange of Sacrifices: West Africa in the Medieval World of Goods." *The Medieval Globe* 3, no. 2 (2017): 97–124.

Hackel, Heidi Brayman. "Rhetorics and Practices of Illiteracy or the Marketing of Illiteracy." In *Reading and Literacy in the Middle Ages and Renaissance*, edited by Ian Frederick Moulton, 169–83. Turnhout, BE: Brepols, 2004.

Hanawalt, Barbara, and Michal Kolbialka, eds. *Medieval Practices of Space*. Minneapolis: University of Minnesota Press, 2000.

Harding, Vanessa. "Reading Plague in Seventeenth-century London." *Social History of Medicine* 32, no. 2 (2019): 267–86.

Hardingham, Glenn James. "The Regimen in Late Medieval England." PhD dissertation, University of Cambridge, 2005.

Harley, J.B. *The New Nature of Maps: Essays in the History of Cartography*, edited by Paul Laxton. Baltimore, MD: Johns Hopkins University Press, 2001.

Harris, Jonathan Gil. *Foreign Bodies and the Body Politic: Discourses of Social Pathology in Early Modern England.* Cambridge: Cambridge University Press, 1998.

Harris, Kate. "Patrons, Buyers and Owners: The Evidence for Ownership, and the Role of Book Owners in Book Production and the Book Trade." In *Book Production and Publishing in Britain 1375–1475*, edited by Jeremy Griffiths and Derek Pearsall, 163–200. Cambridge: Cambridge University Press, 1989.

Harrison, Mark. "Disease, Diplomacy and International Commerce: The Origins of International Sanitary Regulation in the Nineteenth Century." *Journal of Global History* 1, no. 2 (2006): 197–217.

Hartley, Brandon. "War and Tolerance: Catholic Polemic in Lyon during the French Religious Wars." PhD dissertation, University of Arizona, 2007.

Hartog, François. *Regimes of Historicity: Presentism and Experiences of Time*. Translated by Saskia Brown. New York: Columbia University Press, 2015.

Headley, John M. "Geography and Empire in the Late Renaissance: Botero's Assignment, Western Universalism, and the Civilizing Process." *Renaissance Quarterly* 53, no. 4 (2000): 1119–55.

Healy, Margaret. "Defoe's Journal and the English Plague Writing Tradition." *Literature and Medicine* 22, no. 1 (2003): 25–44.

– "Discourses of the Plague in Early Modern London." In *Epidemic Disease in London: Collection of Working Papers Given at the Symposium 'Epidemic Disease in London: from the Black Death to*

Cholera' Held at the Institute of Historical Research, edited by J.A.I. Champion, 19–34. London: Centre for Metropolitan History, 1993.
– *Fictions of Disease in Early Modern England: Bodies, Plagues and Politics*. Houndsmills, UK: Palgrave Macmillan, 2001.
Hecker, J.F.C. *The Black Death of the Fourteenth Century*. Translated by B.G. Babington. London: A. Schloss, 1833.
Hedeman, Anne D. *The Royal Image: Illustrations of the Grandes Chroniques de France, 1274–1422*. Berkeley: University of California Press, 1991.
Heinrichs, Erik A. *Plague, Print, and the Reformation: The German Reform of Healing*. London and New York: Routledge, 2018.
Heller, Henry. *The Conquest of Poverty: The Calvinist Revolt in Sixteenth Century France*. Leiden, NL: Brill, 1986.
Henderson, John. "Charity and Welfare in Early Modern Tuscany." In *Health Care and Poor Relief in Counter Reformation Europe*, edited by Ole Peter Grell, Andrew Cunningham, and Jon Arrizabalaga, 56–84. London: Routledge, 1999.
Herman, Nicholas. "Excavating the Page: Virtuosity and Illusionism in Italian Book Illumination, 1460–1520." *Word & Image: A Journal of Verbal/Visual Enquiry* 27, no. 2 (2011): 190–211.
Herring, Francis. *Certaine Rules, Directions or Advertisements for This Time of Pestilentiall Contagion*. London: William Iones, 1625.
Heywood, C.J. "Sir Paul Rycaut, A Seventeenth-Century Observer of the Ottoman State: Notes for a Study." In *English and Continental Views ofthe Ottoman Empire, 1500–1800*, edited by Ezel Kural Shaw and C.J. Heywood, 31–59. Los Angeles: University of California Press, 1972.
Higgins, Iain Macleod. *Writing East: The 'Travels' of Sir John Mandeville*. Philadelphia: University of Pennsylvania Press, 1997.
Hill, Thomas. *Joyful Jewell*. London: J. Allde, 1579.
Hobart, Brenton. "L'Imaginaire de la Peste dans la Littérature Française de la Renaissance." PhD dissertation, Harvard University, 2012.
– *La Peste à la Renaissance. L'imaginaire d'un fléau dans la littérature au XVIe siècle*. Paris: Classiques Garnier, 2020.
Hobbes, Thomas. *Eight Bookes of the Peloponnesian Warre Written by Thucydides ... Interpreted with Faith and Diligence Immediately out of the Greeke by Thomas Hobbes*. London: Henry Seile, 1629.
Hodges, Nathaniel. *Loimologia, or an Historical Account of the Plague in London in 1665*. Translated by John Quincy. London: E. Bell, 1720.
– *Loimologia, sive Pestis nuperæ apud Populum Londinensem grassantis Narratio Historica*. London: Gul. Godbid, 1672.

Hodnett, Edward. *English Woodcuts, 1480–1535*. London: Printed for the Bibliographical Society at the Oxford University Press, 1935.

Holt, Mack P. *The French Wars of Religion, 1562–1629*. 2nd edition. Cambridge: Cambridge University Press, 2005.

Honkapohja, Alpo. *Alchemy, Medicine, and Commercial Book Production: A Codicological and Linguistic Study of the Sloane Manuscript Group*. Turnhout, BE: Brepols, 2017.

– "Tracing the Early Modern John of Burgundy: Manuscripts and Lexicon." In *Genre in Medical English, 1500–1820: Sociocultural Contexts of Production and Use*, edited by Irma Taavitsainen, Turo Hiltunen, Jeremy Smith, and Carla Suhr. Cambridge: Cambridge University Press, 2022 (forthcoming).

Honkapohja, Alpo, and Lori Jones. "From *Practica Phisicalia* to *Mandeville's Travels*: Untangling the Misattributed Identities and Writings of John of Burgundy." *Notes and Queries* 67, no. 1 (2020): 18–27.

Horden, Peregrine. "Ritual and Public Health in the Early Medieval City." In *Body and City: Histories of Urban Public Health*, edited by Sally Sheard and Helen Power, 17–40. Aldershot, UK: Ashgate, 2000.

Horobin, Simon, and Aditi Nafde, eds. *Pursuing Middle English Manuscripts and their Texts: Essays in Honour of Ralph Hanna*. Turnhout, BE: Brepols, 2017.

Horrox, Rosemary, trans. and ed. *The Black Death*. Manchester, UK: Manchester University Press, 1994.

Houël, Nicolas. *Traité de la peste, auquel est amplement discouru de l'origine, cause, signes, preservation et curation d'icelle*. Paris: Galiot du Pré, 1573.

Housley, Norman. *Crusading and the Ottoman Threat, 1453–1505*. Oxford: Oxford University Press, 2013.

Houssemaine, Nicolas de. *Régime singulier contre la peste*. Troyes, FR: Jehan Lecoq, 1520.

– *Ung regime singulier co[n]tre peste*. Lyon, FR: Thibaud Payen, <1530.

Houston, Alan, and Steve Pincus. "Introduction: Modernity and Later Seventeenth-Century England." In *A Nation Transformed: England after the Restoration*, edited by Alan Houston and Steve Pincus, 1–19. Cambridge: Cambridge University Press, 2001.

Houston, Robert Allan. *Literacy in Early Modern Europe: Culture and Education 1500–1800*. New York: Longman, 2002.

Hutton, Patrick H. *History as an Art of Memory*. Hanover, NH: University Press of New England, 1993.

I.D. *Salomon's Pest-house, Or Tower-royall.* London: for Henry Holland, 1636.

Ingram, Dale. *An Historical Account of the Several Plagues that Have Appeared in the World Since the Year 1346.* London: R. Baldwin, 1755.

Isom-Verhaaren, Christine. *Allies with the Infidel: The Ottoman and French Alliance in the Sixteenth Century.* London: I.B. Tauris, 2011.

J.V. *Golgotha; Or, A Looking-Glass for London, and the Suburbs Thereof Shewing the Causes, Nature and Efficacy of the Present Plagues.* London: printed for J.V., 1665.

Jackson, Peter. *The Mongols and the West: 1221–1410.* New York: Routledge, 2005.

Jacobi, Johannes. *Regime de lepidimie.* Lyon, FR: Guillaume Le Roy, c. 1476.

Jacquart, Danielle. "La perception par les contemporains de la peste de 1348." In *L'homme face aux calamités naturelles dans l'Antiquité et au Moyen Âge.* Actes du 16ème colloque de la Villa Kérylos, Beaulieu-sur-Mer, 14–15 October 2005, 237–47. Paris: Académie des Inscriptions et Belles-Lettres, 2006.

– "Theory, Everyday Practice, and Three Fifteenth-Century Physicians." *Osiris* 6 (1990): 140–60.

Jardine, Nick. "Etics and Emics (Not to Mention Anemics and Emetics) in the History of the Sciences." *History of Science* 42, no. 3 (2004): 261–78.

Jaucourt, Louis de. "Peste." In *Encyclopédie, ou dictionnaire raisonné des sciences, des arts et des métiers*, edited by Denis Diderot and Jean le Rond d'Alembert, volume 12, 452–9. Paris: Sociétés Typographiques, 1751–72.

Jenner, Mark S.R. "Plague on a Page: Lord Have Mercy Upon Us in Early Modern London." *The Seventeenth Century* 27, no. 3 (2012): 255–86.

Jenner, Mark S.R., and Patrick Wallis, eds. *Medicine and the Market in England and Its Colonies, c. 1450-c. 1850.* Basingstoke, UK: Palgrave Macmillan, 2007.

Jennings, Stuart B. "The Anatomy of a Civil War Plague in a Rural Parish: East Stoke, Nottinghamshire, 1646." *Midland History* 40, no. 2 (2015): 201–19.

– "'A Stinking, Miserable, Infected Town': Plague and Death in a Civil War Garrison, Newark, 1640–1649." *Midland History* 28 (2003): 51–70.

Jillings, Karen. "Medical Advice for the Masses? Scotland's First Printed Vernacular Medical Work." In *Fresche fontanis: Studies in the Culture of Medieval and Early Modern Scotland*, edited by Janet Hadley

Williams and J. Derrick McClure, 307–16. Cambridge: Cambridge Scholars Publishing, 2013.
– *Scotland's Black Death: The Foul Death of the English.* Stroud, UK: Tempus, 2003.
Johns, Adrian. *Piracy: The Intellectual Property Wars from Gutenberg to Gates.* Chicago, IL: University of Chicago Press, 2009.
– *The Nature of the Book: Print and Knowledge in the Making.* Chicago, IL: University of Chicago Press, 1998.
Jones, Claire. "Discourse Communities and Medical Texts." In *Medical and Scientific Writing in Late Medieval English*, edited by Irma Taavitsainen and Päivi Pahta, 23–36. Cambridge: Cambridge University Press, 2004.
– "Vernacular Literacy in Late-Medieval England: The Example of East Anglian Medical Manuscripts. PhD dissertation, University of Glasgow, 2000.
Jones, Colin. "Languages of Plague in Early Modern France." In *Body and City: Histories of Urban Public Health,* edited by Sally Sheard and Helen Power, 41–9. Aldershot, UK: Ashgate, 2000.
– "Plague and Its Metaphors in Early Modern France." *Representations* 53 (1996): 97–127.
Jones, Lori. "'Apostumes, Carbuncles, and Botches': Visualizing the Plague in Late Medieval and Early Modern Medical Treatises." In *Asclepius, the Paintbrush, and the Pen: Representations of Disease in Medieval and Early Modern Art and Literature*, edited by Massimo Ciavolella and Rinaldo F. Canalis, 173–200. Turnhout, BE: Brepols, 2021.
– "Bubo Men? Repurposing Medieval Therapeutic Anatomic Illustrations for Plague in the Fifteenth and Sixteenth Centuries." In *Death and Disease in the Medieval and Early Modern World: Perspectives from Across the Mediterranean and Beyond*, edited by Lori Jones and Nükhet Varlık. York, UK: York Medieval Press, 2022 (forthcoming).
– "The Diseased Landscape: Medieval and Early Modern Plague-Scapes." *Landscapes* 17, no. 2 (2016): 108–23.
– "Experience over Education or Education over Experience? Pre-Modern Medical Writing on the Plague." In *Transforming Medical Education: Historical Case Studies of Teaching, Learning, and Belonging in Medicine*, edited by Delia Gravus and Susan Lamb, 86–111. Montreal and Kingston: McGill-Queen's University Press, 2022.
– "Itineraries and Transformations: John of Burgundy's Plague Treatise." *Bulletin of the History of Medicine* 95, no. 3 (2021): 277–314.

Jones, Peter Murray. "Information and Science." In *Fifteenth-Century Attitudes: Perceptions of Society in Late Medieval England*, edited by Rosemary Horrox, 97–111. Cambridge: Cambridge University Press, 1994.

– "Medical Literacies and Medical Culture in Early Modern England." In *Medical Writing in Early Modern English*, edited by Irma Taavitsainen and Päivi Pahta, 30–43. Cambridge: Cambridge University Press, 2011.

Joubert, Laurent. *Traitté de la peste*. Translated by Guillaume des Innocens. Lyon, FR: Jean Lertout, 1581.

Joubert, M. *Reflexions sur l'idée outrée qu'on donne de la contagion de la peste*. Grenoble, FR: Gaspard Giroud, 1721.

Jouyse, David. *Examen du livre de Lamperiere sur le sujet de la peste*. Rouen, FR: D. Geuffroy, 1622.

Jütte, Robert. *Poverty and Deviance in Early Modern Europe*. Cambridge: Cambridge University Press, 1994.

Kacki, Sacha. "Black Death: Cultures in Crisis." In *Encyclopedia of Global Archaeology*, edited by Claire Smith. Cham, CH: Springer, 2020. https://doi.org/10.1007/978-3-319-51726-1_2858-1.

Kamitus [Johannes Jacobi]. *Regimen contra pestilentiam*. Paris: Ulrich Gering, c. 1480.

Kansteiner, Wolf. "Finding Meaning in Memory: A Methodological Critique of Collective Memory Studies." *History and Theory* 41, no. 2 (2002): 179–97.

Keiser, George R. "Two Medieval Plague Treatises and Their Afterlife in Early Modern England." *Journal of the History of Medicine and Allied Sciences* 58, no. 3 (2003): 292–324.

– "Vernacular Herbals: A Growth Industry in Late Medieval England." In *Design and Distribution of Late Medieval Manuscripts in England*, edited by Margaret Connolly and Linne R. Mooney, 292–307. York, UK: York Medieval Press, 2008.

Keller, Marcel, Maria A. Spyrou, Christiana L. Scheib, Gunnar U. Neumann, Andreas Kröpelin, Brigitte Haas-Gebhard, Bernd Päffgen, et al. "Ancient *Yersinia pestis* Genomes from Across Western Europe Reveal Early Diversification during the First Pandemic (541–750)." *Proceedings of the National Academy of Sciences* 116, no. 25 (2019): 12363–72.

Kellwaye, Simon. *A Defensative Against the Plague*. London: John Windet, 1593.

Kemp, W. *A Brief Treatise of the Nature, Causes, Signs, Preservation From, and Cure of the Pestilence, Collected by W. Kemp, Mr. of Arts.* London: D. Kemp, 1665.

Kempshall, M.S. *The Common Good in Late Medieval Political Thought.* Oxford: Oxford University Press, 1999.

Kerwin, William. "Writing the Plague in English Prose Satire." In *Representing the Plague in Early Modern England*, edited by Rebecca Totaro and Ernest B. Gilman, 37–53. New York: Routledge, 2010.

Khanmohamadi, Shirin A. *In Light of Another's World: European Ethnography in the Middle Ages.* Philadelphia: University of Pennsylvania Press, 2014.

Kinglake, Alexander William. *Kinglake's Eothen.* London: Clarendon Press, 1906.

Kinzelbach, Annemarie. "Infection, Contagion, and Public Health in Late Medieval and Early Modern German Imperial Towns." *Journal of the History of Medicine and Allied Sciences* 61, no. 3 (2006), 369–89.

Klebs, Arnold C., and Karl Sudhoff. *Die Ersten Gedruckten Pestschriften.* Munich, DE: Verlag der Munchener Druck, 1926.

Klebs, Arnold C., Karl Sudhoff, and E. Droz. *Remèdes contre la peste: fac-similés, notes et liste bibliographique des incunables sur la peste.* Paris: E. Droz, E. Nourry, 1925; Reprint, Geneva, CH: Slatkine Reprints, 1978.

Klein, Kerwin Lee. *From History to Theory.* Berkeley: University of California Press, 2011.

Knecht, R.J. *The French Wars of Religion 1559–1598.* 3rd edition. New York: Routledge, 2014.

Knolles, Richard. *The Generall Historie of the Turkes, from the First Beginning of that Nation to the Rising of the Othoman Familie.* London: Adam Islip, 1603.

Koch, Tom. *Disease Maps: Epidemics on the Ground.* Chicago, IL: University of Chicago Press, 2011.

Kochhar, Rajesh. "The Truth behind the Legend: European Doctors in Pre-Colonial India." *Journal of Biosciences* 24, no. 3 (1999): 259–68.

Kümin, Beat, ed. *Political Space in Pre-Industrial Europe.* New York: Routledge, 2009.

Kupperman, Karen Ordahl. "Fear of Hot Climates in the Anglo-American Colonial Experience." *The William and Mary Quarterly* 41, no. 2 (1984): 213–40.

Kurath, Hans, ed. *Middle English Dictionary.* Ann Arbor: University of Michigan Press, 1989.

Lamperiere, Jean de. *L'Ombre de Nécrophore*. Rouen: D. Ferrant, 1622.
– *Traité de la peste*. Rouen, FR: D. Du Petit-Val, 1620.
Lauvergnat-Gagnière, Christiane. "Claude Nourry, imprimeur populaire?" *Bulletin de l'Association d'étude sur l'humanisme, la réforme et la renaissance* 11, no. 1 (1980): 84–91.
Lavezzo, Kathy. *Angels on the Edge of the World: Geography, Literature, and English Community, 1000–1534*. Ithaca, NY: Cornell University Press, 2006.
Lefebvre, Henri. *La production de l'espace*. Paris: Éditions Anthropos, 1974.
– *Writings on Cities*. Translated by Eleonore Kofman and Elizabeth Lebas. Oxford: Blackwell, 1996.
Le Forestier, Thomas. *Le regime contre epidemie et pestilence intitulé au povres*. Rouen, FR: Jacques le Forestier, 1495.
– *Tractatus contre pestilentiam thenasmonem et dissinteriam*. Rouen, FR: Guillaume le Talleur, 1490.
Leguay, Jean-Pierre. *La pollution au Moyen Age: dans le royaume de France et dans les grands fiefs*. Paris: Editions Jean-Paul Gisserot, 1999.
Leitch, Stephanie. *Mapping Ethnography in Early Modern Germany: New Worlds in Print Culture*. New York: Palgrave Macmillan, 2010.
Lehmhaus, Lennart, ed. *Defining Jewish Medicine: Transfer of Medical Knowledge in Premodern Jewish Cultures and Traditions*. Wiesbaden, DE: Harrassowitz, 2021.
Le Lievre, Esaie. *Epydimyomachie ou combat de la peste avec le reglement Politique*. Paris: Robert Coulombel, 1582.
Lennard-Brown, Sarah Marion. "Almshouses of London and Westminster: Their Role in Lay Piety and the Relief of Poverty, 1330–1600." PhD dissertation, Birkbeck College University of London, 2020.
Leonardo, Dalia M. "'Cut Off This Rotten Member': The Rhetoric of Heresy, Sin, and Disease in the Ideology of the French Catholic League." *The Catholic Historical Review* 88, no. 2 (2002): 247–62.
Leong, Elaine. "Transformative Itineraries and Communities of Knowledge in Early Modern Europe: The Case of Lazare Rivière's 'The Practice of Physick.'" In *Civic Medicine: Physician, Polity, and Pen in Early Modern Europe*, ed. J. Andrew Mendelsohn, Annemarie Kinzelbach, and Ruth Schilling, 257–79. London and New York: Routledge, 2020.
Le Roux, Nicolas. *Les guerres de religion 1559–1629*. Paris: Belin, 2014.
Lev, Efraim. *Jewish Medical Practitioners in the Medieval Muslim World: A Collective Biography*. Edinburgh, UK: Edinburgh University Press, 2021.

Lévy, Jacques. *L'espace légitime: sur la dimension géographique de la fonction politique.* Paris: Presses de la Fondation Nationale de Sciences Politiques, 1994.

Lévy, Jacques, and Michel Lussault. "Espace." In *Dictionnaire de la géographie et de l'espace des sociétés,* 325–33. Paris: Belin, 2003.

Lewis, Martin W., and Kären E. Wigen. *The Myth of Continents: A Critique of Metageography.* Berkeley: University of California Press, 1997.

Lilley, Keith D., ed. *Mapping Medieval Geographies: Geographical Encounters in the Latin West and Beyond, 300–1600.* Cambridge: Cambridge University Press, 2014.

Linte, Guillaume. "'Hot Climates' and Disease: Early Modern European Views of Tropical Environments." In *Disease and the Environment in the Medieval and Early Modern Worlds*, edited by Lori Jones. London: Routledge, 2022 (forthcoming).

Little, Lester K. "Life and Afterlife of the First Plague Pandemic." In *Plague and the End of Antiquity: The Pandemic of 541–750,* edited by Lester K. Little, 3–32. Cambridge: Cambridge University Press, 2007.

– ed. *Plague and the End of Antiquity: The Pandemic of 541–750.* Cambridge: Cambridge University Press, 2007.

– "Plague Historians in Lab Coats." *Past & Present* 213, no. 1 (November 2011): 267–90.

Lodge, Thomas. *A Treatise of the Plague.* London: for Edward White and N.L., 1603.

Luborsky, Ruth Samson, and Elizabeth Morley Ingram. *A Guide to English Illustrated Books, 1536–1603.* 2 volumes. Tempe, AZ: Medieval and Renaissance Texts and Studies, 1998.

Luce, Siméon. *Chroniques de J. Froissart*, tome 4, *1346–1356*. Paris: Mme Ve. Jules Renouard, 1873.

Lusignan, Serge. *Essai d'histoire sociolinguistique: Le français picard au Moyen Âge.* Paris: Classiques Garnier, 2012.

Lussault, Michel. *L'homme spatial. La construction sociale de l'espace humain.* Paris: Seuil, 2007.

MacLean, Gerald. *The Rise of Oriental Travel.* Houndmills, UK: Palgrave, 2004.

Malcolm, Noel. "Positive Views of Islam and of Ottoman Rule in the Sixteenth Century: The Case of Jean Bodin." In *The Renaissance and the Ottoman World*, edited by Anna Contadini and Claire Norton, 197–217. Farnham, UK: Ashgate, 2013.

Manget, Jean-Jacques. *Traité de la peste et des moyens de s'en préserver.* Lyon, FR: Frères Bruyset, 1722.

Marshall, Louise. "God's Executioners: Angels, Devils and the Plague in Giovanni Sercambi's Illustrated Chronicle (1400)." In *Disaster, Death and the Emotions in the Shadow of the Apocalypse, 1400–1700*, edited by J. Spinks and C. Zika, 177–99. London: Palgrave Macmillan, 2016.
– "Manipulating the Sacred: Image and Plague in Renaissance Italy." *Renaissance Quarterly* 47, no. 3 (1994): 485–532.
Martin, G.H., trans. and ed. *Knighton's Chronicle 1337–1396*. Oxford: Clarendon Press, 1995.
Matheson, Lister M. "The Dialect of the Hammond Scribe." In *Sex, Aging, and Death in a Medieval Medical Compendium. Trinity College Cambridge MS R.14.52, Its Texts, Language, and Scribe*, 2 volumes, edited by M. Teresa Tavormina, volume 1, 65–94. Tempe, AZ: ACMRS, 2006.
– "John of Burgundy: Treatises on Plague." In Tavomina, ed., *Sex, Aging, and Death*, volume 2, 569–606.
– "Médecin sans Frontières? The European Dissemination of John of Burgundy's Plague Treatise." *ANQ: A Quarterly Journal of Short Articles, Notes and Reviews* 18, no. 3 (2005): 19–31.
Mayer, Robert. "The Reception of *A Journal of the Plague Year* and the Nexus of Fiction and History in the Novel." *ELH* 57, no. 3 (1990): 529–55.
McCandless, Peter. *Slavery, Disease, and Suffering in the Southern Lowcountry.* Cambridge: Cambridge University Press, 2011.
McCleery, Iona. "From the Edge of Europe to Global Empire: Portuguese Medicine Abroad (Thirteenth to Sixteenth Centuries)." In *Travels and Mobilities in the Middle Ages: From the Atlantic to the Black Sea*, edited by Marianne O'Doherty and Felicitas Schmieder, 55–90. Turnhout, BE: Brepols, 2015.
McConchie, R.W. "Some Reflections on Early Modern Printed Title-Pages." *Varieng: Studies in Variation, Contacts and Change in English* 14 (2013). http://www.helsinki.fi/varieng/series/volumes/14/mcconchie/index.html.
McCormick, Michael. "Gregory of Tours on Sixth-Century Plague and Other Epidemics." *Speculum* 96, no. 1 (2021): 38–96.
– "Rats, Communications, and Plague: Toward an Ecological History." *Journal of Interdisciplinary History* 34, no. 1 (2003): 1–25.
McFarlane, Colin. "Governing the Contaminated City: Infrastructure and Sanitation in Colonial and Post-Colonial Bombay." *International Journal of Urban and Regional Research* 32, no. 2 (2008): 415–35.

McGovern, Jonathan. "The Compters at Poultry and Wood Street in Early Modern London." *The London Journal*, 5 April 2021. https://doi.org/10.1080/03058034.2021.1885132.

McJannet, Linda. "'History Written by the Enemy': Eastern Sources about the Ottomans on the Continent and in England." *English Literary Renaissance* 36, no. 3 (2006): 396–429.

McKenzie, Donald Francis. *Bibliography and the Sociology of Texts.* Cambridge: Cambridge University Press, 1999.

McKitterick, David. "University Printing at Oxford and Cambridge." In *The Cambridge History of the Book in Britain*, volume 4, edited by John Barnard and D.F. McKenzie, 189–205. Cambridge: Cambridge University Press, 2002.

McLaren, Mary-Rose. *The London Chronicles of the Fifteenth Century: A Revolution in English Writing. With an Annotated Edition of Bradford, West Yorkshire Archives MS 32D86/42.* Cambridge: D.S. Brewer, 2002.

McNeill, John Robert. *Mosquito Empires: Ecology and War in the Greater Caribbean, 1620–1914.* Cambridge: Cambridge University Press, 2010.

Mead, Richard. *Discourse on the Plague, The Ninth Edition Corrected & Enlarged.* London: Printed for A. Millar & J. Brindly, 1744.

– *A Short Discourse Concerning Pestilential Contagion and the Methods Used to Prevent It.* London: Sam. Buckley and Ralph Smith, 1720.

Meier, Mischa. "The 'Justinianic Plague': An 'Inconsequential Pandemic'? A Reply." *Medizinhistorisches Journal* 55 (2020): 172–99.

Melvin-Koushki, Matthew. "Taşköprīzāde on the (Occult) Science of Plague Prevention and Cure." *Nazariyat Journal for the History of Islamic Philosophy and Sciences* 6, no. 2 (2020): 133–68.

Merrens, H. Roy, and George D. Terry. "Dying in Paradise: Malaria, Mortality, and the Perceptual Environment in Colonial South Carolina." *The Journal of Southern History* 50, no. 4 (1984): 533–50.

Merritt, J.F., ed. *Imagining Early Modern London: Perceptions and Portrayals of the City from Stow to Strype, 1598–1720.* Cambridge: Cambridge University Press, 2001.

Mézeray, François Eudes de. *Histoire générale des Turcs, second tome.* Paris: Sebastien Cramoisy, 1663.

Michaud, Francine. "La peste, la peur et l'espoir: le pèlerinage jubilaire de romeux marseillais en 1350." *Le Moyen Âge* 104 (1998): 399–434.

Mikhail, Alan. "The Nature of Plague in Late Eighteenth-Century Egypt." *Bulletin of the History of Medicine* 82, no. 2 (2008): 249–75.

Millar, Bonnie. "LeRoy, Guillaume (c. 1450–c. 1529)." In *The Late Medieval Age of Crisis and Renewal, 1300–1500: A Biographical Dictionary*, edited by Clayton J. Drees, 286–7. Westport, CT: Greenwood Press, 2001.

Miller, Kathleen. *The Literary Culture of Plague in Early Modern England*. London: Palgrave Macmillan, 2016.

Minnis, Alistair. *Medieval Theory of Authorship: Scholastic Literary Attitudes in the Later Middle Ages*. 2nd Edition. Philadelphia: University of Pennsylvania Press, 1988.

Mizauld, Antoine. *Singuliers et secours contre la peste, souventesfois experime[n]tez & approuvez ta[n]t en certaine preservatio[n] que parfaicte guarison*. Paris: M. Breuille, 1562.

Monteyne, Joseph. *The Printed Image in Early Modern London: Urban Space, Visual Representation, and Social Exchange*. Aldershot, UK: Ashgate, 2007.

Mooney, Linne R. "Locating Scribal Activity in Late Medieval London." In *Design and Distribution of Late Medieval Manuscripts in England*, edited by Margaret Connolly and Linne R. Mooney, 183–204. York, UK: York Medieval Press, 2008.

– "The Scribe." In *Sex, Aging, and Death in a Medieval Medical Compendium. Trinity College Cambridge MS R.14.52, Its Texts, Language, and Scribe*, 2 volumes, edited by M. Teresa Tavormina, volume 1, 55–64. Tempe, AZ: ACMRS, 2006.

– "A Scribe of Lydgate's *Troy Book* and London Book Production in the First Half of the Fifteenth Century." In *Pursuing Middle English Manuscripts and their Texts: Essays in Honour of Ralph Hanna*, edited by Simon Horobin and Aditi Nafde, 19–42. Turnhout, BE: Brepols, 2017.

Moore, Helen. "Gathering Fruit: The 'Profitable' Translations of Thomas Paynell." In *Tudor Translation*, edited by Fred Schurink, 39–57. Houndsmills, UK: Palgrave Macmillan, 2011.

Mordechai, Lee, and Merle Eisenberg. "Rejecting Catastrophe: The Case of the Justinianic Plague." *Past & Present* 244, no. 1 (2019): 3–50.

Morozova, Irina, Artem Kasianov, Sergey Bruskin, Judith Neukamm, Martyna Molak, Elena Batieva, Aleksandra Pudło, Frank J. Rühli, and Verena J. Schuenemann. "New Ancient Eastern European *Yersinia pestis* Genomes Illuminate the Dispersal of Plague in Europe." *Philisophical Transactions B* 375, no. 1812 (2020). http://dx.doi.org/10.1098/rstb.2019.0569.

Morsel, Joseph. "Traces? Quelles traces? Réflexions pour une histoire non passéiste." *Revue historique* 4, no. 680 (2014): 813–68.

Moryson, Fynes. *An Itinerary Containing His Ten Yeeres Travell.* 2 Volumes. Glasgow, UK: MacLehose and Sons, 1907.

Mosser, Daniel W. "'Chaucer's Scribe,' Adam and the Hengwrt Project." In *Design and Distribution of Late Medieval Manuscripts in England*, edited by Margaret Connolly and Linne R. Mooney, 11–40. York, UK: York Medieval Press, 2008.

Moulton, Thomas. *This is the Myrour or Glasse of Helthe.* London: Robert Wyer, <1530.

– *This is the Myrour or Glasse of Helth.* London: William Myddleton, c. 1545.

– *This is the Myrour or Glasse of Helthe.* London: Thomas Colwell, c. 1566.

Mouysset, Sylvie. "La peste de 1628 en Rouergue." *Annales du Midi: revue archéologique, historique et philologique de la France méridionale* 105, no. 203 (1993): 329–48.

Mulhall, John. "Confronting Pandemic in Late Antiquity: The Medical Response to the Justinianic Plague." *Journal of Late Antiquity* 14, no. 2 (2021).

– "Plague before the Pandemics: The Greek Medical Evidence for Bubonic Plague before the Sixth Century." *Bulletin of the History of Medicine* 93, no. 2 (2019): 151–79.

Mundy, Peter. *The Travels of Peter Mundy, In Europe and Asia, 1608–1667*, edited by Sir Richard Carnac Temple. Cambridge: Hakluyt Society, 1907.

Murphy, Neil. "Plague Ordinances and the Management of Infectious Diseases in Northern French Towns, c. 1450–1560." In *The Fifteenth Century XII: Society in an Age of Plague*, edited by Linda Clarke and Carole Rawcliffe, 139–60. Woodbridge, UK: Boydell Press, 2013.

Naphy, William G. *Plagues, Poisons, and Potions: Plague-Spreading Conspiracies in the Western Alps, c. 1530–1640.* Manchester, UK: Manchester University Press, 2002.

Nancel, Nicolas de. *Discours tresample de la Peste.* Paris: Denis du Val, 1581.

Newcomb, Lori. "Chapbooks." In *Oxford History of Popular Print Culture, vol 1: Cheap Print in Britain and Ireland to 1660*, edited by Joad Raymond, 471–86. Oxford: Oxford University Press, 2011.

Newfield, Timothy P. "A Cattle Panzootic in Early Fourteenth-Century Europe." *American Historical Review* 57, no. 2 (2009): 155–90.

– "Early Medieval Epizootics and Landscapes of Disease: The Origins and Triggers of European Livestock Pestilences, 400–1000 CE." In *Landscapes and Societies in Medieval Europe East of the Elbe: Interactions between Environmental Settings and Cultural Transformations*, edited by S. Kleingärtner, T.P. Newfield, S. Rossignol, and D. Wehner, 73–113. Toronto: Pontifical Institute of Medieval Studies, 2013.

Nicolay, Nicolas de. *Les quatre premiers livres des navigations et peregrinations Orientales*. Lyon, FR: Gvillavme Roville, 1568.

Nichols, J.G., ed. *Chronicle of the Grey Friars of London*. Camden Society Old series, volume 53. London: Camden Society, 1852.

Nicholls, David. "Protestants, Catholics and Magistrates in Tours, 1562–1572: The Making of a Catholic City During the Religious Wars." *French History* 8, no. 1 (1994): 14–33.

Nicoud, Marilyn. *Les régimes de santé au Moyen Âge: naissance et diffusion d'une écriture médicale (XIIIe–XVe siècle)*. Rome: École Française de Rome, 2007.

Nutton, Vivian. "Humoralism." In *Companion Encyclopedia of the History of Medicine*, edited by W.F. Bynum and Roy Porter, volume 1, 281–91. London: Routledge, 1993.

– "John Caius, Historian." In *Professors, Physicians and Practices in the History of Medicine: Essays in Honor of Nancy Siraisi*, edited by Gideon Manning and Cynthia Klestinec, 69–83. Cham, CH: Springer, 2017.

– "The Reception of Fracastoro's Theory of Contagion: The Seed That Fell among Thorns?" *Osiris* 6 (1990): 196–234.

– "The Seeds of Disease: An Explanation of Contagion and Infection from the Greeks to the Renaissance." *Medical History* 27, no. 1 (1983): 1–34.

– "With Benefit of Hindsight: Girolamo Mercuriale and Simone Simoni on Plague." *Medicina & Storia* 6, no. 11 (2006): 5–19.

O'Doherty, Marianne. *The Indies and the Medieval West: Thought, Report, Imagination*. Turnhout, BE: Brepols, 2013.

Ong, Walter J. *Orality and Literacy: The Technologizing of the Word*. London: Routledge, 2002.

Orders Thought Meet by his Majestie and and his Privie Councell. London: Bonham Norton and John Bill, 1625.

Ormrod, W.M. "The Politics of Pestilence: Government in England after the Black Death." In *The Black Death in England*, edited by W.M. Ormrod and P.G. Lindley, 147–81. Stamford, UK: Paul Watkins, 1996.

Ornato, Ezio. *La face cachée du livre médiéval*. Rome: Viella, 1997.

Orton, David. "'The Long Black Rat': Assessing the a priori Feasibility of Rattus rattus as a European Plague Reservoir during the First and Second Pandemics." Presentation at *Society for Medieval Archaeology Annual Conference: The Long Black Death: New Perspectives*, York, UK, 5 July 2019.

Oxford Dictionary of National Biography. http://www.oxforddnb.com.

Pade, Marianne. "The Renaissance: Scholarship, Criticism, and Education." In *A Handbook to the Reception of Thucydides*, edited by Christine Lee and Neville Morley, 26–42. Chichester, UK: John Wiley and Sons, 2014.

– "Thucydides' Rennaissance Readers." In *Brill's Companion to Thucydides*, edited by Antonis Tsakmakis and Antonios Rengakos, 779–810. Leiden, NL: Brill, 2006.

Pahta, Päivi, and Maura Ratia. "Treatises on Specific Topics." In *Early Modern English Medical Texts: Corpus Description and Studies*, edited by Irma Taavitsainen and Päivi Pahta, 73–99. Amsterdam: John Benjamins, 2010.

Palmer, Richard. "'Ad una sancta perfettione': Health Care and Poor Relief in the Republic of Venice in the Era of the Counter-Reformation." In *Health Care and Poor Relief in Counter Reformation Europe*, edited by Ole Peter Grell, Andrew Cunningham, and Jon Arrizabalaga, 85–95. London: Routledge, 1999.

– "Girolamo Mercuriale and the Plague of Venice." In *Girolamo Mercuriale: medicina e cultura nell'Europa del Cinquecento: atti del convegno Girolamo Mercuriale e lo spazio scientifico e culturale del Cinquecento: Forlì, 8-11 novembre 2006*, edited by Vivian Nutton and Alessandro Arcangeli, 51–65. Florence, IT: Leo S. Olschki, 2008.

Panel, G. *Trois Opuscules sur la Peste de Rouen de 1668*. Rouen, FR: Imprimerie Léon, 1911.

Pansier, Pierre. "Les médecins juifs à Avignon aux XIIIme, XIVme et XVme siècles." *Janus* 15 (1910): 421–51.

Panzac, Daniel. *La peste dans l'empire ottoman 1700–1850*. Leuven, BE: Peeters, 1985.

Paré, Ambroise. *Traicté de la peste, de la petite Verolle & Rougeolle: avec une brefve description de la Lepre*. Paris: André Wechel, 1568.

Parey, Ambrose. *A Treatise of the Plague, Contayning the Causes, Signes, Symptomes, Prognosticks, and Cure Thereof*. London: R.Y and R.C., 1630.

Parker, John. *Books to Build an Empire: A Bibliographic History of English Overseas Interest to 1620*. Amsterdam: Nico Israel, 1965.

Partridge, Stephen, and Erik Kwakkel, eds. *Author, Reader, Book: Medieval Authorship in Theory and Practice.* Toronto: University of Toronto Press, 2012.

Paynel, Thomas. *A Moche Profitable Treatise Against the Pestilence Translated into E[n]glyshe.* London: Thomas Berthelet, 1534.

– *De morbo Gallico.* London: Thomas Berthelet, 1533.

Pearsall, Derek. "The Tribulations of Scribes." In *Pursuing Middle English Manuscripts and their Texts: Essays in Honour of Ralph Hanna*, edited by Simon Horobin and Aditi Nafde, 1–17. Turnhout, BE: Brepols, 2017.

Pearson, M.N. "The Thin End of the Wedge: Medical Relativities as a Paradigm of Early Modern Indian-European Relations." *Modern Asian Studies* 29, no. 1 (1995): 141–70.

Peckham, Robert, ed. *Empires of Panic: Epidemics and Colonial Anxieties.* Hong Kong: Hong Kong University Press, 2015.

Pelling, Margaret. "Skirting the City? Disease, Social Change and Divided Households in the Seventeenth Century." In *Londinopolis, c. 1500–c. 1750: Essays in the Cultural and Social History of Early Modern London*, edited by Paul Griffiths and Mark S.R. Jenner, 154–75. Manchester, UK: Manchester University Press, 2000.

Pennycook, Alistair. "Borrowing Others' Words: Text, Ownership, Memory, and Plagiarism." *TESOL Quarterly* 30, no. 2 (1996): 201–30.

Pestalozzi, Jérome Jean. *Avis de precaution contre la maladie contagieuse de Marseille.* Lyon, FR: Frères Bruyset, 1721.

Peter, Jean-Pierre. "Disease and the Sick at the End of the Eighteenth Century." In *Biology of Man in History*, edited by Robert Forster and Orest Ranum, translated by Elborg Forster and Patricia M. Ranum, 81–124. Baltimore, MD: The Johns Hopkins University Press, 1975.

Pettegree, Andrew, Malcolm Walsby, and Alexander Wilkinson, eds. *French Vernacular Books: Books Published in the French Language before 1601/Livres vernaculaires français: Livres imprimés en français avant 1601*, volume 1, A–G. Leiden, NL: Brill, 2007.

Pfau, Aleksandra. "Lepers in the Streets: Movement of Lepers in Fourteenth- and Fifteenth- Century France." Presentation at the International Medieval Congress, Kalamazoo, MI, 9 May 2019.

Phayer, Thomas. *The Regiment of Life Wherunto is Added a Treatyse of the Pestilence, with the Booke of Children Newly Corrected and Enlarged by T. Phayer.* London: Edward Whitchurche, 1546.

Physician in York. *A Treatise of the Plague.* York, UK: for James Osborn, 1721.

Phillips, J.S.R. *The Medieval Expansion of Europe*. 2nd edition. Oxford: Clarendon Press, 1998.

Pippidi, Andrei. *Visions of the Ottoman World in Renaissance Europe*. Oxford: Oxford University Press, 2012.

Poinar, Hendrik. "Synergies of Genetic and Historical Interpretations of Infectious Disease." In *Death and Disease in the Medieval and Early Modern World: Perspectives from Across the Mediterranean and Beyond*, edited by Lori Jones and Nükhet Varlık. York, UK: York Medieval Press, 2022 (forthcoming).

Pomata, Gianna. "*Praxis Historialis*: The Uses of *Historia* in Early Modern Medicine." In *Historia: Empiricism and Erudition in Early Modern Europe*, edited by Gianna Pomata and Nancy G. Siraisi, 105–46. Cambridge, MA: MIT Press, 2005.

Porter, Dorothy. *Health, Civilization, and the State: A History of Public Health from Ancient to Modern Times*. London: Routledge, 1999.

Potel, Guillaume. *Traicté de la peste advenue en ceste ville de Paris, l'an mil, 1596, 1606, 1619 et 1623, avec les remèdes*. Paris: Nicolas Callemont, 1624.

Procopius. *History of the Wars*. Translated by H.B. Dewing. London: Heinemann, 1914.

Pullan, Brian. "Plague and Perceptions of the Poor in Early Modern Italy." In *Epidemics and Ideas: Essays on the Historical Perception of Pestilence*, edited by Terence Ranger and Paul Slack, 101–23. Cambridge: Cambridge University Press, 1995.

Pye, George. *A Discourse of the Plague wherein Dr. Mead's Notions are Consider'd and Refuted*. London: J. Darby, 1721.

Quarles, John. *Londons Disease, and Cure: Being a Soveraigne Receipt Against the Plague, for Prevention Sake*. London: Edward Crouch, 1665.

Quincy, John. *An Essay on the Different Causes of Pestilential Diseases, and How They Become Contagious*. London: Printed for E. Bell and J. Osborn, 1720.

Ranchin, François. *Opuscvles, ou Traictés divers et curievx en medecine*. Lyon, FR: Pierre Ravavd, 1640.

Rand, Kari Anne. "The Elusive Canutus: An Investigation into a Medieval Plague Tract." *Leeds Studies in English* new series XLI (2010): 186–99.

Rascovan, Nicolás, Karl-Göran Sjögren, Kristian Kristiansen, Rasmus Nielsen, Eske Willerslev, Christelle Desnues, and Simon Rasmussen. "Emergence and Spread of Basal Lineages of Yersinia pestis during the Neolithic Decline." *Cell* 176, no. 1 (2019): 295–305.

Rasmussen, Simon, Morten Erik Allentoft, Kasper Nielsen, Ludovic Orlando, Martin Sikora, Karl-Göran Sjögren, Anders Gorm Pedersen, et al. "Early Divergent Strains of *Yersinia pestis* in Eurasia 5,000 years ago." *Cell* 163 no. 3 (2015): 571–82.

Raspe, Lucia. "The Black Death in Jewish Sources: A Second Look at 'Mayse Nissim.'" The *Jewish Quarterly Review* 94, no. 3 (2004): 471–89.

Ratia, Maura. "Bills of Mortality of the Seventeenth-Century London Plague Epidemics: An Analysis of the Genre." In *Genre in Medical English, 1500–1820: Sociocultural Contexts of Production and Use*, edited by Irma Taavitsainen, Turo Hiltunen, Jeremy Smith, and Carla Suhr. Cambridge: Cambridge University Press, 2022 (forthcoming).

– "Investigating Genre Through Title-Pages: Plague Treatises of the Stuart Period in Focus." *Varieng: Studies in Variation, Contacts and Change in English* 14 (2013), http://www.helsinki.fi/varieng/series/volumes/14/ratia.

Ratia, Maura, and Carla Suhr. "Medical Pamphlets: Controversy and Advertising." In *Medical Writing in Early Modern English*, edited by Irma Taavitsainen and Päivi Pahta, 180–203. Cambridge: Cambridge University Press, 2011.

Raven, James. *The Business of Books: Booksellers and the English Book Trade 1450–1850*. New Haven, CT: Yale University Press, 2007.

Rawcliffe, Carole. *Leprosy in Medieval England*. Woodbridge, UK: Boydell Press, 2006.

– *Medicine and Society in Later Medieval England*. Stroud, UK: Alan Sutton, 1995.

– "The Profits of Practice: The Wealth and Status of Medical Men in Later Medieval England." *Social History of Medicine*, Volume 1, no 1 (1988): 61–78.

– *Urban Bodies: Communal Health in Late Medieval English Towns and Cities*. Woodbridge, UK: Boydell Press, 2013.

Rawcliffe, Carole, and Claire Weeda, eds. *Policing the Urban Environment in Premodern Europe*. Amsterdam: Amsterdam University Press, 2019.

Raymond, Joad, ed. "The Newspaper, Public Opinion, and the Public Sphere in the Seventeenth Century." *Journal of Prose Studies* 21, no. 2 (1998): 109–36.

– *Oxford History of Popular Print Culture, Volume 1: Cheap Print in Britain and Ireland to 1660*. Oxford: Oxford University Press, 2011.

Reeves, William, ed. *Life of Saint Columba, Founder of Hy. Written by Adamnan, Ninth Abbot of that Monastery.* Edinburgh, UK: Edmonston and Douglas, 1874.

Renouard, Philippe. *Répertoire des imprimeurs parisiens, libraires, fondeurs de caractères et correcteurs d'imprimerie depuis l'introduction de l'imprimerie à Paris (1470) jusqu'à la fin du seizième siècle.* Paris: J. Laget, 1965.

Revel, Jacques. "Autour d'une épidémie ancienne: la peste de 1666–1670." *Revue d'histoire moderne et contemporaine* 17, no. 4 (1970): 953–83.

Ricaut, Sir Paul. *The History of the Present State of the Ottoman Empire.* 6th edition. London: Charles Brome, 1686.

Riley, Henry Thomas, ed. *Thomas Walsingham, quondam monachi S. Albani, historia anglicana.* 2 Volumes. London: Longman, Green, Longman, Roberts, and Green, 1862.

Robin, Vincent. *Advis sur la peste recognue quelque endroit de la Bourgogne avec chois des remedes propres pour la preservation & guerison de cette maladie.* Dijon, FR: Nicolas Spirinx, 1628.

Robson, Charles. *Newes from Aleppo, A letter Written to T.V.B. of D. Vicar of Cockfield in Southsex.* London: for M.S., 1628.

Rochas, Henry de. *Discours tresutile sur la maladie contagieuse de ce temps.* Paris: Nicolas Bourdin, 1619.

Rochas d'Ayglun, Henry de. *Examen ou raisonnment sur la cause de la peste cy-devant incognuë.* Toulouse, FR: Jean Baude, 1652.

Roger, Euan. "'To Be Shut Up': New Evidence for the Development of Quarantine Regulations in Early-Tudor England." *Social History of Medicine* 33, no. 4 (2020): 1077–96.

Roland, Meg. "'After poyetes and astronomyers': English Geographical Thought and Early English Print." In *Mapping Medieval Geographies: Geographical Encounters in the Latin West and Beyond, 300–1600,* edited by Keith D. Lilley, 127–51. Cambridge: Cambridge University Press, 2014.

Rolfe, Kirsty. "Fatal and Memorable: Plague, Providence and War in English Texts, 1625–6." *The Seventeenth Century* 35, no. 3 (2020): 293–314.

Roosen, Joris, and Daniel R. Curtis. "Dangers of Noncritical Use of Historical Plague Data." *Emerging Infectious Diseases* 24, no. 1 (2018): 103–110.

Rose, Philip. *A Theorico-practical, Miscellaneous, and Succinct Treatise of the Plague.* London: T. Jauncy, 1721.

Rouse, Richard H., and Mary A. Rouse. *Manuscripts and their Makers: Commercial Book Producers in Medieval Paris 1200–1500*. Turnhout, BE: Brepols, 2000.

Rubys, Claude de. *Discours sur la contagion de peste qui a esté ceste presente annee en la ville de Lyon*. Lyon, FR: Jean d'Ogerolles, 1577.

– *Histoire veritable de la ville de Lyon*. Lyon, FR: Bonaventurs Nugo, 1604.

Runciman, Steven. *The Fall of Constantinople 1453*. Cambridge: Cambridge University Press, 2012.

Rusnock, Andrea A. *Vital Accounts: Quantifying Health and Population in Eighteenth-Century England and France*. Cambridge: Cambridge University Press, 2002.

Russell, Patrick. *A Treatise of the Plague: Containing an Historical Journal, and Medical Account, of the Plague, at Aleppo, In the Years 1760, 1761, and 1762*. London: for G.G.J. and J. Robinson, 1791.

Said, Edward. *Orientalism*. New York: Vintage Book, 1978.

Sainct-Hillier, I.S. de. *Loimologie contenant les causes, signes, prognosticques, & remedes contre la Peste*. Pont-a-Mousson, FR: pour Jean le Geant, 1623.

Sargeant, Michael G. "What Do the Numbers Mean? A Textual Critic's Observations on Some Patterns of Middle English Manuscript Transmission." In *Design and Distribution of Late Medieval Manuscripts in England*, edited by Margaret Connolly and Linne R. Mooney, 205–44. York, UK: York Medieval Press, 2008.

Scase, Wendy. "Introduction: Essays in Manuscript Geography." *Essays in Manuscript Geography: Vernacular Manuscripts of the English West Midlands from the Conquest to the Sixteenth Century*, edited by Wendy Scase, 1–10. Turnhout, BE: Brepols, 2007.

Schlatter, Richard. "Thomas Hobbes and Thucydides." *Journal of the History of Ideas* 6, no. 3 (1945): 350–62.

Schmid, B.V., Ulf Büntgen, W. Ryan Easterday, Christian Ginzler, Lars Walløe, Barbara Bramanti, and Nils Chr Stenseth. "Climate-Driven Introductions of the Black Death and Successive Plague Reintroductions into Europe." *Proceedings of the National Academy of Sciences* 112 (2015): 3020–5.

Schurink, Fred. "Introduction." In *Tudor Translation*, edited by Fred Schurink, 1–17. Houndsmills, UK: Palgrave Macmillan, 2011.

Scott, Kathleen L. "Newly Discovered Booklets from a Reconstructed Middle English Manuscript." In *English Manuscript Studies 1100–1700, Volume 14 Regional Manuscripts 1200–1700*, edited by A.S.G. Edwards, 112–30. London: British Library, 2008.

Seifert, Lisa, Ingrid Wiechmann, Michaela Harbeck, Astrid Thomas, Gisela Grupe, Michaela Projahn, Holger C. Scholz, and Julia M. Riehm. "Genotyping *Yersinia pestis* in Historical Plague: Evidence for Long-Term Persistence of *Y. pestis* in Europe from the 14th to the 17th Century." *PLOS ONE* 11, no. 1 (2016): e0145194. https://doi.org/10.1371/journal.pone.0145194.

Semmens, Justine. "Plague, Propaganda and Prophetic Violence in Sixteenth-Century Lyon." In *Aspects of Violence in Renaissance Europe*, edited by Jonathan Davies, 83–104. London: Ashgate, 2013.

Shakow, Aaron David Abraham. "Marks of Contagion: The Plague, The Bourse, the Word and the Law in the Early-Modern Mediterranean, 1720–62." PhD dissertation, Harvard University, 2009.

Sharpe, W.D., ed. "Isidore of Seville: The Medical Writings. An English Translation with an Introduction and Commentary." *Transactions of the American Philosophical Society*, new series 54, no. 2 (1964): 1–75.

Shatzmiller, Joseph. *Jews, Medicine, and Medieval Society.* Berkeley: University of California Press, 1994.

Shep, Sydney. "Books in Global Perspectives." In *The Cambridge Companion to the History of the Book*, edited by Leslie Howsam, 53–70. Cambridge: Cambridge University Press, 2015.

Siena, Kevin. *Rotten Bodies: Class and Contagion in Eighteenth-Century Britain.* New Haven, CT: Yale University Press, 2019.

Signoli, Michel, Isabelle Séguy, Jean-Noël Biraben, Olivier Dutour, and Paul Belle. "Paleodemography and Historical Demography in the Context of an Epidemic: Plague in Provence in the Eighteenth Century." *Population* 57, no. 6 (2002): 829–54.

Silva, Cristobal. *Miraculous Plagues: An Epidemiology of Early New England Narrative.* Oxford: Oxford University Press, 2011.

Singer, Dorothea Waley. "Some Plague Tractates (Fourteenth and Fifteenth Centuries)." *Proceedings of the Royal Society of Medicine* 9 (1916): 159–212.

– "Survey of Medical Manuscripts in the British Isles Dating from before the Sixteenth Century." *Proceedings of the Royal Society of Medicine* 12 (1919): 96–107.

Singer, Dorothea Waley, and Annie Anderson. *Catalogue of Latin and Vernacular Plague Texts in Great Britain and Eire in Manuscripts Written before the Sixteenth Century.* London: William Heineman Medical Books, 1950.

Siraisi, Nancy. "Anatomizing the Past: Physicians and History in Renaissance Culture." *Renaissance Quarterly* 53, no. 1 (2000): 1–30.

– "Cardano and the History of Medicine." In *Girolamo Cardano: le opere, le fonti, la vita*, edited by Marialuisa Baldi, Guido Canziani, and Giovanni Aquilecchia, 341–62. Milan, IT: F. Angeli, 1999.
– "The Changing Fortunes of a Traditional Text: Goals and Strategies in Sixteenth-Century Latin Editions of the *Canon* of Avicenna." In *The Medical Renaissance of the Sixteenth Century*, edited by A. Wear, R.K. French, and I.M. Loney, 16–41. Cambridge: Cambridge University Press, 1985.
– *History, Medicine, and the Traditions of Renaissance Learning*. Ann Arbor: The University of Michigan Press, 2007.
Skelton, Leona J. *Sanitation in Urban Britain, 1560–1700*. New York: Routledge, 2015.
Skene, Gilbert. *Ane breve descriptioun of the pest quhair in the causis, signis and sum speciall preservatioun and cure thairof ar contenit*. Edinburgh, UK: Robert Lekprevik, 1568.
Slack, Paul. "Books of Orders: The Making of English Social Policy, 1577–1631." *Transactions of the Royal Historical Society* 30 (1980): 1–22.
– "Great and Good Towns 1540–1700." In *The Cambridge Urban History of Britain*, volume 2, *1540–1840*, edited by Peter Clark, 347–76. Cambridge: Cambridge University Press, 2000.
– *The Impact of Plague in Tudor and Stuart England*. London: Routledge & Kegan Paul, 1985.
– "Mirrors of Health and Treasure of Poor Men: The Uses of the Vernacular Medical Literature of Tudor England." In *Health, Medicine and Mortality in the Sixteenth Century*, edited by Charles Webster, 237–74. Cambridge: Cambridge University Press, 1979.
– "Perceptions of Plague in Eighteenth-Century Europe." *The Economic History Review* (2021): 1–19. https://doi.org/10.1111/ehr.13080.
– *Poverty and Policy in Tudor and Stuart England*. London: Longman, 1988.
Slauter, Will. "Write Up Your Dead: The Bills of Mortality and the London Plague of 1665." *Media History* 17, no. 1 (2011): 1–15.
Slavin, Philip. "The Great Bovine Pestilence and Its Economic and Environmental Consequences in England and Wales, 1318–50." *Economic Historical Review* 65, no. 4 (2012): 1239–66.
– "Out of the West: Formation of a Permanent Plague Reservoir in South-Central Germany (1349–1356) and Its Implications." *Past and & Present* (2021). https://doi.org/10.1093/pastj/gtaa028.
Slerca, Anna. "Guillaume de Machaut et Boccace. Le traitement du thème de la peste dans le Jugement du roy de Navarre et dans le Decameron."

In *La mort dans la littérature française du Moyen Âge*, edited by Jean-François Kosta-Théfaine, 399–410. Villers-Cotterêt, FR: Ressouvenances, 2013.

Sloane, Barney. *The Black Death in London*. London: History Press, 2011.

Soll, Jacob. "The Uses of Historical Evidence in Early Modern Europe." *Journal of the History of Ideas* 64, no. 2 (2003): 149–57.

Sprat, Thomas. *The Plague of Athens, Which Hapned in the Second Year of the Peloponnesian Warre. First Describ'd in Greek by Thucydides; Then in Latin by Lucretius; Now Attempted in English*. London: T. Childe and L. Parry, for Henry Brome, 1659.

Spufford, Margaret. *Small Books and Pleasant Histories: Popular Fiction and Its Readership in Seventeenth-Century England*. Cambridge: Cambridge University Press, 1981.

Spyrou, Maria A. "Towards an Understanding of the Early History of the Second Plague Pandemic." Presentation at 9th International Symposium on Biomolecular Archaeology, Toulouse, France, 4 June 2021.

Spyrou, Maria A., Kirsten I. Bos, Alexander Herbig, and Johannes Krause. "Ancient Pathogen Genomics as an Emerging Tool for Infectious Disease Research." *Nature Reviews Genetics* 20 (2019): 323–40.

Spyrou, Maria A., Marcel Keller, Rezeda I. Tukhbatova, Christiana L. Scheib, Elizabeth A. Nelson, Aida Andrades Valtueña, Gunnar U. Neumann, et al. "Phylogeography of the Second Plague Pandemic Revealed through Analysis of Historical *Yersinia pestis* Genomes." *Nature Communications* 10, no. 4470 (2019). https://doi.org/10.1038/s41467-019-12154-0.

Spyrou, Maria A., Rezeda Tukhbatova, Chuan-Chao Wang, Aida Andrades Valtueña, Aditya K. Lankapalli, Vitaly V. Kondrashin, Victor A. Tsybin, et al. "Analysis of 3800-Year-Old *Yersinia pestis* Genomes Suggests Bronze Age Origin for Bubonic Plague." *Nature Communications* 9, no. 1 (2018): 1–10.

Stathakopoulos, Dionysios Ch. *Famine and Pestilence in the Late Roman and Early Byzantine Empire: A Systematic Survey of Subsistence Crises and Epidemics*. Aldershot, UK: Ashgate, 2004.

Stearns, Justin K. *Infectious Ideas: Contagion in Premodern Islamic and Christian Thought in the Western Mediterranean*. Baltimore, MD: Johns Hopkins University Press, 2011.

Stock, Marcus, and Nicola Vöhringer. "Spatial Practices, Medieval/Modern." In *Spatial Practices, Medieval/Modern*, edited by Marcus Stock and Nicola Vöhringer, 7–24. Göttingen, DE: V&R Press, 2014.

Stoclet, Alain J. "*Consilia humana, ops divina, superstitio*: Seeking Succor and Solace in Times of Plague, with Particular Reference to Gaul in the Early Middle Ages." In *Plague and the End of Antiquity: The Pandemic of 541–750*, edited by Lester K. Little, 135–49. Cambridge: Cambridge University Press, 2007.

Stolberg, Michael. "The Student Perspective: Medical Education in Sixteenth- and Early-Seventeenth-Century Padua and Montpellier." In *Transforming Medical Education: Historical Case Studies of Teaching, Learning, and Belonging in Medicine*, edited by Delia Gravus and Susan Lamb, 112–35. Montreal and Kingston: McGill-Queen's University Press, 2022.

Stow, John. *A Survey of London*. London: John Windet, 1603.

Suau, Jean. *Traitez contenans la pure et vraye doctrine de la peste*. Paris: Didier Millor, 1586.

Sublet, Jacqueline. "La peste prise aux rêts de la jurisprudence: le traité d'Ibn Ḥağar al-'Asqalānī sur la peste." *Studia Islamica* 33 (1971): 141–9.

Subrahmanyam, Sanjay. "On World Historians in the Sixteenth Century." *Representations* 91 (2005): 26–57.

Sudhoff, Karl. "Pestschriften aus den ersten 150 Jahren nach der Epidemie des 'schwarzen Todes' 1348." *Archiv für Geschichte der Medizin* (1907–27): 2–19.

Sullivan, Erin. "Physical and Spiritual Illness: Narrative Appropriations of the Bills of Mortality." In *Representing the Plague in Early Modern England*, edited by Rebecca Totaro and Ernest B. Gilman, 76–94. New York: Routledge, 2010.

Swanson, Maynard W. "The Sanitation Syndrome: Bubonic Plague and Urban Native Policy in the Cape Colony, 1900–1909." *The Journal of African History* 18, no. 03 (1977): 387–410.

Taavitsainen, Irma. "Scriptorial 'House-styles' and Discourse Communities." In *Medical and Scientific Writing in Late Medieval English*, edited by Irma Taavitsainen and Päivi Pahta, 23–36. Cambridge: Cambridge University Press, 2009.

Taavitsainen, Irma, Peter Murray Jones, Päivi Pahta, Turo Hiltunen, Ville Marttila, Maura Ratia, Carla Suhr, and Jukka Tyrkkö. "Medical Texts in 1500–1700 and the Corpus of *Early Modern English Medical Texts*." In *Medical Writing in Early Modern English*, edited by Irma Taavitsainen and Päivi Pahta, 9–29. Cambridge: Cambridge University Press, 2011.

Talbot, C.H., and E.A. Hammond. *The Medical Practitioners in Medieval England: A Biographical Register*. London: Wellcome Historical Medical Library, 1965.

Tavernier, Jean-Baptiste. *Les six voyages de Monsieur Jean-Baptiste Tavernier … qu'il a fait en Turquie, en Perse, et aux Indes*. Paris: Gervais Clouzier et Claude Barbin, 1676.

Taylor, John. *The Fearefull Summer: Or, Londons Calamitie*. London: Elizabeth Purslowe, 1636.

Thaisen, Jacob. "Trinity Gower D Scribe's Two *Canterbury Tales* Manuscripts." In *Design and Distribution of Late Medieval Manuscripts in England*, edited by Margaret Connolly and Linne R. Mooney, 41–60. York, UK: York Medieval Press, 2008.

Thayre, Thomas. *An Excellent and Best Approoued Treatise of the Plague*. London: Thomas Archer, 1625.

Thévenot, Jean de. *Relation d'un voyage fait au Levant*. Paris: Louis Billaine, 1665.

Thomas, Keith. *Religion and the Decline of Magic: Studies in Popular Beliefs in Sixteenth- and Seventeenth-Century England*. London: Weidenfeld & Nicolson, 1971.

Thompson, E.P. *Customs in Common: Studies in Traditional Popular Culture*. New York: New Press, 1993.

Thomson, George. *Loimotomia, or the Pest Anatomized*. London: Nath. Crouch, 1666.

Thucydides. *The History of the Peloponnesian War*. http://classics.mit.edu/Thucydides/ pelopwar.2.second.html.

Thyr, Nicholas. "The End of an Era: Later Medieval Views on an Early Medieval Plague." Presentation at the International Medieval Congress, Kalamazoo, MI, 10 May 2021.

Tolan, John Victor. *Saracens: Islam in the Medieval European Imagination*. New York: Columbia University Press, 2002.

Tomasch, Sylvia, and Sealy Gilles, eds. *Text and Territory: Geographical Information in the European Middle Ages*. Philadelphia: University of Pennsylvanian Press, 1998.

Tomić, Zlata Blažina, and Vesna Blažina. *Expelling the Plague: The Health Office and the Implementation of Quarantine in Dubrovnik, 1377–1533*. Montreal and Kingston: McGill-Queen's University Press, 2015.

Tonry, Kathleen. *Agency and Intention in English Print, 1476–1526*, Texts and Transitions series, volume 7. Turnhout, BE: Brepols, 2016.

Totaro, Rebecca, trans. and ed. *The Plague in Print: Essential Elizabethan Sources, 1558–1603*. Pittsburgh, PA: Duquesne University Press, 2010.

Totaro, Rebecca, and Ernest B. Gilman, eds. *Representing Plague in Early Modern England.* New York: Routledge, 2010.

Touati, François-Olivier. *Maladie et société au Moyen Âge: la lèpre, les lépreux et les léproseries dans la province ecclésiastique de Sens jusqu'au milieu du XIVe siècle.* Brussels, BE: De Boeck Université, 1998.

Tuetey, Alexandre, ed. *Journal d'un Bourgeois de Paris, 1405–1449.* Paris: H. Champion, 1881.

Twyne, Thomas. *A New Counsell Against the Pestilence.* London: John Charlewood, 1578.

Tyrkkö, Jukka. "A Physical Dictionary (1657): The First English Medical Dictionary." In *Selected Proceedings of the 2008 Symposium on New Approaches in English Historical Lexis (HEL-LEX 2),* edited by R.W. McConchie, Alpo Honkapohja, and Jukka Tyrkkö, 171–87. Somerville, MA: Cascadilla Proceedings Project, 2009. http://www.lingref.com/cpp/hel-lex/2008/paper2175.pdf.

Updike, Daniel Berkeley. *Printing Types: Their History, Forms, and Use: A Study in Survivals*, Volume 1. Cambridge, MA: Harvard University Press, 1922.

Vadianus, Joachim. *Ein kurtz und trüwlich underricht wider die sorgklich kranckeyt der Pestilentz.* Basel, CH: Adam Petri, 1519.

Valleriole, François. *Traicté de la peste.* Lyon, FR: Antoine Gryphius, 1556.

Valtueña, Aida Andrades, Alissa Mittnik, Felix M. Key, Wolfgang Haak, Raili Allmäe, Andrej Belinskij, Mantas Daubaras, et al. "The Stone Age Plague and Its Persistence in Eurasia." *Current Biology* 27, no. 23 (2017): 3683–91.

Van Diemerbroeck, Isbrand. *Several Choice Histories of the Medicines Manner and Method Used in the Cure of the Plague.* London: Matthew Keinton, 1666.

– *A Treatise Concerning the Pestilence.* Translated by Thomas Stanton. London: for J. Downing and T. Warner, 1722.

Van Linschoten, J.H. *The Voyage of John Huyghen van Linschoten to the East Indies.* 2 volumes. London: for the Hakluyt Society, 1885.

Various. *A Collection of Very Valuable and Scarce Pieces Relating to the Last Plague in the Year 1665.* London: J. Roberts, 1721.

Varlık, Nükhet. "Between Local and Universal: Translating Knowledge in Early Modern Ottoman Plague Treatises." In *Knowledge in Translation: Global Patterns of Scientific Exchange, 1000–1800 CE*, edited by Patrick Manning and Abigail Owen, 177–90. Pittsburgh, PA: University of Pittsburgh Press, 2018.

– "Beyond Eurocentric Histories of Plague." *Early Science and Medicine* 22, no. 4 (2017): 361–73.
– "New Science and Old Sources: Why the Ottoman Experience of Plague Matters." *The Medieval Globe* 1, no. 1 (2014): 193–228.
– "'Oriental Plague' or Epidemiological Orientalism?: Revisiting the Plague Episteme of the Early Modern Mediterranean." In *Plague and Contagion in the Islamic Mediterranean*, edited by Nükhet Varlık, 57–87. Kalamazoo, MI: ARC Humanities Press, 2017.
– *Plague and Empire in the Early Modern Mediterranean World: The Ottoman Experience, 1347–1600*. Cambridge: Cambridge University Press, 2015.
– "Rethinking the History of Plague in the Time of COVID-19." *Centaurus* 62 (2020): 285–93.
– "Why Is Black Death *Black*? European Gothic Imaginaries of 'Oriental' Plague." In *Plague Image and Imagination: from Medieval to Modern Times*, edited by Christos Lynteris, 11–36. London: Palgrave, 2021.
Vigier, Jean. "Traitté de la Peste." In *Œvvres Chirurgicales*. Lyon, FR: Christophle Fourmy, 1658.
Vincent, Thomas. *Gods Terrible Voice in the City of London*. Cambridge: Samuel Green, 1667.
Voigts, Linda Ehrsam. "Plague Saints, Henry VII, and Saint Armel." In *Saints and Cults in Medieval England: Proceedings of the 2015 Harlaxton Symposium*, Harlaxton Medieval Studies XXVII, edited by Susan Powell, 101–23. Donington, UK: Shaun Tyas, 2017.
– "The 'Sloane Group': Related Scientific and Medical Manuscripts from the Fifteenth Century in the Sloane Collection." *The British Library Journal* 16, no. 1 (1990): 26–57.
Voigts, Linda Ehrsam, and Michael R. McVaugh. "A Latin Technical Phlebotomy and Its Middle English Translation." *Transactions of the American Philosophical Society* 74, no. 2 (1984): 1–69.
Voigts, Linda Ehrsam, and Ann Payne. "Medicine for a Great Household (ca. 1500): Berkeley Castle Muniments Select Book 89." In *Studies in Medieval and Renaissance History*, third series, volume XII, edited by Cynthia Cosso and Anne Marie Scott, 87–255. New York: AMS Press, 2016.
Wakelin, Daniel. *Humanism, Reading, and English Literature, 1430–1530*. Oxford: Oxford University Press, 2007.
Wallis, Patrick. "Dreadful Heritage: Interpreting Epidemic Disease at Eyam, 1666–2000." *History Workshop Journal* 61 (2006): 31–56.
Wang, I-Chun. "Imperial Landscape of the Mughal Empire in Early Seventeenth-Century Geographical and Travel Writings." In

Landscape, Seascape, and the Eco-Spatial Imagination, edited by Simon C. Estok, I-Chun Wang, and Jonathan White, 66–81. New York: Routledge, 2016.

Warner, James Christopher. *Henry VIII's Divorce: Literature and the Politics of the Printing Press*. Woodbridge, UK: Boydell Press, 1998.

Wear, Andrew. "Explorations in Renaissance Writings on the Practice of Medicine." In *The Medical Renaissance of the Sixteenth Century*, edited by A. Wear, R.K. French, and I.M. Loney, 118–45. Cambridge: Cambridge University Press, 1985.

– *Knowledge and Practice in English Medicine, 1550–1680*. Cambridge: Cambridge University Press, 2000.

– "Making Sense of Health and the Environment in Early Modern England." In *Medicine in Society: Historical Essays*, 119–47. Cambridge: Cambridge University Press, 1992.

– "Place, Health, and Disease: The *Airs, Waters, Places* Tradition in Early Modern England and North America." *Journal of Medieval and Early Modern Studies* 38, no. 3 (2008): 443–65.

Webster, Charles. *The Great Instauration: Science, Medicine, and Reform, 1626–1660*. Oxford: Peter Lang, 2002.

– "Paracelsus: Medicine as Popular Protest." In *Medicine and the Reformation*, edited by Ole Peter Grell and Andrew Cunningham, 57–77. London: Routledge, 1993.

Wickersheimer, Ernest. *Dictionnaire biographique des médecins en France au Moyen Age*. Geneva, CH: Librairie Droz, 1979. First published 1936 (Paris).

– "Jean Jacme et les régimes de pestilence qui porte son nom." *Archivio di storia della scienza* 6 (1925): 105–112.

Winkler, Albert. "The Approach of the Plague in Switzerland and the Persecution of Jews, 1348–1349." *Swiss American Historical Society Review* 43, no. 3 (2007). https://scholarsarchive.byu.edu/sahs_review/vol43/iss3/2.

– "'The Clamor of the People': Popular Support for the Persecution of Jews in Switzerland and Germany at the Approach of the Black Death, 1348–1350." *Swiss American Historical Society Review* 53, no. 2 (2017): 31–61.

Winslow, C.E.A., and M.L. Duran-Reynals. "Jacme d'Agramont: The First of the Plague Tractates." *Bulletin of the History of Medicine* 22 (1948): 748–66.

Wintle, Michael. "Islam as Europe's 'Other' in the Long Term: Some Discontinuities." *History* 101, no. 344 (2016): 42–61.

Witakowski, Witold, trans. *Pseudo-Dionysius of Tel-Mahre: Chronicle, Part III*. Liverpool, UK: Liverpool University Press, 1996.

Wither, George. *Britain's Remembrancer, Containing a Narration of the Plague Lately Past*. London: John Grismond, 1628.

Withington, Phil. *Society in Early Modern England: The Vernacular Origins of Some Powerful Ideas*. Cambridge: Polity, 2010.

Woolf, Daniel. "Erudition and the Idea of History in Renaissance England." *Renaissance Quarterly* 40, no. 1 (1987): 11–48.

– "Historical Writing in Britain from the Late Middle Ages to the Eve of Enlightenment." In *The Oxford History of Historical Writing*, volume 3, *1400–1800*, edited by Masayuki Sato, Daniel Woolf, Edoardo Tortarolo, and José Rabasa, 473–96. Oxford: Oxford University Press, 2012.

– "Memory and Historical Culture in Early Modern England." *Journal of the Canadian Historical Association/Revue de la Société historique du Canada* 2, no. 1 (1991): 283–308.

Wormold, Frances, and Phyllis M. Gilles. *A Descriptive Catalogue of the Additional Illuminated Manuscripts in the Fitzwilliam Museum Acquired between 1895 and 1979*. Cambridge: Fitzwilliam Museum, 1982.

Wragg, Richard. "A Civic Relationship: The Guild Book of the Barbers and Surgeons of York as an Expression of Professional Status and City Authority." In *Occupying Space in Medieval and Early Modern Britain and Ireland*, edited by Gregory Hulsman and Caoimhe Whelan, 235–52. Oxford: Peter Lang, 2016.

Wrightson, Keith. *Earthly Necessities: Economic Lives in Early Modern Britain*. New Haven, CT: Yale University Press, 2000.

– *Ralph Tailor's Summer: A Scrivener, His City and the Plague*. New Haven, CT: Yale University Press, 2011.

Ydeley, Estienne. *Des secrets souverains et vrais remedes contre la peste*. Lyon, FR: Jean Stratius, 1581.

Yérasimos, Stefanos. *Les voyageurs dans l'Empire ottoman, XIVe–XVIe siècles: bibliographie, itinéraires et inventaire des lieux habités*. Ankara, TR: TTK, 1991.

Ziegler, Michelle. "Black Death and the Future of the Plague." *The Medieval Globe* 1, no. 1 (2014): 259–84.

Zink, Michel, and Katherine Lydon. "The Time of the Plague and the Order of Writing: Jean le Bel, Froissart, Machaut." *Yale French Studies*, special issue, *Contexts: Style and Values in Medieval Art and Literature* (1991): 269–80.

Zuckerman, Arnold. "Plague and Contagionism in Eighteenth-Century England: The Role of Richard Mead." *Bulletin of the History of Medicine* 78, no. 2 (2004): 273–308.

Index

Abbas, Haly (Ali ibn Abbas al-Majusi, physician), 23–4, 123, 162
Aberdeen, 43, 175, 176, 300n69
administrators and councillors, as tract writers. *See* Rochas d'Ayglun, Henry de; Davin, Antoine; Rubys, Claude de
aDNA (ancient DNA), 19, 20, 296n4. *See also* palaeogenetics
Africa: as source of plague, 206, 233, 235, 238, 310n197; plague reservoirs in, 17, 20; sub-Sahara affected by Black Death, 5, 16, 207, 253n27, 311n216
Agramont, Jacme d' (tract writer), 26–8; 32–3, 186, 259n22, 260n30, 297n23
air: cleansing or countering as preventative measure, 32, 36–7, 39, 187–8, 194; corrupted by the poor, 189, 192, 304n125; geographical origins of corruption in, 201–2, 215, 227–8, 232, 296n5; mutated by demons, 147; as poisoned breath, 44; salubrious places, 202, 220, 228, 231, 310n195; source of corruption in, 128, 162, 172, 187, 215, 244. *See also* causes of plague: breath; causes of plague: corrupted air; wind
Airs, Waters, Places: expanded interpretation of, 227–8; influence on tracts, 187, 219, 303n120. *See also* Hippocrates
al-Rāzī (Abū Bakr Muḥammad ibn Zakariyyā' al-Rāzī, physician), 24, 38, 114, 123, 126, 162
Alberti, Bernard (tract writer), 63, 260n35
Albucasis (Abū al-Qāsim Khalaf ibn al-'Abbās al-Zahrāwī al-Ansari, physician), 37
alchemy/alchemical, 39–40, 44, 47, 95, 265n92
Allde, John (printer), 88
American colonies: as plague-free, 228–9
Andernach, Jehan Guinter d' (tract writer), 79, 134–5
André, Pierre (tract writer), 40, 44, 183, 302n99

Apennine Mountains. *See* cause of plague: earthquakes
apostemes, 34, 37, 130. *See also* buboes
apothecaries, as tract writers. *See* Boghurst, William; Garencières, Theophilus de; Houël, Nicolas
Aristotle, 23, 123, 149
astrologers, on plague. *See* Covino, Simon of; Gadbury, John; Meaux, Geoffrey de; Thibault, Jean
astrology: and plague, *see* causes of plague: planetary conjunctions
Asia: as origin of plague, 220, 232, 235, 239. *See also* Levant; Ottoman Empire
Atila. *See* Jacobi, Johannes
Aubert, Jacques (tract writer), 140
Avenzoar (Abū Marwān 'Abd al-Malik ibn Zuhr, physician and surgeon), 114, 122
Averroes (Ibn Rushd, philosopher), 114
Avicenna (physician). *See* Ibn Sīnā

Babington, Benjamin Guy (translator), 120, 158
Baker, Geoffrey le (chronicler), 33
Balmford, James (clergyman): debate with Henoch Clapham, 43
barber-surgeons. *See* surgeons
Barbette, Paul (tract writer), 77–8, 277n117
Barralis, B. (tract writer), 276n116
Basle, 84, 92, 210, 277n117
Baux, Pierre (tract writer), 47, 50, 156, 161–2, 164–6, 233–4
Beaufort, Margaret (countess of Richmond and Derby, mother of King Henry VII of England), 68–9, 72, 102–3
Belon du Mans, Pierre (travel writer). *See* travel writing (early modern)
Berthelet, Thomas (printer), 59–62, 100
Bertrand, Jean-Baptiste (tract writer), 157, 202
Béziers, 184
biblical references: in plague tracts, 42, 114–15, 121, 124, 148–9, 186
bills of mortality, 3, 8, 145, 147, 291n131, 305n133, 315n28; as geographical information, 190–3, 231; as historical information, 142–3, 152–3, 235, 241
Bishop of Arusiens. *See* Jacobi, Johannes
Black Death (c. 1346–53), 16; debates about nature of by historians, 19; as historical touchstone, 6, 13, 127–9; plague tracts written during, 5, 21, 23–8, 55, 63; portrayed as unprecedented, 5, 121–6. *See also* palaeogenetics; *Yersinia pestis*
Blasius of Barcelona (tract writer), 37, 64, 66, 70
bloodletting. *See* phlebotomy
Boccaccio, Giovanni (writer), 24, 33, 149–50, 158, 203, 234, 282n32
Boeti, Michel (tract writer), 64
Boghurst, William (tract writer), 74, 78, 143
Bordeaux, 40, 58, 85, 139–40, 210

Bordeaux, John of. *See* Burgundy, John of
Bouillet, Jean (tract writer), 184
Boyer, Jean-Baptiste-Nicolas (tract writer), 4, 156
Bradley, Richard (tract writer), 78, 152–3, 201–2, 231, 242, 320n8
Bradwell, Stephen (tract writer), 48–9, 83, 178, 192
Brasbridge, Thomas (tract writer), 139, 149, 175–6, 178–80, 192, 275n108
breath: as source of contagion, *see* causes of plague: breath
Briet, Guillaume (tract writer), 139–40, 210, 276n115
broadsheets, 78, 117, 141–4, 190–1
Bronze Age, 16, 253n27, 254n36
Brookes, Richard (tract writer), 50–1, 154, 294n174
Browne, Joseph (tract writer), 50, 155, 232, 235
Brownrigg, William (physician), 216, 239
buboes: images of, 84, 94, 112; location of, 34, 130, 211; as sign of plague, 18, 122, 130–1, 156, 172, 239; treatment of, 34–5, 37–8, 42, 82. *See also* signs and symptoms of plague
bubonic plague, 18–19, 239
Bullein, William (tract writer), 80, 192
Burgundy, John of (tract writer), 26, 31–2, 35–7, 48, 126–9, 172–3, 191, 243–4; illuminated/illustrated copies of tract by, 72, 103–4, 112; ownership of tract by, 68–70, 72–4, 107; versions of tract by, 65–6, 101, 106, 134, 173–4. *See also* Multon, Thomas
Busbecq, Ogier Ghiselin de (ambassador), 223

Caffa: as origin of Black Death, 203–4, 206; debunked as origin of Black Death, 204–5
Caillaut, Antoine (printer), 58, 269–70n28
Cairo, 201, 216, 222, 231–2
Caius, John (tract writer), 275n108, 290n107
Calvinists/Calvinism, 195, 197–8, 210, 220, 230
Cambridge, 48, 86, 180
Caslari, Abraham (tract writer), 26–8, 32, 258–9n20, 260n26
Caucasus, 20, 205
causes of plague, 17, 21; alternative theories of, 40; breath, 4, 32, 44–5, 199, 215; comets, 129, 235; corrupted air, 24, 31–2, 49, 81, 119, 162, 210; divine judgment, 4, 31, 41–6, 59, 114, 121, 177–8, 186; earthquakes, 31, 118, 184, 187; environmental, 31, 162, 167, 187–8, 201–2, 215, 218, 220, 226–8; greasing conspiracies, 32, 195–8, 210, 308n168; humoral susceptibility, 31, 164, 191, 285n50; planetary conjunctions, 31, 127–9, 134, 171, 244; wide spectrum of, 32, 49, 81, 210; witches, 115. *See also* air; *Airs, Waters, and Places*; climate; contagion; Wars of Religion
Cauwet, Bauduin (nobleman), 69

Central Asia, 20, 204, 207, 310n198
Charles I (King of England), 155, 189, 280n5
Charles II (King of England), 46, 74
Charles V (Holy Roman Emperor), 135, 230
Charles V (King of France), 53–4, 69, 71, 104–5
Chartreis, Pierre (scribe), 54, 69
Chauliac, Guy de (surgeon), 32, 57–8, 64, 126, 128–30, 170–1, 209, 247; personal experience of plague, 37, 64, 129–30, 170, 172; referred to by later writers, 150–1, 156, 158, 234, 292n148
Chettle, Henry (writer), 151–2
Chevalier, Guillaume (tract writer), 140
Chicoyneau, François (tract writer), 4, 50, 277n117
China, 16, 18, 20, 206–7, 220, 235
chroniclers: and discussion of plague, *see* Baker, Geoffrey le; Grey Friars, at Lynn; Knighton, Henry; Muisis, Gilles Li; Mussis, Gabriele d'; Venette, Jean de; Villani, Giovanni; Villani, Matteo; Walsingham, Thomas
Clapham, Henoch (clergyman), 43, 177
Clarke, Samuel (clergyman), 141
clergy, as tract writers. *See* Brasbridge, Thomas; Gatford, Lionel; Gaudereau, Abbé Martin; Grillot, P. Jean; Lozeillère, Alexis Allaire de; Multon, Thomas; Paynel, Thomas; Ydeley, Estienne
climate, 17, 21, 157, 198, 219–20, 229; linked to sources of plague, 215, 220, 223, 232, 245. See also *Airs, Waters, and Places*
Clot, Antoine Barthélemy (tract writer), 216, 239
clothing, 81, 118, 192, 196, 198
Colin, Sébastien (tract writer), 38, 276n117
College of Physicians (London), 189, 200, 221–2, 306n134. *See also* Herring, Francis; Mead, Richard; Rose, Philip
College of Surgeons (Paris, tract writer), 151
Collins, Samuel (tract writer), 74, 200, 274n95, 280n5
colonialism, 137–8, 213, 218–19, 228–30, 238
Colwell, Thomas (printer), 87–8
comets. *See* causes of plague: comets
common good, 77, 83, 95, 174, 243
consilia, 24–6
Constantinople, 208, 225–6; *émigrés* from, 13, 125, 148, 236, 244; historical plague in, 150, 155, 233; as source of plague, 201, 216, 222, 226, 231, 234
contagion: debates about, 49, 79, 156, 216, 218–19; impetus for prevention measures, 194; as name for plague, 141, 152, 185, 220, 231, 239; on spectrum of causation, 32, 49, 81, 210; and spread of plague, 43, 47, 199, 210, 220
Córdoba, Alfonso de (tract writer), 32, 63, 123, 167, 207
cotton: as source of plague, 215, 220–1, 245
Courcelles, François de (tract writer), 46, 135–6, 194

Covino, Simón of (tract writer), 63, 168
Crannon, epidemic of: compared to Black Death, 115, 122, 280n4
Crestien, Gervaise (physician), 71–2
Crimea. *See* Caffa
cures and treatments, 27, 34–41, 64–5, 82

Damouzy, Pierre de (tract writer), 23–4, 32–3, 63, 122–3, 168, 207
Davin, Antoine (tract writer), 200–1, 276n116
Dawson, Gertrude (printer), 81–3
Defoe, Daniel (writer), 3–6, 11, 79, 241–2
Dekker, Thomas (writer), 178
deliberate spread of plague. *See* causes of plague: greasing conspiracies
Denidel, Antoine (printer), 58
Despars, Jacques (tract writer), 131
Dethick, Sir William (herald), 74, 274n93
dissection: of plague corpses, 48, 50, 95, 265n95
divine punishment, 41, 186, 262n60, 321n21
doctors. *See* physicians, as tract writers
Doesborch, Jan van (printer), 59, 89
Douai, 85, 181, 183
Drouet, Pierre (tract writer), 38–40, 47, 76, 176, 276n115

earthquakes. *See* causes of plague: earthquakes
East Africa, 20
eastern Mediterranean. *See* Ottoman Empire
Egypt: biblical plagues of, 114–15; plague in, 206, 216, 220, 226, 234, 240; as source of plague, 228, 232, 310n197. *See also* Cairo
Elyot, Thomas (writer), 60, 192
Enghien, 136
English Sweating Sickness, 59, 61, 68, 75, 172, 290n107; discussed using plague tract format, 66, 275n108; misdated in plague tracts, 294n173, 294n186; used to historicize plague, 136, 150, 154, 156, 160, 220. *See also* Caius, John; Henry VII; Le Forestier, Thomas; Machlinia, William de; Beaufort, Margaret
environmental causes of plague. *See* causes of plague: environmental
Eurasia, 5–6, 16, 131, 206–7, 235, 254n36, 255n38
Eurocentrism, 17. *See also* Orientalism

Fabre, Pierre-Jean (tract writer), 40, 276n115
fatalistic Turk (i.e., predestination), 4, 222, 226, 234, 245; origins of stereotype, 223
Ferrier, Oger (tract writer), 40, 147–8, 194, 197, 276n114
First Plague Pandemic (c. 541 to eighth century), 5, 16, 254n30, 262n59, 284n41; contemporary writing about, 125–6, 169; referenced by tract writers, 116–17, 149–50, 152, 157, 213, 237, 248; unknown during Black Death, 116, 124–6, 169. *See also*

Islamicate plague-writing tradition; Jaucourt, Louis de
fleas, 17–19, 21
Foligno, Gentile da (tract writer), 26–8, 34, 122, 292n148
Fontenay, 38
Forman, Simon (tract writer), 74, 274n95

Gadbury, John (astrologer), 152, 222
Galen: full works of, 125, 148; and non-naturals, 25; plague purportedly unknown by, 122, 126, 169; references to, 23, 40, 47, 147, 187
Galenic medicine, 25, 27, 30, 44, 148, 162; rejection of, 39–41, 95, 177
Gardin, Louis du (tract writer), 183, 276n114
Garencières, Theophilus de (tract writer), 179
Gatford, Lionel (tract writer), 45–6, 180, 264n77
Gaudereau, Abbé Martin (tract writer), 156, 201, 232, 236, 277n116
genetics, 20. *See also* aDNA; palaeogenetics
Genoa/Genoans, 203–5, 208, 220–1
genome. *See* aDNA; palaeogenetics
Gering, Ulrich (printer), 58, 83, 92, 268n19
Goiffon, Jean-Baptiste (tract writer), 4, 199–200
Golden Horde. *See* Mongols
Göttingen, Johannes von (tract writer), 63
Grand Saint Antoine (ship): role in Plague of Provence disputed, 295n4; as source of plague in Marseille, 161–2, 165, 210, 221, 232
Grandes Chroniques de France, 132
Graunt, John (demographer), 143, 145, 152, 192–3, 235
graves: and aDNA, 19; mass, 21; as source of plague, 193, 227
greasing conspiracies. *See* causes of plague: greasing conspiracies
Great Plague of London (1665), 3, 16, 144–5, 152, 180, 200, 231; plague absent in official records after, 8, 78; as referent for Plague of Provence, 79, 153. See also bills of mortality; Boghurst, William; broadsheets; Collins, Samuel; Gadbury, John; Garencières, Theophilus de; Graunt, John; Hodges, Nathaniel; Kemp, William; Quarles, John; Thomson, George
Greek: lack of knowledge in West, 116, 125, 169; new access to texts in, 117, 148, 214. *See also* Constantinople: *émigrés* from
Gregoras, Nicephorus (historian), 203–4
Gregory I, Pope, 125, 166, 169, 297n17, 298n35
Grelot, Guillaume-Joseph (artist), 224–5
Grey Friars, at Lynn (chronicler), 124, 128; of London (chronicler), 132
Grillot, P. Jean (tract writer), 46, 139, 198, 277n116
Guerin, Jacques (tract writer), 136

Gybson, Thomas (printer), 59, 62, 278n143

Havard, Martin (printer), 75, 92, 108
healthscaping, 218, 220, 224
Hecker, Justus (medical writer), 120, 158, 239–40
Henry VII (King of England), 59, 68, 172
Henry VIII (King of England), 59, 89
Herring, Francis (tract writer), 47, 80, 178, 191, 275n108
Hippocrates: full works of, 125, 148; plague purportedly unknown by, 123, 126, 169; references to, 23, 47, 123, 147, 150, 187. See also *Airs, Waters, Places*
historia. *See* humanism
Hobbes, Thomas (philosopher): and Plague of Athens, 149
Hodges, Nathaniel (tract writer), 46, 78, 178–9, 193, 198, 221–3; referenced by Defoe, 4, 242
Holland: as source of plague in London, 3, 222–3, 231, 238, 242
Houël, Nicolas (tract writer), 140, 276n116
Houssemaine, Nicolas de (tract writer), 44, 76, 181–2, 263n74, 276n114, 277n117
humanism, 14, 117, 138, 148, 157, 159
humoralism/humoural theory, 30–2, 93, 171; and buboes, 34, 122; and Paracelsianism, 39, 47, 95; and plague therapies, 24, 34, 36; and predisposition to plague, 31, 164, 191, 285n50
Ibn al-Khaṭīb (tract writer), 27, 122
Ibn Khātimah (tract writer), 26–8, 122, 206–7
Ibn Sīnā (physician), 24, 27, 123, 126, 162
Ibn al-Wardī (Abū Ḥafs Zayn al-Dīn ‘Umar ibn al-Muẓaffar Ibn al-Wardī, historian), 204, 206
India, 168, 201, 204, 229, 235, 311n211
Indian Plague Commission, 19
Ingram, Dale (tract writer), 78, 155–6
Islamicate plague-writing tradition, 28, 125, 256–7n6, 261n48, 262n59, 284n41
Istanbul. *See* Constantinople

Jackson, Hugh (printer), 87–8
Jacobi, Johannes (tract writer), 53–4, 64, 129, 171, 186–7, 270n52; illuminated version of tract by, 68–9, 102; ownership of tract by, 69; personal experience of plague, 64, 130; tract by in print, 57–62, 75–6, 86, 89, 92, 135, 292n148
Jacobites (i.e., Jacobins or Dominicans): blamed for plague, 185, 303n111
Jacme, Jean. *See* Jacobi, Johannes
Jahangir (Nur-ud-din Muhammad Salim, Mughal Emperor), 229
James II (King of Scotland), 65
James VI and I (King of Scotland and England), 81, 142, 155
Jaucourt, Louis de (encyclopedist): on Oriental plague, 239
Jehannot, Estienne (printer), 58

Jews: pogroms against, 195–6
Joubert, Laurent (tract writer), 139, 150–1,194, 234, 276n114
Joubert, M. (tract writer), 156, 295n189
Jouyse, David (tract writer), 146
Justinianic Plague or Plague of Justinian. *See* First Plague Pandemic

Kamitus. *See* Jacobi, Johannes
Kantakouzenos, John VI (Byzantine Emperor), 125, 204
Kazakhstan, 20
Kele, Richard (printer), 87–9, 278n139
Kellwaye, Simon (tract writer), 78, 175
Kemp, William (tract writer), 114–15, 117–19, 141, 178, 193, 222
Kinglake, Alexander William (travel writer). *See* travel writing (early modern)
Knighton, Henry (chronicler), 128, 132, 170
Knolles, Richard (historian), 237
Kyrgyzstan, 20

Lamperiere, Jean de (tract writer), 146
Late Neolithic, 16
Le Forestier, Thomas (tract writer), 66, 75, 136, 172, 250
Le Lievre, Esaïe (tract writer), 140–1
Lérida (Lleida), 26–7, 186
Levant. *See* Ottoman Empire
Lodge, Thomas (tract writer), 76–7, 192
Lombardy, 210
London: outbreaks in, 43, 45, 47, 61, 89, 118, 132–3, 139, 141, 143; as plagued city, 97, 163, 172, 175–80; as publishing centre, 55, 70, 85–7, 90, 96–7, 110. *See also* bills of mortality; broadsheets; Great Plague of London (1665)
Lord Have Mercy. *See* broadsheets
Loüet, Theobaldi (Theobaldus Loneti, tract writer), 64
Lozeillère, Alexis Allaire de (tract writer), 74, 274n95
Lyon: as generator of plague, 201; plague in, 47, 139–40, 147, 156, 165, 183, 196–8, 210; print industry in, 57, 75, 84–5, 181

Machlinia, William de (printer), 59, 89
Magnus, Albertus (philosopher), 123, 259n23
Mandeville, John. *See* travel writing (medieval)
Manget, Jean-Jacques (tract writer), 156, 232
maritime complexion, 223
Marnef, frères (printer), 75
Marseille, Plague of. See Provence, Plague of
Mead, Richard (tract writer), 80, 155, 193, 243–5; and Daniel Defoe, 4, 242; on foreign origin of plague, 202, 215, 217–21, 228, 232, 245; on historical plague, 235–6; inspires debates about plague spread through trade, 50, 79, 155

Meaux, Geoffrey de (tract writer), 29–30, 63, 123, 168, 170–1
medicines. *See* cures and treatments
Mercuriale, Girolomo (tract writer), 150–1
Mézeray, François Eudes de (historian): on Ottoman plagues, 238
miasma. *See* causes of plague: corrupted air
Milan, 31, 131, 210, 292n131
Mizauld, Antoine (tract writer), 182–3
Mongolia, 20, 204
Mongols, 204–5, 207, 310n198, 319n73. *See also* Pax Mongolica; Tartars; Saracens
Montpellier, 53–4, 85, 128, 136, 163, 165, 173. *See also* University of Montpellier
Moryson, Fynes (travel writer). *See* travel writing (early modern)
Moulton, Thomas. *See* Multon, Thomas
Muisis, Gilles Li (chronicler), 168
Multon, Thomas (tract writer), 42–3, 45, 66, 74, 134, 174; work by in print, 42, 61, 75–6, 86
Mundy, Peter (travel writer). *See* travel writing (early modern)
Mussis, Gabriele d' (chronicler), 33, 203–6
Myddleton, Henry (printer), 89–90
Myddleton, William (printer), 87–90, 278n139

Nancel, Nicolas de (tract writer), 46, 139, 185–6, 243–5, 276n115
Naples, plague of, 200
Nicolay, Nicolas de (geographer), 224, 316n35
Nîmes, 85, 161, 165
Nourry, Claude (printer), 75, 84, 92, 94, 277n126
Nyverd, Jacques (printer), 58

Orders Thought Meet, 209
Oriental plague, myth of, 217–18, 234, 239–40, 248, 318n62
Orientalism: epidemiological, 22; medieval, 208. *See also* Oriental plague, myth of
Orléans, 85
Orléans, Philippe d' (French regent), 156
Orléans, Raoulet d' (royal scribe), 72
Ottoman Empire, 218–19; and Black Death, 203; cleanliness of, 217, 224–6; described as plague-ridden, 201, 215–16, 219–22, 226–8, 231–2, 237–40; European relations with, 230–1; plague coming from, 3, 218–21, 223, 233–4, 236, 242; Plague of Provence arrived from, 157, 210, 221, 232; as "sick man of Europe," 216. *See also* Constantinople; Turks
Oultre, Petrus de (student), 69, 74, 274n92
Oxford, 45, 134, 139, 174–6, 179–80, 232; printing in, 86, 180

Padua, 26, 139, 308n165
palaeogenetics, 16, 20. *See also* aDNA
pandemics (of plague), 16–17; as problematic notion, 17–21. *See also* First Plague Pandemic
panzootic, 17

Paracelsianism, 39–40, 47
Paré, Ambroise (tract writer), 77, 95, 276n116
Paris: plague coming from, 139, 183, 185–6, 244; plague in, 133, 140–1, 163, 165, 167–8, 183, 201; print industry, 58, 70–1, 75, 84–5, 181
Paris Medical Faculty (tract writer). *See* University of Paris, Medical Faculty
Paston, Sir John II (courtier), 69, 74
Pax Mongolica, 206
Paynel, Thomas (tract writer), 59–62, 92, 100, 135
Pestalozzi, Jérome Jean (tract writer), 156
pestis secunda, 20, 234, 285n53
Petrarch (scholar), 122, 168
Petyt, Thomas (printer), 87–90
Phayer, Thomas (tract writer), 44–5, 76, 80, 93, 135, 182; printers of tract by, 89; tract by reprinted, 90, 242
Philip VI (King of France), 26, 63, 69
Philippe, Gaspard (printer), 58
phlebotomy, 24, 34–5, 49, 84, 94, 112
physicians, as tract writers, 27, 64. *See also* Agramont, Jacme d'; Alberti, Bernard; Andernach, Jehan Guinter d'; Barbette, Paul; Barralis, B.; Baux, Pierre; Bertrand, Jean-Baptiste; Blasius of Barcelona; Boeti, Michel; Bouillet, Jean; Boyer, Jean-Baptiste-Nicolas; Bradwell, Stephen; Briet, Guillaume; Brookes, Richard; Browne, Joseph; Bullein, William; Burgundy, John of; Caius, John; Caslari, Abraham; Chevalier, Guillaume; Chicoyneau, François; Clot, Antoine Barthélemy; Colin, Sébastien; Collins, Samuel; Córdoba, Alfonso de; Courcelles, François de; Damouzy, Pierre de; Davin, Antoine; Despars, Jacques; Drouet, Pierre; Fabre, Pierre-Jean; Ferrier, Oger; Foligno, Gentile da; Forman, Simon; Gardin, Louis du; Goiffon, Jean-Baptiste; Göttingen, Johannes von; Guerin, Jacques; Herring, Francis; Hodges, Nathaniel; Houssemaine, Nicolas de; Ibn al-Khaṭīb; Ibn Khātimah; Jacobi, Johannes; Joubert, Laurent; Jouyse, David; Kemp, William; Lamperiere, Jean de; Le Forestier, Thomas; Lodge, Thomas; Loüet, Theobaldi; Manget, Jean-Jacques; Mead, Richard; Meaux, Geoffrey of; Mercuriale, Girolomo; Mizauld, Antoine; Nancel, Nicolas de; Paris Medical Faculty; Phayer, Thomas; Pons, D.M.; Quincy, John; Ranchin, François; Reguardati, Benedetto; Robin, Vincent; Rose, Philip; Sainct-Hillier, I.S. de; Skene, Gilbert; Spierinck, Joannes; Suau, Jean; Thomson, George; Todros, Isaac ben; Tournemire, Jean de; Twyne, Thomas; Valleriole, François; Van Diemerbroeck, Isbrand; Vigier, Jean; Vinario, Raymond Chalin de; Watt, Joachim von
Pickering, Elisabeth (printer), 87–8

plague, 16–21. *See also* aDNA; Africa; American colonies; Asia; Black Death; buboes; bubonic plague; causes of plague; climate; First Plague Pandemic; Oriental plague, myth of; signs and symptoms of plague; *Yersinia pestis*
Plague of Athens: as historical precedent, 115, 118–19, 147–50, 197, 233, 236; as literary trope, 124
plague pits. *See* graves: mass
plague prevention: medical, 24, 27, 34–41, 53, 82, 187; religious, 41–4
planetary conjunctions. *See* causes of plague: planetary conjunctions
Polo, Marco. *See* travel writing (medieval)
Pons, D.M. (tract writer), 49–50
poor, the: associated with plague, 188–95, 212–13, 220, 222, 242
Potel, Guillaume (tract writer), 140, 194, 277n116, 292n148
Poultry Compter, 77, 87–8, 278n138
Powell, William (printer), 87
Pré, Jean de (printer), 58
predestination. *See* fatalistic Turk
printers, 11, 74–5, 83–4, 92–5. *See also* Allde, John; Berthelet, Thomas; Caillaut, Antoine; Colwell, Thomas; Dawson, Gertrude; Denidel, Antoine; Doesborch, Jan van; Gering, Ulrich; Gybson, Thomas; Havard, Martin; Jackson, Hugh; Jehannot, Estienne; Kele, Richard; Machlinia, William de; Marnef, frères; Myddleton, Henry; Myddleton, William; Nourry, Claude; Nyverd, Jacques; Petyt, Thomas; Philippe, Gaspard; Pickering, Elisabeth; Powell, William; Pré, Jean de; Redman, Robert; Roy, Guillaume le; Soquand, Guichard; Toye, Robert; Vele, Abraham; Waley, John; Whitchurch, Edward; Worde, Wynken de; Wyer, Robert
Procopius (Greek scholar), 125, 148–9, 151, 155–6, 169, 233
Provence, Plague of, 3–4, 7, 50, 164–5, 49–50, 156–7, 164–6, 202; as impetus for tract production, 78–80, 153, 184, 201–2, 215; print industry in Marseille, 181. See also *Grand Saint Antoine*
Ptolemy, Claudius (geographer), 23, 123, 214, 313n237
public good. *See* common good

Quarles, John (poet), 78, 179
Quincy, John (tract writer), 46, 79, 154–5, 214, 232

Ranchin, François (tract writer), 46, 91, 111, 276n114
rats, 17, 19, 20
Redman, Robert (printer), 87–8, 278n137
regimen of health (*regimen sanitatis*), 4, 25–6; *Regimen sanitatis Salerni*, 60–1
Reguardati, Benedetto (tract writer), 66, 270n52
religious enemies, 46, 196–8. *See also* Calvinists/Calvinism; greasing conspiracies

Rhazes. *See* al-Rāzī
Robin, Vincent (tract writer), 183
Robson, Charles (travel writer). *See* travel writing (early modern)
Rochas d'Ayglun, Henry de (tract writer), 183, 276n116
Rose, Philip (tract writer), 4, 79, 202, 231
Rouen: and plague, 144, 146, 183, 194, 210, 309n172; printing industry in, 85
Roy, Guillaume le (printer), 57–9, 92
Rubys, Claude de (tract writer), 139, 150–1, 183, 234, 276n116; on deliberate spread of plague (greasing), 197, 210, 308n168; and religious enemies, 46, 196–8
Rufus of Ephesus (physician), 283n37
Russell, Patrick (physician), 313n4
Russian Empire: effect on Western European plague mentalities, 252n15; plague epidemics in, 8, 16, 18, 230, 240; war with Ottoman Empire, 216
Rycaut, Sir Paul (diplomat), 227, 238

Sainct-Hillier, I.S. de (tract writer), 151, 276n114
Saracens: and Black Death, 203, 205–6, 231, 235, 239; definition of, 310n198; prophetic destruction of, 127
Scythians, 204–5
Sedan, 135–6
Shibasaburō, Kitasato (bacteriologist), 19
Siberia, 20
signs and symptoms of plague, 18–19; described by lay writers, 33; described (or not) by tract writers, 33–4, 82, 122–3, 130, 156, 239–40, 247, 264n91, 294n174; during First Pandemic, 259n21, 298n36; as familiar, 116, 129, 131, 149, 152–4, 293n150; in Islamicate writing, 284n41; as unusual/unfamiliar, 5, 126
Skene, Gilbert (tract writer), 43–4, 175–6, 300n69
Solomon, Jacob b. (physician), 269n44
Soquand, Guichard (printer), 58
Spierinck, Joannes (tract writer), 65
Sprat, Thomas (writer), 149–50
Suau, Jean (tract writer), 40, 276n115
sudor anglicus. *See* English sweating sickness
surgeons: as tract owners, 70, 73–4; as tract writers. *See* André, Pierre; Chauliac, Guy de; College of Surgeons; Guerin, Jacques; Ingram, Dale; Le Lievre, Esaïe; Paré, Ambroise; Potel, Guillaume; Thayre, Thomas; Vigier, Jean

Tartars: and Black Death, 203–6, 231, 235; definition of, 198
Tartary, 232
Tavernier, Jean-Baptiste (travel writer). *See* travel writing (early modern)
Taylor, John (poet), 178
Thayre, Thomas (tract writer), 48, 75–6, 80, 143, 178, 275n108

Thévenot, Jean de (travel writer). *See* travel writing (early modern)
Thibault, Jean (tract writer), 135
Third Plague Pandemic, 16–18, 21
Thomson, George (tract writer), 40, 48, 78, 201, 231; illustration in tract by, 95, 113
Thucydides: as historical referent, 122, 147–51, 155, 197, 233, 236; work available in Latin or vernacular, 149–50; writing becomes trope, 282n32
Tian Shan mountains, 20
Todros, Isaac ben (tract writer), 64–5
Toulouse, 64; greasers executed in, 309n170; plague in, 156, 165, 183, 201, 302n99, 302n102; as printing centre, 84–5, 181
Tournai, 65, 168
Tournemire, Jean de (Johannes de Tornamira, tract writer), 64, 69, 129–30, 133, 173
Tours, 139, 185–6; Gregory of, 125, 157, 169; print industry in, 85
Toye, Robert (printer), 88, 278n139
trade: debated role in plague transmission, 50, 155, 232, 234; and plague, 8, 19, 71, 196
travel writing (early modern), 223–4; and impressions of Ottoman Empire, 216–17; 224–8
travel writing (medieval), 208
treatments. *See* cures and treatments
Turkey. *See* Ottoman Empire
Turkish fatalism. *See* fatalistic Turk
Turks, 206, 218, 222, 229, 231. *See also* fatalistic Turk; Orientalism: epidemiological; Ottoman Empire
Twyne, Thomas (tract writer), 76, 176

University of Montpellier: production of tracts at, 34, 63–4, 122, 131; and rivalry with Paris, 15, 127. *See also* Baux, Pierre; Córdoba, Alfonso de; Jacobi, Johannes; Joubert, Laurent; Oultre, Petrus de; Pons, D.M.; Ranchin, François; Tournemire, Jean de
University of Paris, Medical Faculty (tract writer), 26, 63, 131, 268n21; on astrological causes of plague, 126–7; and fear of approaching plague, 167–8; on geography of plague, 202–3; production and circulation of plague tract by, 26, 28, 63–4, 69, 72, 105, 121; ridiculed by Justus Hecker, 158; and rivalry with Montpellier, 15; on traditional versus modern knowledge, 123; treatment recommendations by, 36; on winds, 129, 187. *See also* Barralis, B.; Damouzy, Pierre de; Despars, Jacques
Utrecht, 136

Vadianus. *See* Watt, Joachim von
Vallériole, François (tract writer), 77, 276n115. *See also* Lodge, Thomas
Van Diemerbroeck, Isbrand (tract writer), 77
Van Linschoten, Jan Huyghen (travel writer), 229

Vele, Abraham (printer), 89–90
Venette, Jean de (chronicler), 124, 170, 206
Venice, 57, 151, 230, 259; Black Death and, 204; greasers in, 210; printed tract from, 84
Vigier, Jean (tract writer), 151
Villani, Giovanni (chronicler), 203
Villani, Matteo (chronicler), 149–50, 220, 234–5, 256n4, 286n56
Vinario, Raymond Chalin de (tract writer), 34, 64, 126, 194, 292n148, 299n48; on astrological causes of plague, 34, 127, 129; on environmental causes of plague, 186–7, 213–14; personal experience with plague, 48, 64
Vincent, Thomas (tract writer), 180; Volga River, 20

Waley, John (printer), 88
Walsingham, Thomas (chronicler), 128, 170
warfare: as cause of plague, *see* Wars of Religion
Wars of Religion, 46, 186, 195–6, 230, 244
Watt, Joachim von (tract writer), 84, 94
weather: and plague, 24, 32, 215. *See also* climate
Whitchurch, Edward (printer), 89
wind, 119; as carrier of plague, 23, 31, 129, 185, 187, 202; as precursor to plague, 32; from south as dangerous, 24, 187, 303n120. *See also* air
Wither, George (poet), 141–2
Worde, Wynken de (printer), 59, 89
Wyer, Robert (printer), 86–9, 94, 174. *See also* Multon, Thomas

Ydeley, Estienne (priest), 42–3, 94, 277n116
Yersin, Alexandre (bacteriologist), 19
Yersinia pestis (*Y. pestis*), 7, 16–21; aDNA of, 19–20; branches and strains of, 18, 20–1, 254n30; debates about role in Black Death, 19; ecology of, 17–19; geographic origins of, 20; polytomy of, 20. *See also* palaeogenetics; plague
York, 86, 179–80, 190, 201; anonymous physician in, 79, 180, 201; Archbishop of, 168; Barber-Surgeons of, 70, 72, 272n76; Margaret of, 65
Yorkshire, North Riding of, 55, 70, 73